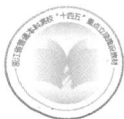

首批国家级一流本科课程"系统解剖学（全英文）"配套教材

浙江省普通本科高校"十四五"重点立项建设教材

供八年制、"5+3"一体化临床医学等专业学生及MBBS留学生用

U0738837

Systematic Anatomy

系统解剖学

(2nd Edition)

（第二版）

主　编　张晓明　刘海岩

副主编　姜华东　罗道枢　高　璐　方马荣　崔怀瑞

ZHEJIANG UNIVERSITY PRESS

浙江大学出版社

·杭州·

图书在版编目（CIP）数据

系统解剖学 = Systematic Anatomy（2nd Edition）：
英文 / 张晓明，刘海岩主编. -- 2版. 杭州 ： 浙江
大学出版社，2025. 4. -- ISBN 978-7-308-26029-9

Ⅰ. R322

中国国家版本馆 CIP 数据核字第 20250TN028 号

系统解剖学（第二版）

张晓明　刘海岩　主编

责任编辑	张凌静 （zlj@zju.edu.cn）	
责任校对	徐　瑾	
封面设计	周　灵	
出版发行	浙江大学出版社	
	（杭州市天目山路148号　邮政编码310007）	
	（网址：http://www.zjupress.com）	
排　　版	杭州晨特广告有限公司	
印　　刷	浙江省邮电印刷股份有限公司	
开　　本	787mm×1092mm　1/16	
印　　张	23.75	
字　　数	683千	
版 印 次	2025年4月第2版　2025年4月第1次印刷	
书　　号	ISBN 978-7-308-26029-9	
定　　价	88.00元	

编 委 会

主编简介

张晓明,男,浙江绍兴人,教授,博士研究生导师,国家级课程思政教学名师,首批国家级一流课程负责人,浙江省解剖学会理事长。从事解剖学教学和科研工作30余年。担任教育部首期来华留学生全英文教学师资培训班负责人,国家自然基金、多个省市自然基金评委及会评专家,专业SCI期刊审稿专家;现任教育部101计划基础医学核心教材共同主编,《解剖学报》和《解剖学杂志》编委。

刘海岩,男,教授,博士研究生导师,吉林大学白求恩医学部副学部长,吉林省解剖学会副理事长,吉林省神经科学学会副理事长。从事解剖学教学和科研工作25年,聚焦于神经退行性疾病、脑损伤等的发病机制及新治疗靶点的研究,主持国家自然科学基金项目、吉林省科技厅项目等各类科研项目10余项;主编、参编教材多部。

副主编简介

姜华东,男,浙江嵊州市人。主持中国红十字会项目1项,主参省级、校级虚拟仿真项目2项,教育部课程思政教学团队成员,主编《局部解剖学》(浙江大学出版社)。

罗道枢,男,福州市闽侯县人。福建医科大学博士研究生,主要研究方向为神经病理性疼痛机制。目前主持国家级课题1个,发表学术论文30多篇。

高　璐,女,复旦大学基础医学院博士研究生,主要负责本科教学。参与、主持国家级、上海市一流课程5项,获国家级教学比赛奖4项,参编教材8部,发表教学论文9篇。

方马荣,男,兰溪市人。浙江大学教授、博士研究生导师,研究方向为脑脊髓损伤的分子机制。主持国家自然科学基金项目6项,发表SCI论文100余篇。

崔怀瑞,男,蚌埠人。温州医科大学教授。研究方向为临床解剖。参与国家级课题3项,主持省级一流课程、课题4项;主编、副主编教材3部;发表学术论文20余篇。

前　言

　　"系统解剖学"是面向临床医学专业开设的专业必修课程,也是临床医学专业的主干课程。随着我国高等医学教育改革的不断深入,对于八年制及"5+3"一体化临床医学专业学生和 MBBS(Bachelor of Medicine and Bachelor of Surgery,医学学士和外科学士)留学生而言,当前国内外该课程的全英文教材内容过于繁杂,且内容不够系统,不适合作为课堂用书使用,更适合作为参考工具书使用,因此本书编委会试图编写一本适合当前国内招收八年制及"5+3"一体化临床医学专业学生和 MBBS 学生的医学院校使用的全英文的系统解剖学教材,即一本按照人体各系统来阐述分析正常器官形态结构和位置毗邻关系的简明教材。《系统解剖学》(英文版)第一版问世后,深受大家欢迎,读者对本书内容、插图和编排提出了诸多宝贵的意见和反馈。在此基础上,我们对第一版教材做了大幅度的修订与改版。在内容上,除了做必要的更新和补充外,鉴于多数院校未开设"神经解剖学"课程,本修订版教材中特别增加了"外周神经系统"和"中枢神经系统"两章。同时,在第一版教材黑白标本插图的基础上,增加了以二维码形式呈现的彩图、视频、音频等数字化新形态内容。此外,优化编委团队结构,遴选增补教学经验丰富的解剖学专家,使本书内容更具编写特色和教学特色,更加契合对医学生基础知识应用、临床前思维和科学创新精神的培养目标。

　　在"新医科"建设背景下,本教材以习近平新时代中国特色社会主义思想为指导,深入学习贯彻党的二十大精神,全面贯彻党的教育方针,围绕"健康中国"战略,优化教材内容。习近平总书记强调,要把保障人民健康放在优先发展的战略位置,坚持"人民至上、生命至上",为医学教育改革指明了方向、提供了遵循。本教材以本课程实验对象——"无语良师"和临床案例为核心载体,从"人格修养、家国情怀、国际视野、求是创新"四个维度出发,在专业知识的讲授中无形地融合"祖国医学历史""身边爱国名医"和"科学创新成果"等主题,并深入挖掘人文思政元素,使学生感受到"无语良师"的生命热度与人性伟大,激发其学习动力,培养具有家国情怀、国际视野、仁心仁术、求是创新的卓越医学人才,为全面提高医学人才的培养质量,推进"健康中国"建设、保障人民健康提供强有力的人才保障。

　　最后,我们诚恳地希望并期待业内专家、学者、老师和同学们不吝指导,及时指出本教材存在的不足之处,以便编者在今后的版本中进行充分的修订和完善。

编委会

2025 年 1 月

CONTENTS

系统解剖学（全英文）
慕课（MOOC）

Introduction

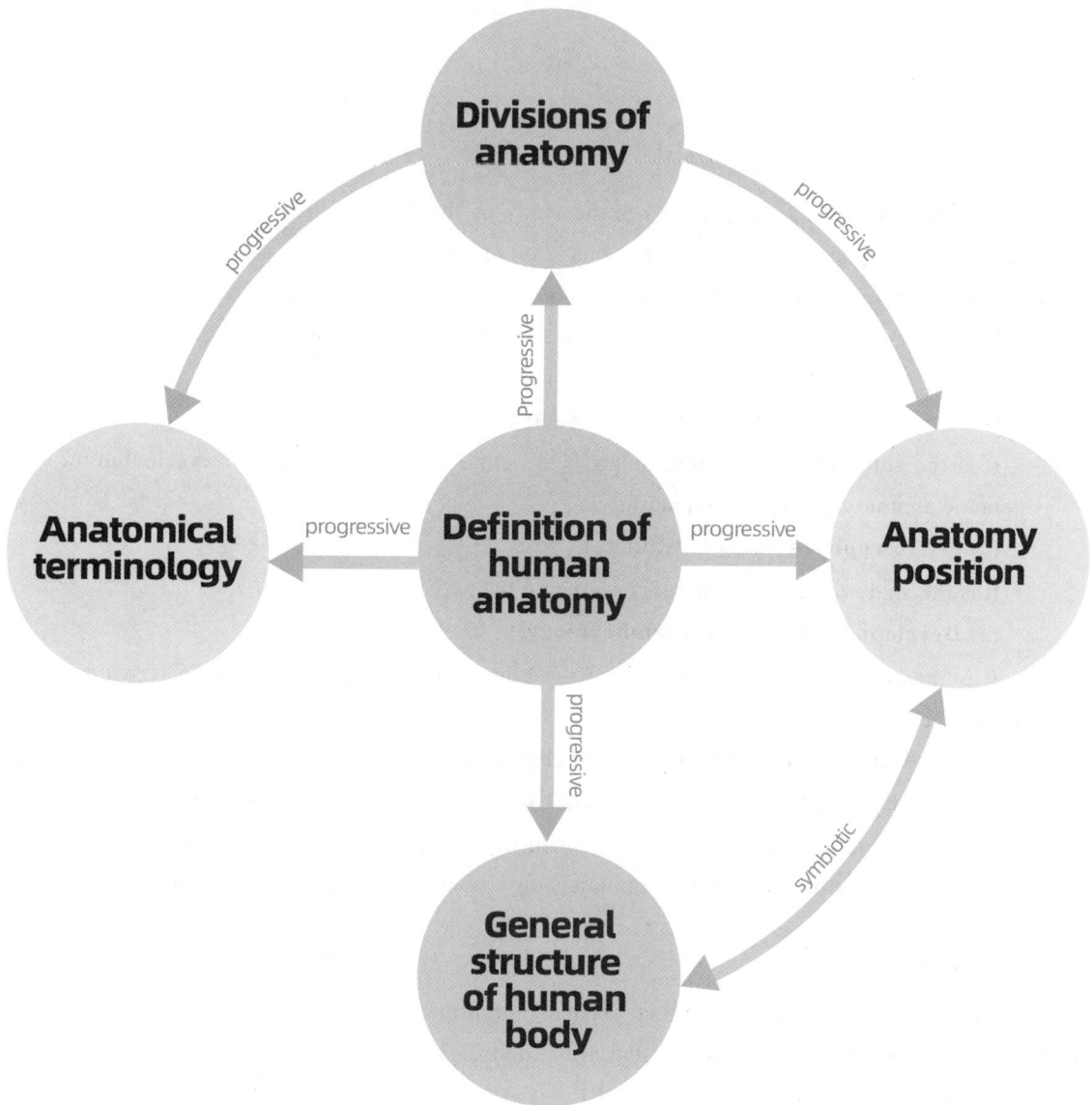

Divisions of anatomy

progressive

progressive

Progressive

Anatomical terminology

progressive

Definition of human anatomy

progressive

Anatomy position

progressive

General structure of human body

symbiotic

Introduction

Human anatomy (人体解剖学) is the study of the body's structure, encompassing gross morphology and spatial interrelations. For medical students, it is one of the most crucial foundational courses in the preclinical curriculum.

Based on different methods and purposes of study, divisions of anatomy are as follows:

(1) Gross anatomy (macroscopic anatomy)

It is the study of macroscopic or gross structure visible to the naked eye, including systematic anatomy and regional anatomy.

(2) Microscopic anatomy (histology)

It is the study of minute structures requiring the use of the microscope.

(3) Developmental anatomy (embryology)

It is the study of the development of the human body from its beginning (fertilized ova, stem cells) to maturity.

(4) Applied anatomy (practical or surgical anatomy)

It typically involves the examination of human anatomical structures that are particularly pertinent to medicine, notably in surgical procedures and clinical diagnoses.

The general structure of the human body comprises cells, tissues, organs, and systems.

(1) Cells

Cells are enclosed by a distinct plasma membrane, the cytoplasm, which contains several membrane-bound structures that are called organelles, and surrounds the nucleus. A body consists of innumerable cells.

(2) Tissues

Most cells exist as cellular aggregates with similar functions in a coordinated manner, termed tissues. They can be classified into epithelial tissue, connective tissue, muscular tissue, and nervous tissue.

(3) Organs

Organs are structural units composed of a variety of tissues that can perform a certain function.

(4) Systems

The main systems of the human body are as follows:

Locomotor system (运动系统). This system comprises bones (osteology), joints (arthrology), and muscles (myology). Osteology delves into the study of bones that provide support to the body and its organs. Arthrology focuses on the joints of the body, while myology explores the muscular system, encompassing muscle structure, function, and diseases. With the description of the muscles, it also includes that of fasciae, intimately connected tissues.

Alimentary system (消化系统). This system involves mechanical and chemical processes providing nutrients through the mouth, the esophagus, the stomach, the intestines, and the digestive glands.

Respiratory system (呼吸系统). The lungs and the respiratory tract facilitate the inhalation of oxygen and the expulsion of carbon from the body.

Urinary system (泌尿系统). The kidneys, ureters, bladder and urethra perform the function of filtering blood and eliminating waste from the body.

Reproductive system (生殖系统). This system consists of the internal and external genitalia required for the production of offspring.

Circulatory system (循环系统). It includes the cardiovascular system and the lymphatic system.

Cardiovascular system (心血管系统). Comprising the heart and blood vessels (arteries, capillaries, and veins), the cardiovascular system circulates blood throughout the body. It delivers oxygen and nutrients to organs (cells) and carries away waste products.

Lymphatic system (淋巴系统). Consisting of lymphatic vessels and lymph glands, the lymphatic system supports the cardiovascular system and the immune system by supplying and draining lymph fluid.

Nervous system (神经系统). This system collects and processes information from the senses via nerves to the brain. It communicates instructions to muscles and organs, regulating physiological activities.

Endocrine system (内分泌系统). This system provides chemical communication within the body through hormones.

Immune system (免疫系统). This system defends the body against disease-causing agents.

Anatomical Terminology

The anatomical position serves as the standard reference point for describing the various parts of the body and their locations in anatomy. It is essential to learn this position as most directional terminology in anatomy refers to the body in this standardized posture.

(1) Anatomical position (解剖学姿势)

The body is assumed to stand erect with the face and toes directed forward, the eyes looking straight ahead. The heels and toes are together, and the upper limbs hang by the sides of the body with the palms facing forward.

(2) The relational planes and sections for the whole body (Fig.0-1)

1) The median plane is a vertical plane which divides the body into the left and right parts. The two parts are equal.

2) The sagittal plane is a vertical plane that is parallel with the median plane, which divides the body into the left and right parts.

3) The coronal (frontal) plane is a vertical plane, which divides the body into the anterior and posterior parts.

4) The horizontal (transverse) plane divides the body into the superior and inferior parts.

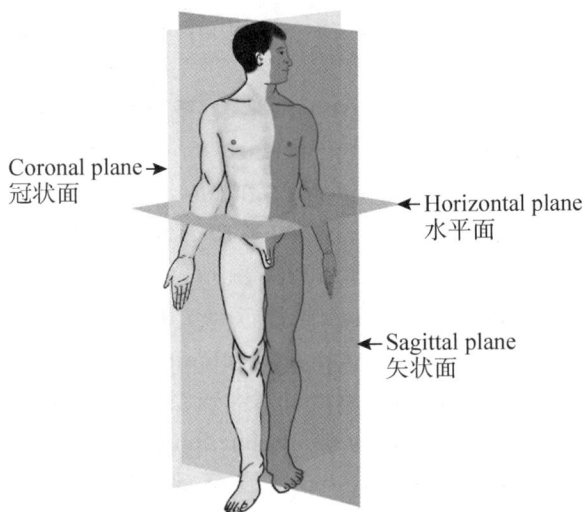

Fig.0-1　Planes of the body

(3) Axes

Axes consist of the vertical axis, sagittal axis and coronal axis.

(4) Terms of direction

1) Anterior (ventral) and posterior (dorsal). They refer to the front or back of the body or limbs.

2) Medial and lateral. Structures nearer to or farther from the median plane are referred to as medial or lateral respectively, e.g., ulnar (medial) and radial (lateral), tibial (medial) and fibular (lateral).

3) Superior (cranial) and inferior (caudal). Structures nearer to the head are superior, whereas structures closer to the feet are inferior.

4) Proximal and distal. In the case of the limbs, the words proximal (near) and distal (far) refer to the relative distance from the body.

5) Internal (inner) and external (outer). They indicate the distance from the center of

an organ or a cavity.

6) Superficial and deep. They are strictly confined to the description of the relative depth between adjacent structures.

(5) Pay Our Respects to Silent Mentors

Silent Mentors are individuals who generously donate their bodies for medical education and research after death. These donors play a crucial role in the training of healthcare professionals, including medical students, surgeons, and anatomists. By allowing students to learn anatomy through hands-on experience with real human bodies, Silent Mentors contribute to the advancement of medical knowledge and the improvement of medicine. Let us honor and pay tribute to the profound generosity and altruism of Silent Mentors.

Silent Mentors enhance medical education, particularly in the study of human anatomy. Silent Mentors provide medical students with an opportunity for hands-on dissection, allowing them to gain a deeper understanding of the human body's structure. The Silent Mentor Program is founded on ethical considerations, emphasizing the dignity of the donors and the respect for them. Donors and their families are often informed about the educational impact that their contribution will have on future healthcare providers.

Interacting with Silent Mentors humanizes the medical profession for students. It instills empathy and a sense of responsibility toward individuals who have entrusted their bodies for educational purposes. The impact of Silent Mentors goes beyond the anatomy lab. The knowledge and insights gained from dissection experiences stay with medical students throughout their careers, influencing their clinical practice and patient care.

The Silent Mentor Program embodies a distinctive, curriculum-integrated approach to ideological education in the teaching of human anatomy. It emphasizes the values of respect, gratitude, and professionalism in medical education, enabling future healthcare professionals to learn from the ultimate teachers—Silent Mentors. These mentors ignite students' motivation to learn and nurture their spirit through the principles of "Cherishing Life, Saving Life, Willing to Dedicate, and Boundless Compassion", guiding them to develop into exceptional medical professionals.

（浙江大学医学院　张晓明）

The Locomotor System

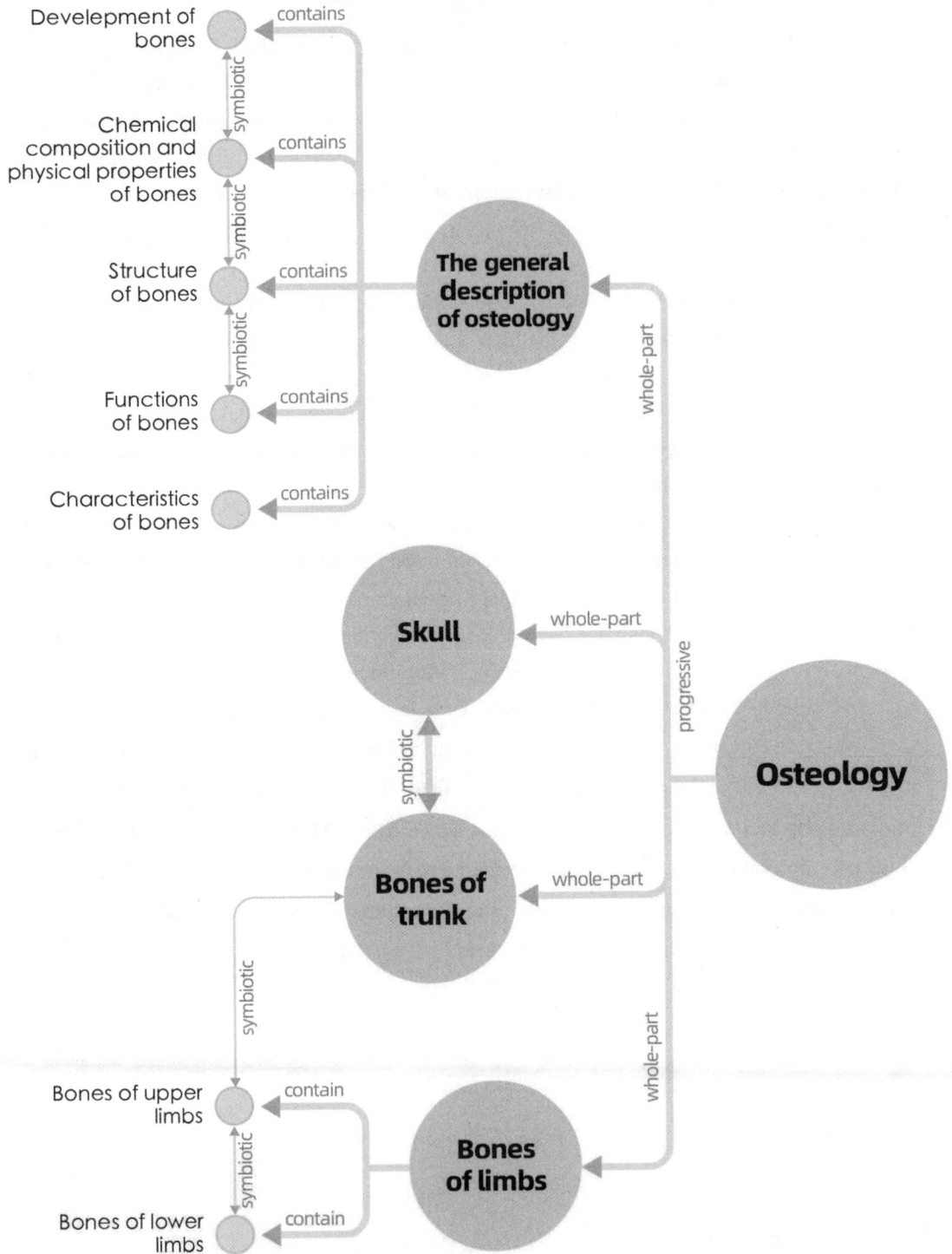

Develepment of bones ← contains

Chemical composition and physical properties of bones ← contains

Structure of bones ← contains ← **The general description of osteology**

Functions of bones ← contains

Characteristics of bones ← contains

symbiotic (between bone items)

Skull ← whole-part

symbiotic

Bones of trunk ← whole-part ← **Osteology**

whole-part / progressive

Bones of upper limbs ← contain

symbiotic

Bones of lower limbs ← contain ← **Bones of limbs** ← whole-part

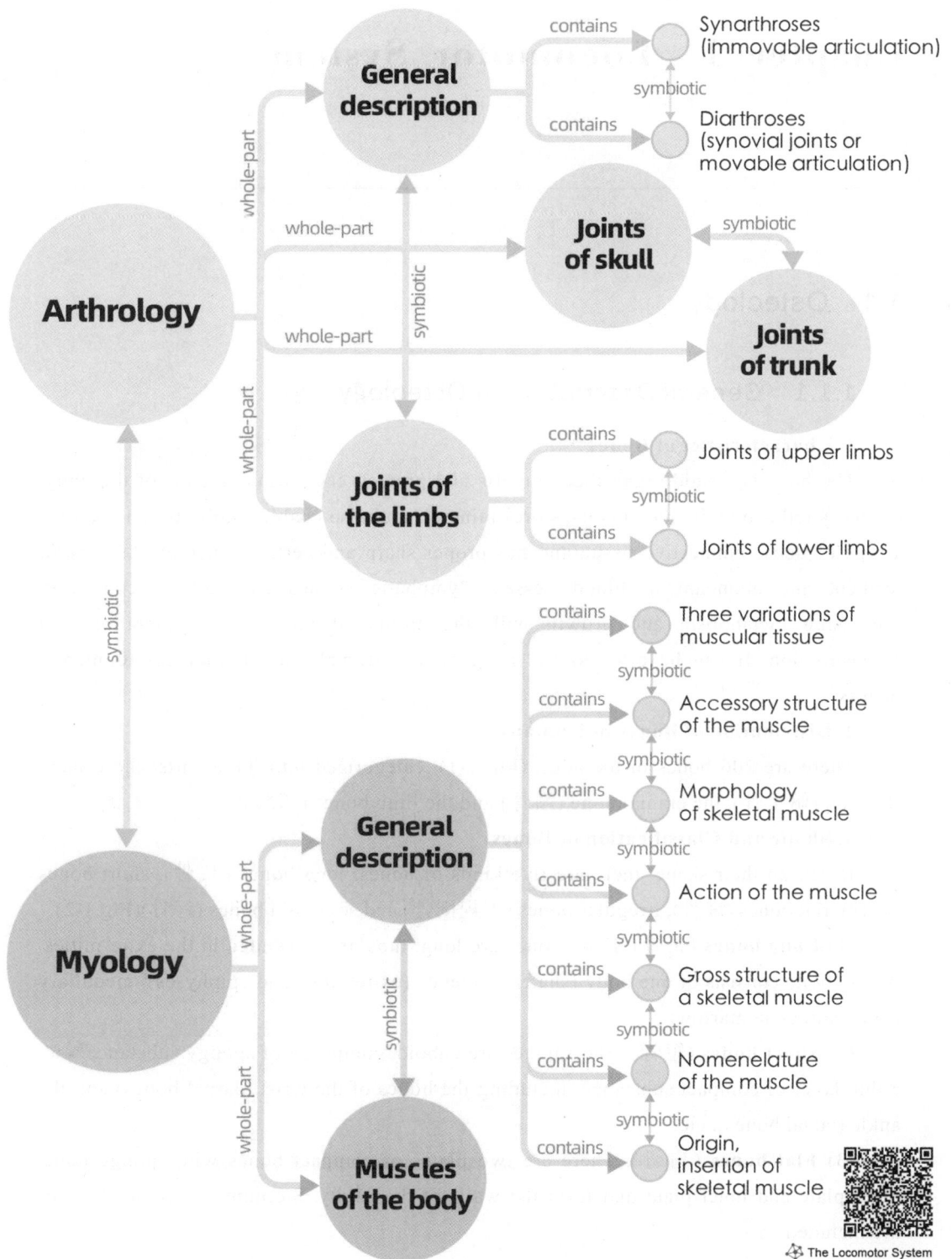

General description

contains → Synarthroses (immovable articulation)

symbiotic

contains → Diarthroses (synovial joints or movable articulation)

whole-part

Arthrology

whole-part → Joints of skull ← symbiotic

symbiotic

whole-part → Joints of trunk

whole-part

Joints of the limbs

contains → Joints of upper limbs

symbiotic

contains → Joints of lower limbs

symbiotic

Myology

whole-part

General description

contains → Three variations of muscular tissue

symbiotic

contains → Accessory structure of the muscle

symbiotic

contains → Morphology of skeletal muscle

symbiotic

contains → Action of the muscle

symbiotic

contains → Gross structure of a skeletal muscle

symbiotic

contains → Nomenelature of the muscle

symbiotic

contains → Origin, insertion of skeletal muscle

symbiotic

whole-part

Muscles of the body

The Locomotor System

Chapter 1　Locomotor System

1.1　Osteology

1.1.1　General Description of Osteology

1. Characteristics of Bones

The bone is a rigid organ that supports and protects the various organs of the body, produces red and white blood cells, stores minerals and also enables mobility. The bone is a type of dense connective tissue and has proper sharp and certain functions. It is hard, resilient and abundant in blood vessels, lymphatic vessels and nerves, constantly processing metabolism and growth with the ability of repairing, regeneration and reconstruction. It can be affected by the genetic, external and internal environmental factors.

2. Distribution of Bones in Humans

There are 206 bones in the adult (Fig. 1-1), categorized into three parts: the truncal skeleton (躯干骨), the cranial bone (颅骨) and the limb bones (四肢骨).

3. Shape and Classification of Bones

Based on their shape, there are five kinds of bones: long bones (长骨), short bones (短骨), flat bones (扁骨), irregular bones (不规则骨) and sesamoid bones (籽骨)(Fig.1-2).

(1) **Long bones** (长骨). Long bones are long, tubular, distributed in the extre-mities. A long bone consists of one body (shaft), two ends (extremities and epiphyses), medullary cavity and bone marrow.

(2) **Short bones** (短骨). Short bones are cuboid, composed of spongy substance with a thin layer of compact substance, including the bones of the wrist (carpal bones) and the ankle (tarsal bones), etc.

(3) **Flat bones** (扁骨). There are two plates of compact bones with sponge bone, outer plate and inner plate that form the walls of the cavity. Sternum and parietal bones are included.

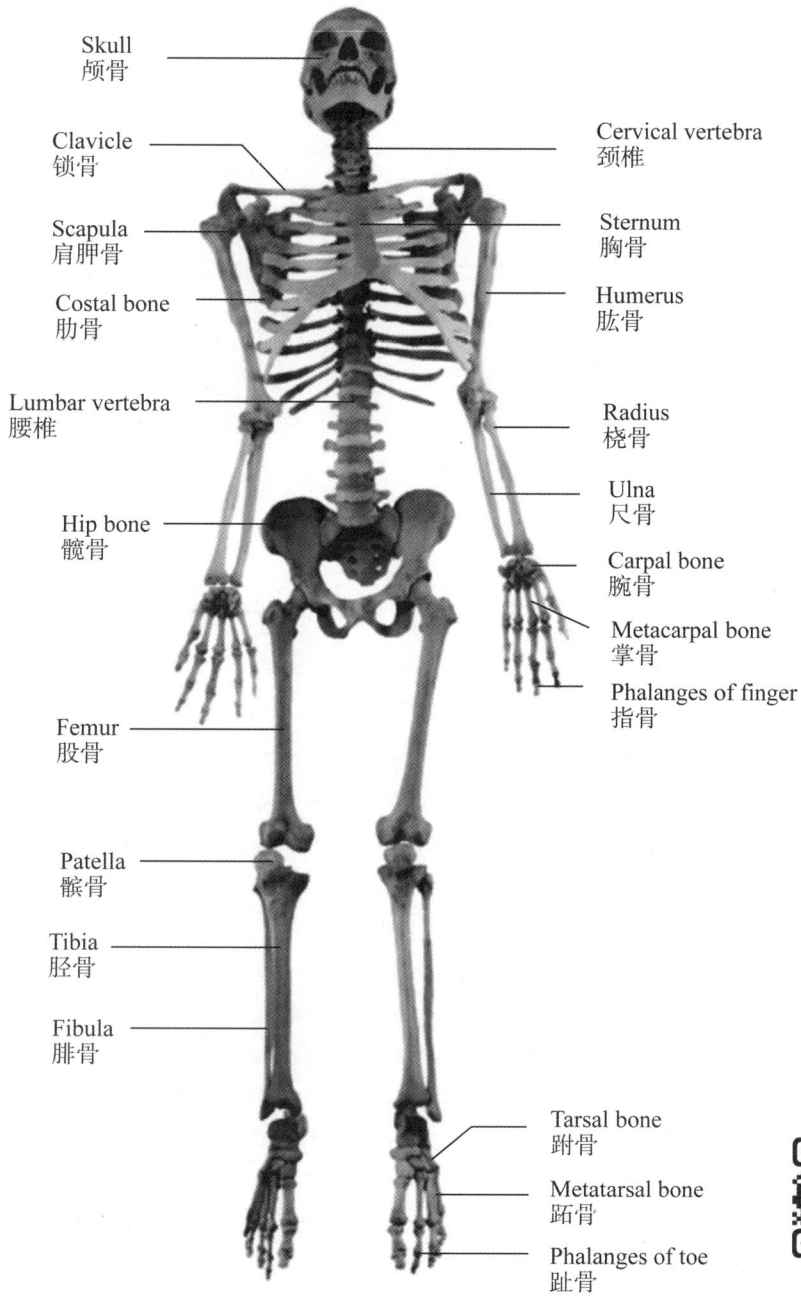

Skull
颅骨

Clavicle
锁骨

Scapula
肩胛骨

Costal bone
肋骨

Lumbar vertebra
腰椎

Hip bone
髋骨

Femur
股骨

Patella
髌骨

Tibia
胫骨

Fibula
腓骨

Cervical vertebra
颈椎

Sternum
胸骨

Humerus
肱骨

Radius
桡骨

Ulna
尺骨

Carpal bone
腕骨

Metacarpal bone
掌骨

Phalanges of finger
指骨

Tarsal bone
跗骨

Metatarsal bone
跖骨

Phalanges of toe
趾骨

Fig.1-1　The skeleton (anterior aspect)

(4) **Irregular bones** (不规则骨). Irregular bones do not fit into the above categories. Their shapes are irregular and complicated with many centers of ossification, and some contain bony sinuses. Irregular bones include the spine, the pelvis, and some cranial bones.

(5) **Sesamoid bones** (籽骨). Sesamoid bones are embedded in tendons. The patella is the largest sesamoid bone.

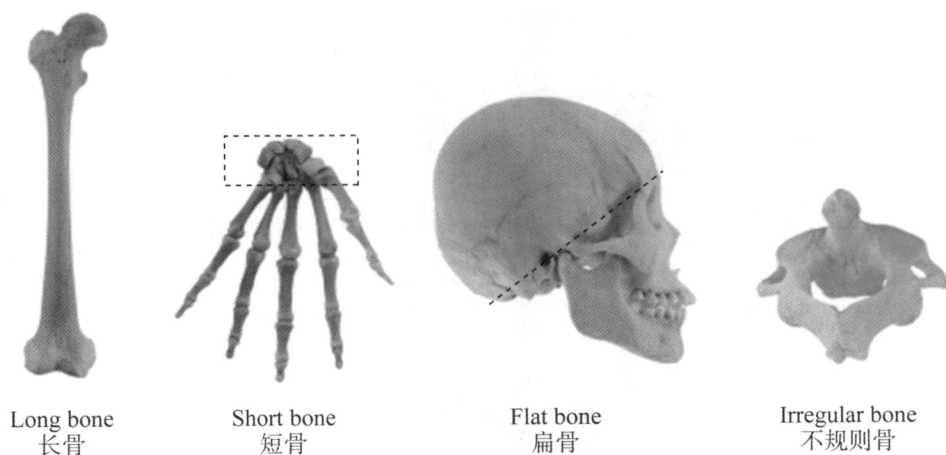

| Long bone
长骨 | Short bone
短骨 | Flat bone
扁骨 | Irregular bone
不规则骨 |

Fig.1-2　Morphological classification of bones

4. Structure of Bones

(1) **Bony substance** (骨质). One bone is composed of two kinds of bony subs-tance: One is dense in texture, termed compact tissue; the other consists of slender fibers and lamellae, which join to form a reticular structure, called cancellous tissue.

1) Compact bone (骨密质). The compact tissue is always placed on the exterior of the bone. The difference in structure between the compact tissue and the cancellous tissue depends merely upon the different amount of solid matter. It can resist stresses and bend.

2) Spongy bone (骨松质). Sponge bone is composed of a large number of bone trabeculae interwoven with each other, in a spongy shape. Bone trabeculae are arranged in the same direction as that of the pressure and tension on the bone.

(2) **Periosteum** (骨膜). It envelops the external surface of the bones, except the joint surface (articular cartilage). It consists of two layers which are the fibrous membrane (outer layer) and vascular membrane (inner layer) of elastic fibers of the finer kind with osteoblasts and osteoclasts, forming dense membranous networks. It is important for the bone regeneration, growth and repair.

(3) **Bone marrow** (骨髓). The bone marrow is a soft pulpy tissue that not only fills up the cylindrical cavities in the bodies of the long bones, but also occupies the space of the cancellous tissue and extends into the larger bony canals (Haversian canals) which contain blood vessels. There are two kinds of marrow as follows.

1) Red bone marrow (红骨髓). It is found in the ends of long bones and cancellous bones of flat and short bones in adults with red color. The red marrow consists of a small

quantity of connective tissue, blood vessels, and numerous cells, a few of which are fat cells, but the great majority is roundish nucleated cells, the true "marrow cells" of Kolliker. It is capable of making blood cells.

2) Yellow bone marrow (黄骨髓). It is found in the medullary cavity of the long bones in adults with yellow color. It consists of a basis of connective tissue supporting numerous blood vessels and cells, most of which are fat cells but some are "marrow cells", and don't have the ability of making blood cells in general. In critical situations, yellow bone marrow may be reactivated to make blood cells (Fig.1-3).

Blood cells have but a short life. The red cells live for about 120 days, while the white cells live far shorter than the red ones. At birth, the cancellous bone and the medullary cavities of long bones are filled

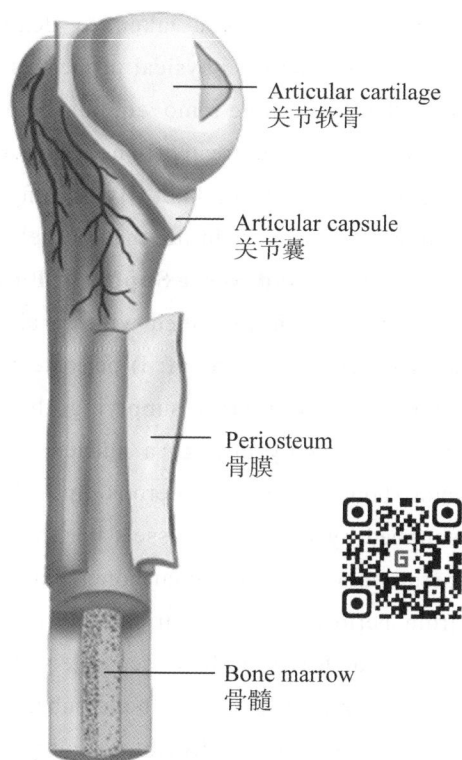

Articular cartilage
关节软骨

Articular capsule
关节囊

Periosteum
骨膜

Bone marrow
骨髓

Fig.1-3   Structure of the bone

with the red marrow. By the sixth year, the red marrow in the medullary cavities is gradually replaced by the yellow marrow. In about the 18th year, the red marrow is almost entirely replaced by the yellow one in the bones of limbs. A puncture on iliac crest (or spinous process of iliac bone, or sternum) to examine the marrow is a useful method to make a diagnosis of some blood diseases.

5. Chemical Composition and Physical Properties of Bones

Living bones are plastic tissues with organic and inorganic components. Bones have an organic framework of fibrous tissue and cells, among which inorganic salts are deposited. The organic material (the main one is collagen) accounts for 30%－40% of the dry weight of the bone, while the inorganic material, mineral salts (the main one is calcium phosphate), 60%－70%. In mature living bones, water takes up about one-fifth of the weight. The organic material gives the bones resilience and toughness; the inorganic salts give them hardness and rigidity, making them opaque to X-rays. The physical properties of the bones depend upon the chemical components which change with age. In the infants and the children, the organic components are relatively more than those in the adults, so their bones are softer, and are easier to be deformed. But in elders, the inorganic components are comparatively more, and bone fracture happens more often in the aged people. A test can be taken to demonstrate the relationship between the chemical components and the physical properties of the bones. By submerging a bone in a mineral acid, the salts can be removed, but the organic material remains and still displays in detail the shape of the untreated bone. Such a specimen is flexible. For example, a decalcified fibula can be tied in a knot. By burning a bone with fire, the organic material is removed and the bone is more brittle than porcelain, and crumbled and fractured easily.

6. Blood and Nerve Supply of Bones

The bone is furnished with an abundance of fine arterioles. In the long bones, the arterial supply consists of: i) periosteal twigs entering the shaft at many points; ii) twigs from articular arteries supplying the epiphyses; iii) the nutrient artery entering the medullary cavity through a nutrient foramen, supplying the shaft and the marrow. The short bones receive numerous fine blood vessels from the periosteum. Flat bones are supplied by numerous vessels which enter the bone at various points from the covering periosteum. Large irregular bones like the scapula and hip bone receive superficial vessels from periosteum and nutrient arteries. The blood is drained by veins which run with arteries or leave the bone separately. Lymphatic vessels are abundant in the periosteum, and are present within the bone substances. Numerous nerve fibers accompany the blood vessels of bones, and distribute widely to periosteum, bone substance and arteries.

7. Development of Bones

Bones develop from the mesoderm. During about the eighth gestational week, two patterns of ossification begin to occur. One is the process of calcification, followed by ossification in a cartilage model, referred to as the cartilage bone, and the other is what takes place in connective fibrous membrane without intervention of cartilage formation, and the bone formed in such a way is referred to as membrane bone. Some bones develop from a single ossific center, while others, including the long bones, have two or more centers of ossification. For the latter, the primary centers form the shaft or diaphysis. The extremities and certain processes remain cartilaginous for a time, and then eventually the secondary centers of ossification appear, forming the epiphysis. After a time the epiphyses are separated from the shaft by a thin layer of cartilage, forming the epiphysial cartilage. An increase in the length of the bone takes place at the epiphysial cartilage, followed by ossification. Eventually the epiphysial cartilage becomes entirely ossified, and the epiphyses join with shaft. When this has taken place, no further increase in the length of the bone can occur. Skeleton develops as a unit, and various bones tend to keep pace with one another, so that a radiographic examination of the limited portion of the body may help the doctor understand the condition of the entire skeleton.

The centers of ossification for the shaft of the long bone and many primary centers for the others appear at about the eighth week of the fetal life. Most epiphyses in the limbs begin to ossify during childhood, one or two years earlier in girls than in boys. Most of the epiphyses become completely ossified during the $18^{th}-20^{th}$ years. The development of the skeleton is finished entirely in the 25th year.

The normal development and maintenance of the bones can be affected by many factors; an adequate dietary intake and absorption of calcium, phosphorus, vitamine A, C and D and a balanced interplay between somatotrophic hormone, thyroxin, estrogens and androgens etc.

8. Functions of Bones

The functions of bones can be summed up as follows: i) the rigid supporting framework of the body; ii) the levers for muscles; iii) the protection of certain impor-tant organs or viscera (e. g. the brain and spinal cord, heart and lungs etc.); iv) the sites for making blood cells (erythrocytes, granulocytes, monocytes and platelets); and v) the bank of calcium and phosphorus.

1.1.2 Bones of the Trunk

Bones of the trunk include the vertebrae, the rib and the sternum, which formed the vertebral column and the rib cage.

1. Vertebral Column (脊柱)

The vertebral column (Fig. 1-4) is a flexuous and flexible column, comprised of a series of bones called vertebrae.

The vertebrae are thirty-three in number, and are grouped under the names: cervical vertebra (颈 椎), thoracic vertebra (胸 椎), lumbar vertebra (腰椎), sacral vertebra (骶椎), and coccygeal vertebra (尾 椎). According to the regions they occupy, there are seven in the cervical region, twelve in the thoracic, five in the lumbar, five in the sacral, and four in the coccygeal.

(1) **General features of the typical vertebrae**. Each vertebra is an irregular bone with a complex structure (Fig. 1-5). It is composed of a ventral body, a dorsal vertebral arch, two pedicles, one laminae, and seven processes.

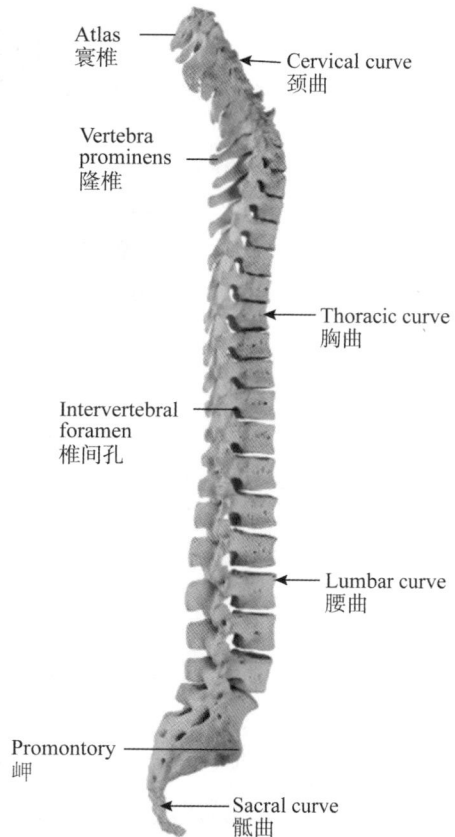

Fig.1-4 The vertebral column

Vertebral body
椎体

Superior costal fovea
上肋凹

Superior
articular process
上关节突

Spinous process
棘突

Vertebral pedicle
椎弓根

Vertebral foramen
椎孔

Transverse process
横突

Vertebral arch
椎弓

Superior aspect
上面观

Superior
articular process
上关节突

Transverse
costal fovea
横突肋凹

Spinous process
棘突

Superior costal fovea
上肋凹

Vertebral body
椎体

Inferior costal fovea
下肋凹

Inferior
articular process
下关节突

Right lateral aspect
右侧面观

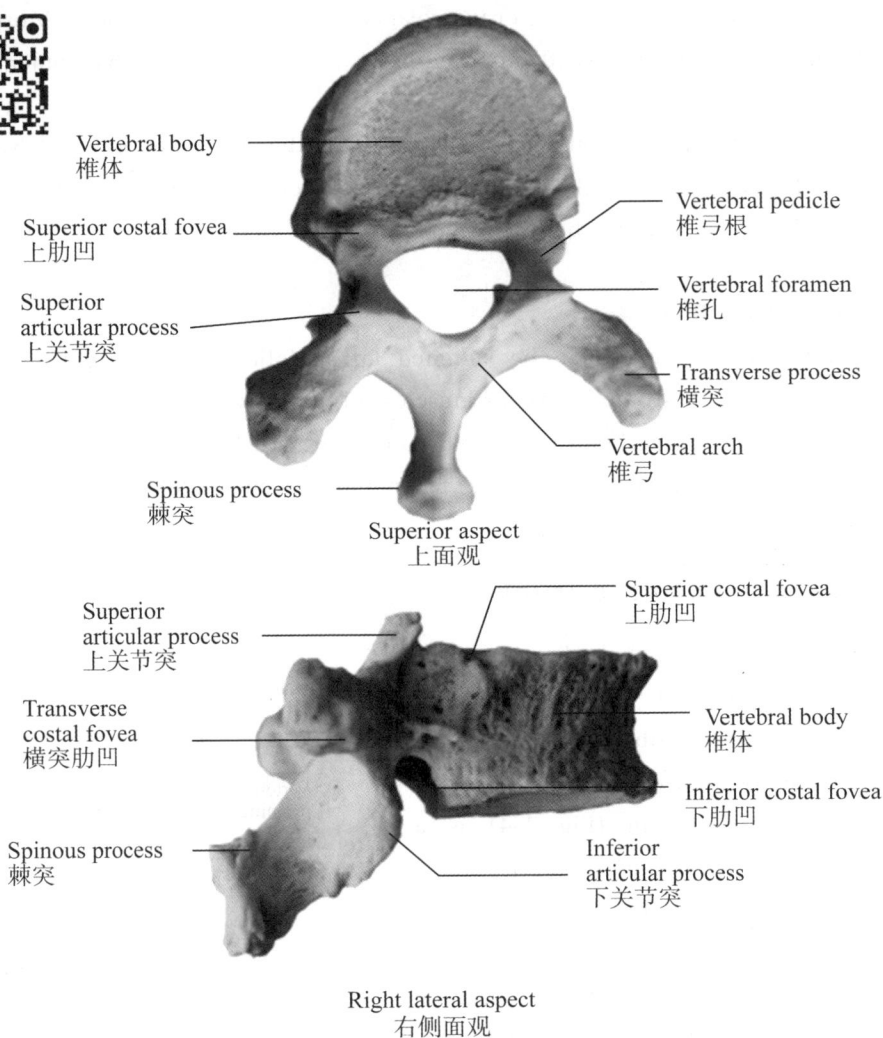

Fig.1-5　General features of the typical vertebrae

1) Vertebral body (椎体). The body is the largest part of a vertebra, and is more or less cylindrical in shape. The interior of the vertebral body is filled with cancellous bone and the compact bone exterior is thin. Its upper and lower surfaces are flattened and rough, and give attachment to the intervertebral fibrocartilages, and each presents a rim around its circumference. In front, the body is convex from side to side and concave from above downward. In the back, it is flat from above downward and slightly concave from side to side. Its anterior surface presents a few small apertures, for the passage of nutrient vessels; on the posterior surface is a single large, irregular aperture, or occasionally more than one, for the exit of the basi-vertebral veins from the body of the vertebrae.

2) Vertebral arch (椎弓). The vertebral arch consists of a pair of pedicles and a lamina

of vertebral arch. The pedicles are the constricted parts that attach tightly to the vertebral body and form vertebral foramen (椎孔) with vertebrae body. The vertebral arch supports seven processes: two superior articular processes, two inferior articular processes, two transverse processes and one spinous processes.

(2) **Main characteristics of vertebrae in each part**

1) Cervical vertebrae (颈椎)(Fig.1-6). As the smallest of the moveable vertebrae, it can be readily distinguished from those of the thoracic or lumbar regions by the presence of a foramen in each transverse process. The first, the second, and the seventh cervical vertebrae present exceptional features and must be separately described.

2) Transverse foramen (横突孔). It can be readily distinguished from those of the thoracic or lumbar regions by the presence of a foramen in each transverse process that passes through the vertebral artery.

3) Spinous processes (棘突). They are short and bifid.

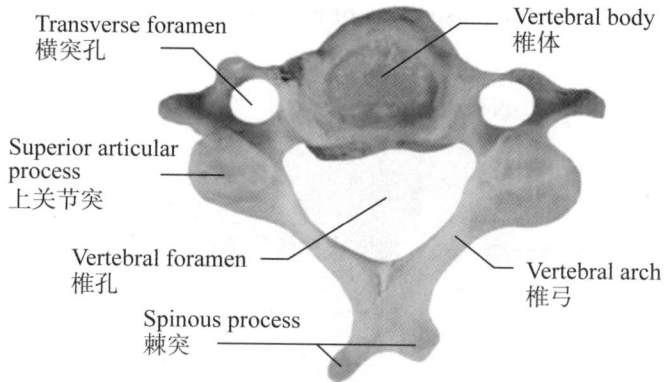

Transverse foramen 横突孔

Vertebral body 椎体

Superior articular process 上关节突

Vertebral foramen 椎孔

Vertebral arch 椎弓

Spinous process 棘突

Fig.1-6　General morphology of cervical vertebrae

The first cervical vertebrae (Fig.1-7). It is named the atlas because it supports the skull. Its chief peculiarity is that it has no body, whose expected position is occupied by the dens, a cranial protuberance from the axis. This is because the body of the atlas has fused with that of the next vertebra. Without spinous process, it is ring-like, and consists of an anterior arch, a posterior arch and two lateral masses.

Superior articular process
上关节突

Anterior tubercle
前结节

Dental fovea of atlas
齿突凹

Transverse foramen
横突孔

Groove for vertebral a.
椎动脉沟

Vertebral foramen
椎孔

Posterior tubercle
后结节

Posterior arch
后弓

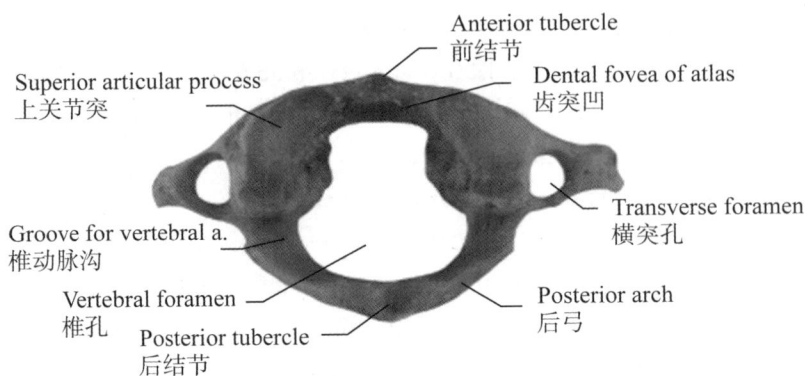

Fig.1-7　The atlas (a.: artery)

The second cervical vertebrae (Fig. 1-8). It is named the axis because it forms the pivot upon which the first vertebra, carrying the head, rotates. It has a dens or odontoid which process exhibits a slight constriction or neck, where it joins the body.

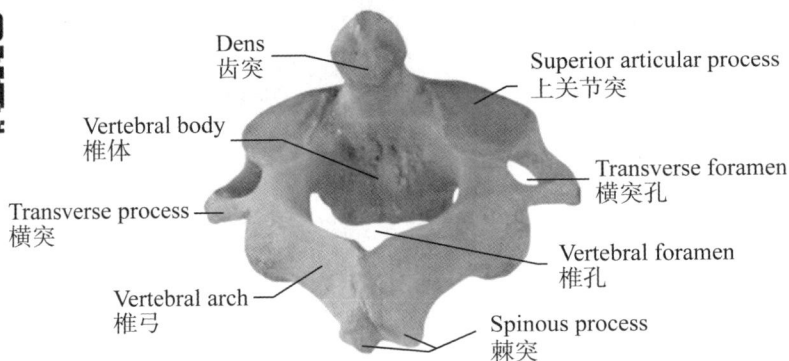

Dens
齿突

Superior articular process
上关节突

Vertebral body
椎体

Transverse foramen
横突孔

Transverse process
横突

Vertebral foramen
椎孔

Vertebral arch
椎弓

Spinous process
棘突

Fig.1-8　The axis

The seventh cervical vertebrae (Fig. 1-9). Known as the vertebra prominens, it is the longest spinous process and can easily be felt out.

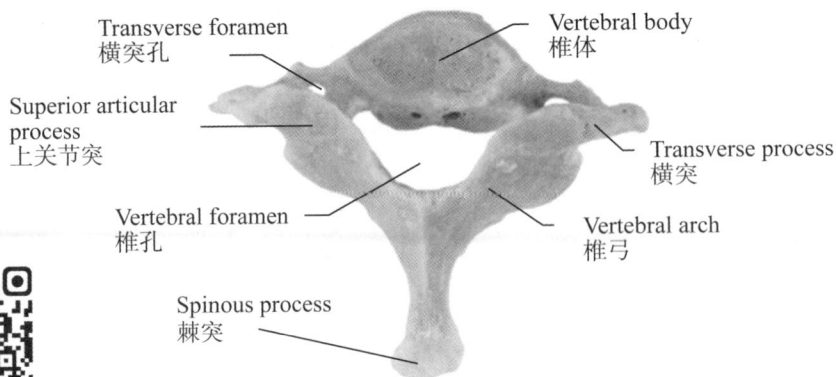

Transverse foramen
横突孔

Vertebral body
椎体

Superior articular process
上关节突

Transverse process
横突

Vertebral foramen
椎孔

Vertebral arch
椎弓

Spinous process
棘突

Fig.1-9　The seventh cervical vertebrae

4) Thoracic vertebrae (胸椎) (Fig. 1-10). The body of the thoracic vertebrae is typically heart-shaped, and increases in size from upper downwards and bears increasing weight. These vertebrae are characterized by two costal facets on each side of their bodies for articulation with the head of the ribs and by facets on their transverse processes (apart from those of the lower two vertebrae) for the tubercle of the ribs. The spines are long and downward sloping, and the articular facets of articular processes are relatively vertical. The vertebral foramen is nearly circular and smaller than that in the other regions.

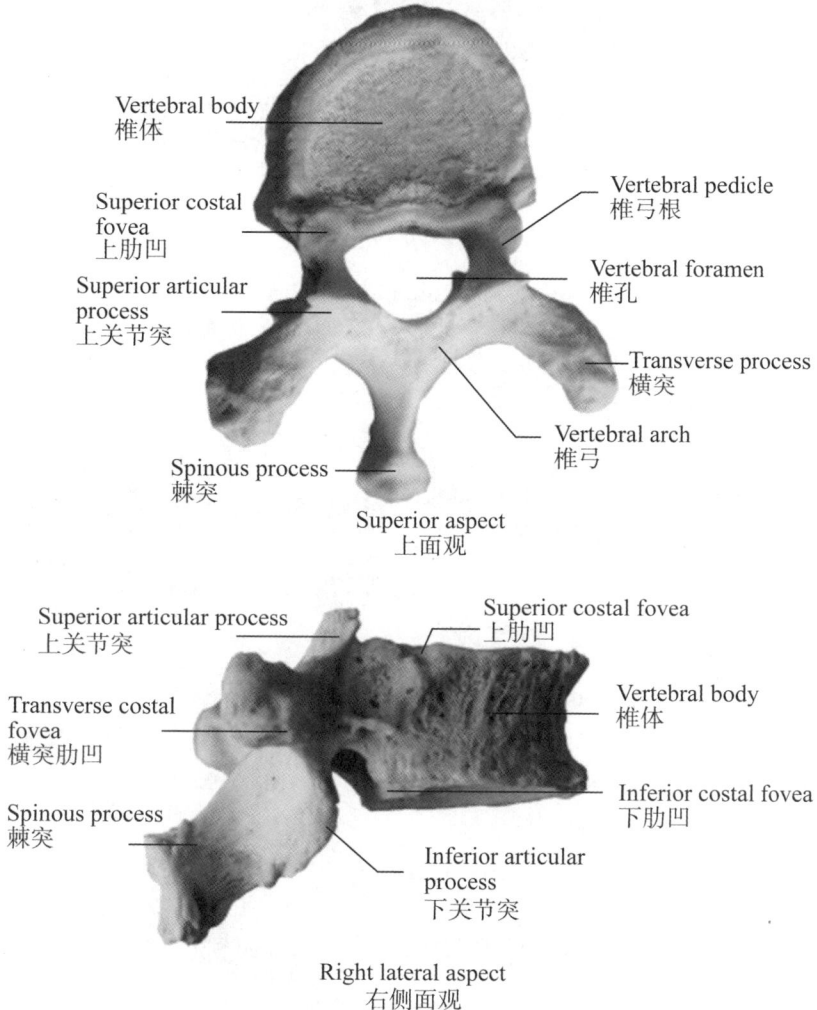

Vertebral body 椎体
Superior costal fovea 上肋凹
Superior articular process 上关节突
Spinous process 棘突
Vertebral pedicle 椎弓根
Vertebral foramen 椎孔
Transverse process 横突
Vertebral arch 椎弓
Superior aspect 上面观

Superior articular process 上关节突
Transverse costal fovea 横突肋凹
Spinous process 棘突
Superior costal fovea 上肋凹
Vertebral body 椎体
Inferior costal fovea 下肋凹
Inferior articular process 下关节突
Right lateral aspect 右侧面观

Fig.1-10   Thoracic vertebrae

5) Lumbar vertebrae (腰椎)(Fig.1-11).The lumbar vertebrae are the largest segments of the movable part of the vertebral column, and can be distinguished by the strong body, and square and horizontal spines. The fifth lumbar vertebra is the largest, characterized by

its body being much deeper in front than in the back, which accords with the prominence of the sacrovertebral articulation; by the smaller size of its spinous process; by the wide interval between the inferior articular processes; and by the thickness of its transverse processes, which spring from the body as well as from the pedicles.

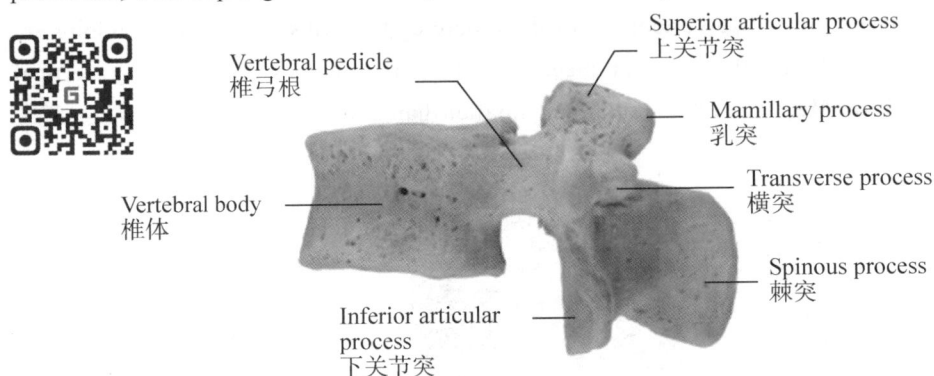

Fig.1-11   Lumbar vertebrae

6) Sacrum vertebrae (骶椎)(Fig.1-12). The sacrum is a large, triangular fusion of five vertebrae, situated in the lower part of the vertebral column and at the upper and back parts of the pelvic cavity, where it is inserted like a wedge between the two hip bones; its upper part or base articulates with the last lumbar vertebra, its apex with the coccyx.

Promontory of sacrum(岬). Its upper part or base articulates with the last lumbar vertebra. It is curved upon itself and placed very obliquely, its base projecting forward and forming the prominent sacrovertebral angle when articulated with the last lumbar vertebra; its central part is projected backward, so as to give increased capacity to the pelvic cavity.

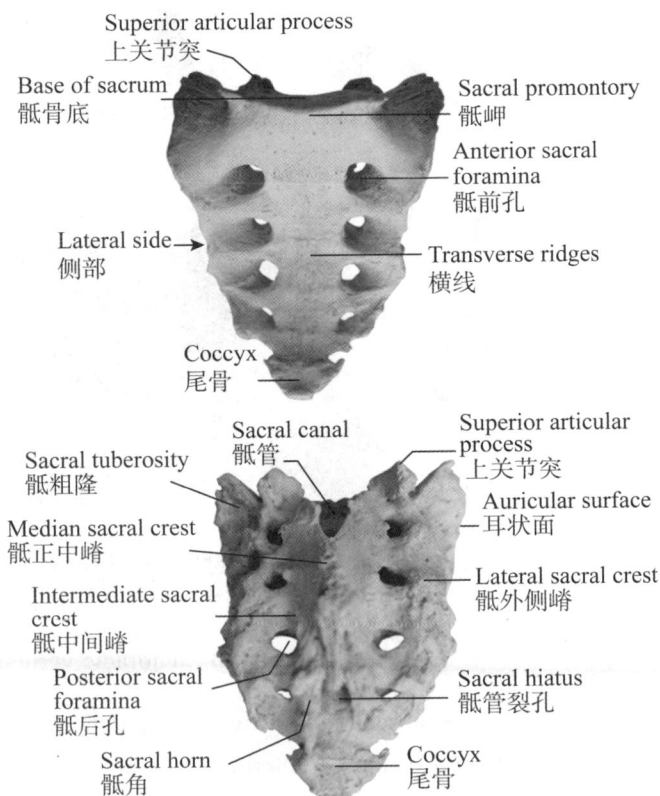

Fig.1-12   The sacrum

The sacropelvic surface (盆面) is concave from above downward, and slightly so from side to side. At the ends of the ridges are the anterior sacral foramina, four in number on either side (through which anterior branches of the sacral nerve pass). The large area between the right and left foramina is formed by the flat pelvic aspects of the sacral bodies.

The dorsal surface (背面) is convex and narrower than the pelvic. There are four pairs of posterior sacral foramina (through which posterior branches of the sacral nerve pass).

The lateral surface (外侧面), broad above, but narrowed into a thin edge below, is a fusion of transverse processes and costal elements. The upper half presents an ear-shaped surface, *the auricular surface* (耳状面), covered with cartilage in the fresh state, for articulation with the ilium.

The apex of sacrum (尖) is the inferior aspect of the fifth sacral vertebral body, with its oval facet connected to the coccyx.

The sacral canal (骶管) forms with the vertebral foramina of each sacral vertebra connected to the vertebral canal, and the lower end of the sacral canal hiatus.

2. Costal Bones (肋骨)

The 12 pairs of ribs are elastic arches of bone formed by the sternum and the distal parts of the ribs and their costal cartilages, which form the thoracic cage with the 12 thoracic vertebrae.

(1) The first 7 ribs

They are connected behind with the vertebral column, and in front, through the intervention of the costal cartilages, with the sternum, called true or vertebro-sternal ribs.

(2) The remaining 5 ribs

They are false ribs, of these, the first three(8, 9 & 10) have their cartilages attached to the cartilage of the rib above (vertebro-chondral); the last two are free at their anterior extremities and are termed floating ribs. The 8, 9 & 10 ribs join together one by one to form the costal costal arch by means of the costal cartilages.

(3) Shape of a typical rib (Fig.1-14)

Posterior extremity. The posterior or vertebral extremity presents for examina-tion a head, neck, and tubercle. *Costal head* (肋头) is marked by a kidney-shaped articular surface, divided by a horizontal crest into two facets on the bodies of two adjacent thoracic vertebræ; the upper facet is the smaller; to the crest is attached the interarticular ligament. *Costal neck* (肋颈) is the flattened portion which extends lateralward from the head; it is about 2.5 cm long, and is placed in front of the transverse process of the lower of the two vertebrae with which the head articulates. On the posterior surface of the junction of the neck and body, nearer to the lower than the upper border, there is an eminence, *costal tubercle* (肋结节), which consists of an articular and a non-articular portion.

Shaft of a rib. The body or shaft is thin and flat with two surfaces, an external and an internal, and two borders, a superior and an inferior. The external surface is convex, smooth, and marked, a little in front of the tubercle, by a prominent line, directed downward and lateralward; this gives attachment to a tendon of the iliocostalis, and is called *costal angle* (肋角). Between the shaft and the inferior border is a groove, the costal groove, for the intercostal vessels and nerves. The shaft is curved, bent at the angle of the rib and twists about its long axis.

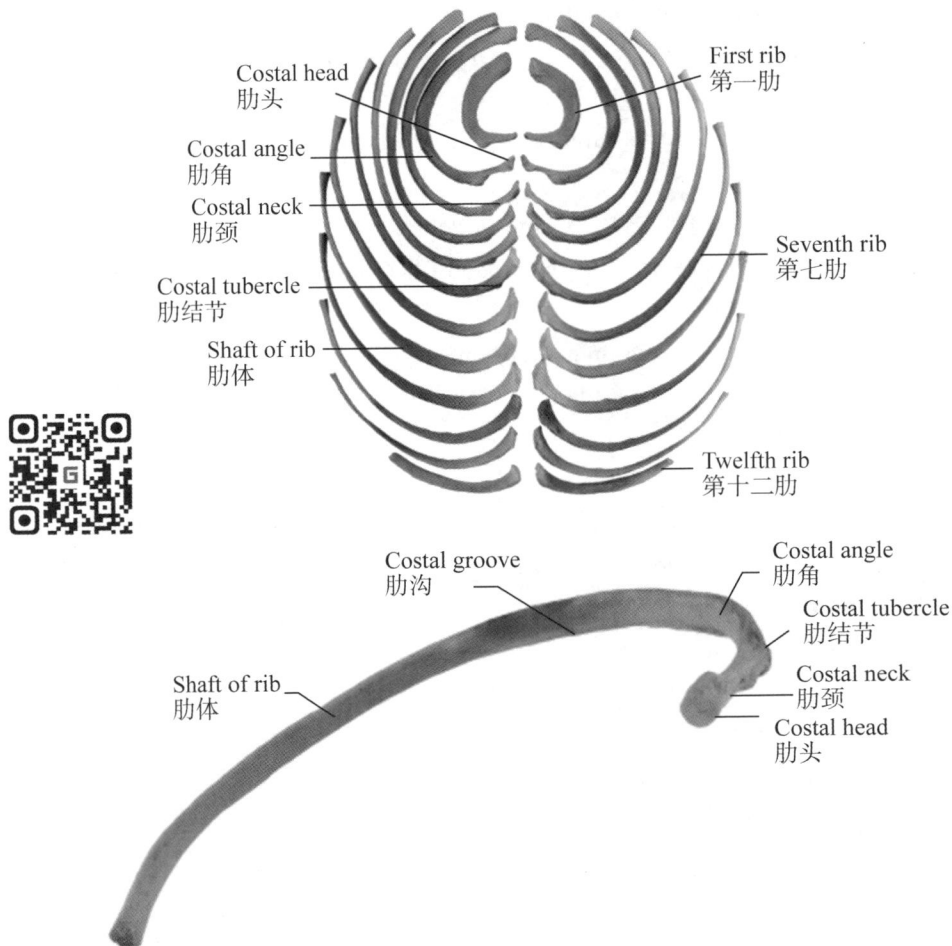

Fig.1-13　The rib

3. Sternum (胸骨)

Sternum (Fig.1-14) refers to an elongated, flattened bone, forming the middle portion of the anterior wall of the thorax.

Subdivision. It consists of three parts: the manubrium of sternum, the body of sternum, and the xiphoid process.

Manubrium of sternum (胸骨柄). The manubrium is of a somewhat quadrangular form, broad and thick above, narrow below at its junction with the body. The anterior and posterior surfaces are smooth in appear-ance. The suprasternal (jugular) notch is medially located at the upper broadest part of the manubrium. This notch can be felt between the two clavicles (collarbones). On the lateral side of this notch are the right and left clavicular notches.

Clavicular notch 锁切迹
Jugular notch 颈静脉切迹
First costal notch 第一肋切迹
Sternal angle 胸骨角
Manubrium sterni 胸骨柄
Body of sternum 胸骨体
Xiphoid process 剑突

Fig.1-14   The sternum

Body of sternum (胸骨体). The body, considerably longer, narrower, and thinner than the manubrium, attains its greatest breadth close to the lower end. Sternal angle is located at the point where the body joins the manubrium. It marks the position of the second rib.

Xiphoid process (剑突). The xiphoid process is the smallest and most variable of the three pieces. It is thin and elongated, cartilaginous in structure in youth, but more or less ossified at its upper part in the adult. The xiphoid process joins the inferior part of the sternal body at the xiphisternal joint.

1.1.3   Bones of the Skull (颅骨)

The skull (Figs.1-15 & 1-16) is supported on the summit of the vertebral column, and is of an oval shape, wider behind than in front. It houses the brain, the organs of special sense, and the upper parts of the respiratory and digestive systems. It provides attachments for muscles of the head and neck. It is composed of a series of flattened or irregular bones which, with one exception (the mandible), are immovably jointed together. It divides into two parts: *the cerebral cranium* (脑颅骨), which lodges and protects the brain, consists of eight bones (occipital, two parietals, frontal, two temporals, sphenoidal and ethmoidal), and *facial cranium* (面颅骨), the skeleton of the face, of fifteen bones (two nasals, two maxillae, two lacrimals, two zygomatics, two palatines, two inferior nasal concha, vomer, mandible and hyoid bone).

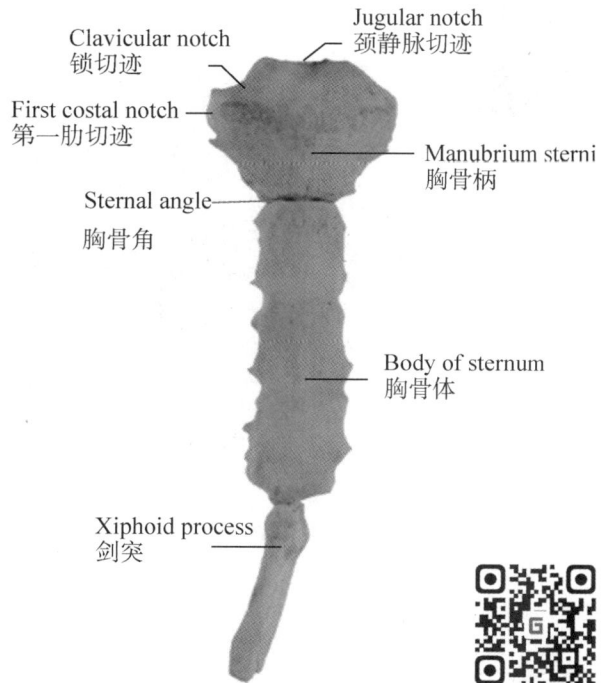

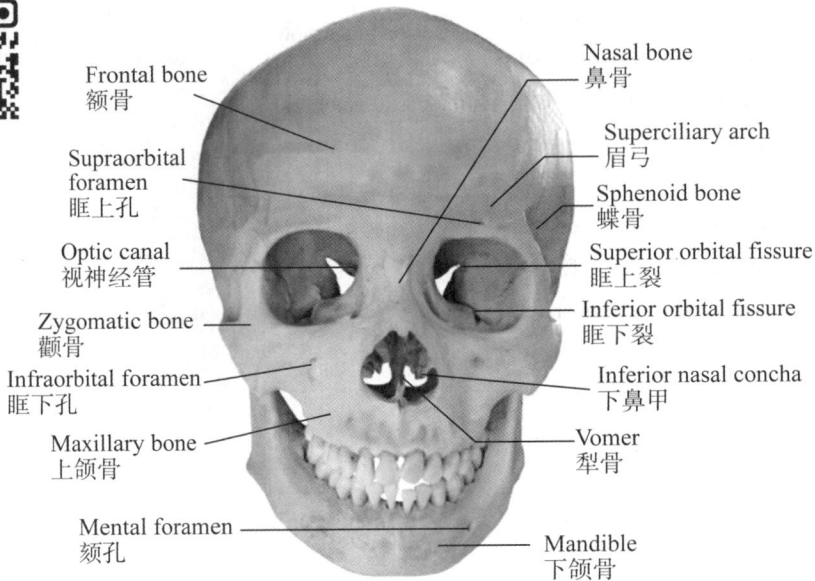

Fig.1-15　The skull (anterior aspect)

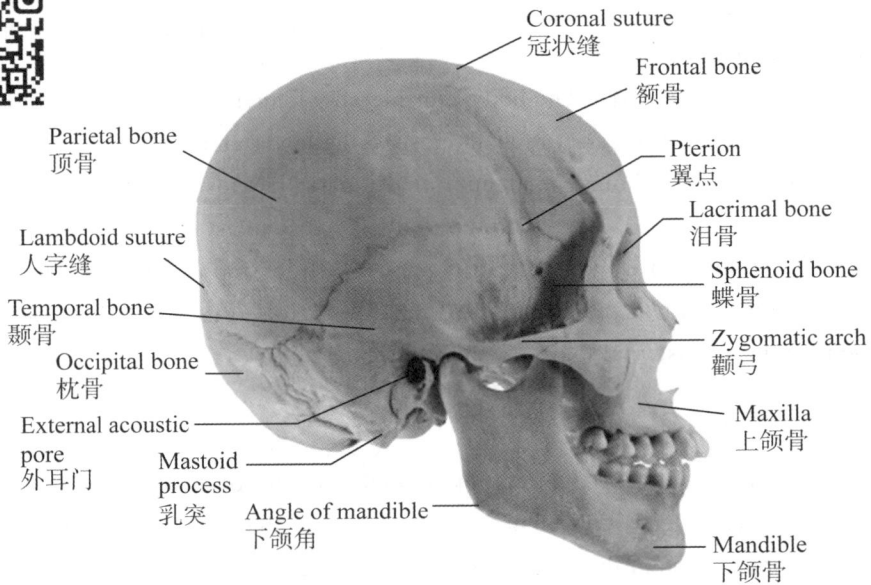

Fig.1-16　The skull (lateral aspect)

1. Cerebral Cranium (脑颅骨)

(1) **The frontal bone** (额骨). It resembles a cockle-shell in form, and consists of two portions—a vertical portion, the squama, corresponding with the region of the forehead; and an orbital or horizontal portion which enters the formation of the roofs of the orbital

and nasal cavities. It has three parts (squamous part, nasal part and orbital part) and contains two cavities (the frontal sinuses).

(2) **The occipital bone** (枕骨). Situated at the back and lower parts of the cranium, it is trapezoid in shape and curved on itself. It is pierced by a large oval aperture, the foramen magnum, through which the cranial cavity communicates with the vertebral canal. It has four parts: the basilar, squamous parts and two lateral parts.

(3) **The temporal bones** (颞骨). They are situated at the sides and base of the skull. Each consists of four parts: the squamous, the petromastoid, tympanic parts, and the styloid process.

(4) **The sphenoid bone** (蝶骨). It is situated at the base of the skull in front of the temporals and basilar parts of the occipital. It somewhat resembles a butterfly with its wings extended, and divides into a median portion or body (sphenoid sinus inside), two great and two small wings extending outward from the sides of the body, and two pterygoid processes which project from it below.

(5) **The ethmoid bone** (筛骨). It is situated at the anterior part of the base of the cranium, between the two orbits, at the roof of the nose, and contributes to each of these cavities. It consists of four parts: a horizontal or cribriform plate, forming part of the base of the cranium; a perpendicular plate, constituting part of the nasal septum; and two lateral labyrinths that contain the ethmoidal sinuses.

2. Facial Cranium (面颅骨)

(1) **The maxilla** (上颌骨). They are the largest bones of the face, excepting the mandible, and form, by their union, the upper jaw. Each assists in forming the boundaries of three cavities: the roof of the mouth, the floor and the lateral wall of the nose and the floor of the orbit. It also enters the formation of two fossae, the infratemporal and pterygopalatine, and two fissures, the inferior orbital and pterygomaxillary. Each maxilla has a body that contains the maxilla sinuses, and four processes: the zygomatic, frontal, alveolar and palatine processes.

(2) **The palatine bone** (腭骨). Situated at the back part of the nasal cavity between the maxilla and the pterygoid process of the sphenoid, it contributes to the walls of three cavities: the floor and lateral wall of the nasal cavity, the roof of the mouth, and the floor of the orbit; it enters into the formation of two fossae, the pterygopalatine and pterygoid fossae; and one fissure, the inferior orbital fissure. The palatine bone somewhat resembles letter L, and consists of a horizontal and a vertical part and three outstanding processes: the pyramidal process, the orbital and sphenoidal processes, which surmount the vertical part, and are separated by a deep notch, the sphenopalatine notch.

(3) **The mandible** (下颌骨). As the largest and strongest bone of the face, it supports the mandibular teeth within the alveolar process. It consists of a curved, horizontal

portion, the body, and two perpendicular portions, the rami, which unite with the ends of the body nearly at angles.

(4) **The hyoid bone** (舌骨). Shaped like a horseshoe, it is suspended from the tips of the styloid processes of the temporal bones at the level of the fourth cervical vertebra by the stylohyoid ligaments. It consists of five segments: a body, two greater cornua, and two lesser cornua.

(5) **The nasal bones** (鼻骨). They are two small oblong bones, varying in size and form in different individuals; they are placed side by side in the middle and the upper parts of the face, and form, by their junction, "the bridge" of the nose. Each has two surfaces and four borders.

1.1.4　Bones of the Limbs

The bones of the upper and lower limbs are attached to the trunk and constitute respectively the shoulder and pelvic girdles. Because of the erect standing and labor, the bones of the upper limbs are lighter and smaller in shape and size. The bones of lower limbs are heavy and strong enough to bear the weight of the body and to provide movement of the whole body.

1. Bones of the Upper Limbs

The bones of the upper limb include the scapula, clavicle, humerus, radius and ulna, the eight bones forming the carpus, five metacarpals and fourteen phalanges.

(1) **The shoulder girdle of the upper limbs**

It is formed by the scapulae and clavicles, and is imperfect in front and behind. In front, however, it is completed by the upper end of the sternum, with which the medial ends of the clavicles articulate. Behind, it is widely imperfect, with the scapulae being connected to the trunk by muscles only.

1) Clavicle (锁骨) (Fig.1-17). It is a doubly curved long bone that connects the arm (upper limb) to the body (trunk), located directly above the first rib. It has one shaft and two ends. It acts as a strut to keep the scapula in place so the arm can hang freely. It has a rounded medial end and a flattened lateral end. The medial end is quadran-gular and articulates with the clavicular notch of the manubrium to form the sternoclavicular joint. The lateral end is flat from above downward, forming the acromioclavicular joint.

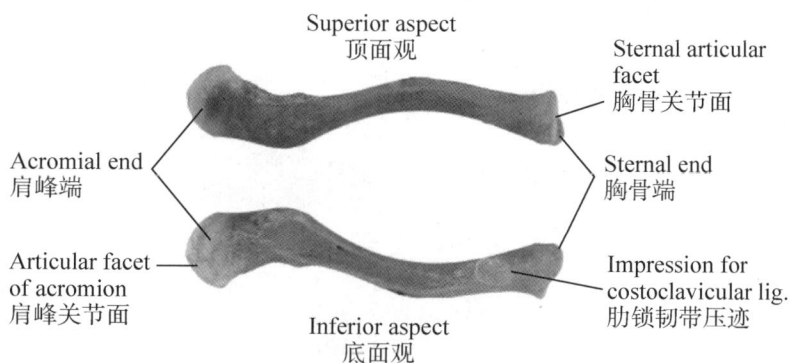

Fig.1-17   The clavicle (lig.: ligament)

2) Scapula (肩胛骨) (Fig.1-18). It refers to a wide, flat, triangular bone lying on the thoracic wall covering parts of the second to the seventh ribs. The front of the scapula (also known as the costal or ventral surface) has a subscapular fossa (肩胛下窝), to which the subscapularis muscle attaches. The back of the scapula (also called the dorsal or posterior surface) is subdivided into two unequal parts by the spine of scapula (肩胛冈). The portion above the spine is called the supraspinous fossa (冈上窝), and that below it the infraspinous fossa (冈下窝). There are three borders of the scapula. The superior border is the shortest and thinnest; it is concave, and extends from the medial angle to the base of the coracoid process. At its lateral part is a deep, semicircular notch, the scapular notch. The axillary border (or "lateral border") is the thickest of the three. The medial border (also called the vertebral border or medial margin) is the longest. There are three angles. The superior angle is covered by trapezius. The inferior angle is covered by latissimus dorsi. The lateral or glenoid angle is broad and bears *the glenoid cavity* (关节盂) or fossa, which is connected with the humerus as a shoulder joint. There are three process: the spine, the acromion and the coracoid process.

(2) Free bones of the upper limbs

1) The humerus (肱骨) (Fig.1-19). It refers to the long bone in the arm and connects the scapula, the radius and the ulna. The upper extremity consists of a rounded head, a narrow neck, and two short processes (major tubercle and lesser tubercle or tuberosities). The lower extremity consists of two epicondyles (lateral to medial), two processes (trochlea & capitulum), and three fossae (radial fossa, coronoid fossa, and olecranon fossa). As well as its anatomical neck just below the articular surface of the humeral head, and the surgical neck due to its tendency to commonly get fractured, thus often becoming the focus of surgeons.

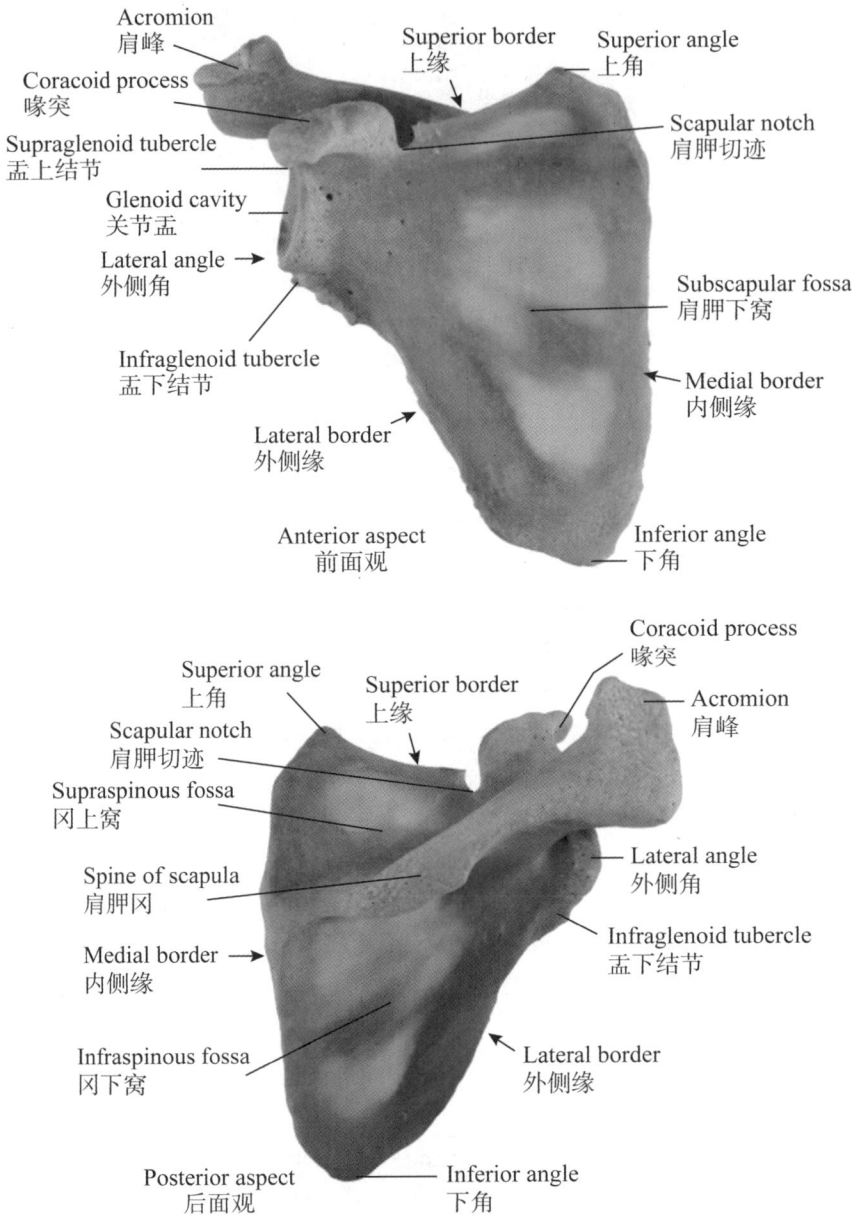

Fig.1-18 The Scapula

2) The radius (桡骨) (Fig.1-20). It refers to the the lateral bone of the forearm, and has one body and two extremities. The shaft widens rapidly towards its distal end, and is convex laterally and concave anteriorly in its distal part. The upper extremity of the radius consists of a somewhat cylindrical head articulating with the ulna and the humerus, and the lower extremity with articular surfaces for the ulna, scaphoid and lunate bones. The distal end of the radius forms radially the styloid process and Lister's tubercle on the ulnar side.

Greater tubercle
大结节

Lesser tubercle
小结节

Crest of
greater tubercle
大结节嵴

Head of humerus
肱骨头

Anatomical neck
解剖颈

Surgical neck
外科颈

Intertubercular sulcus
结节间沟

Deltoid tuberosity
三角肌粗隆

Sulcus for radial n.
桡神经沟

Shaft of humerus
肱骨体

Lateral epicondyle
外上髁

Radial fossa
桡窝

Capitulum
of humerus
肱骨小头

Coronoid fossa
冠突窝

Medial epicondyle
内上髁

Olecranon fossa
鹰嘴窝

Trochlea
of humerus
肱骨滑车

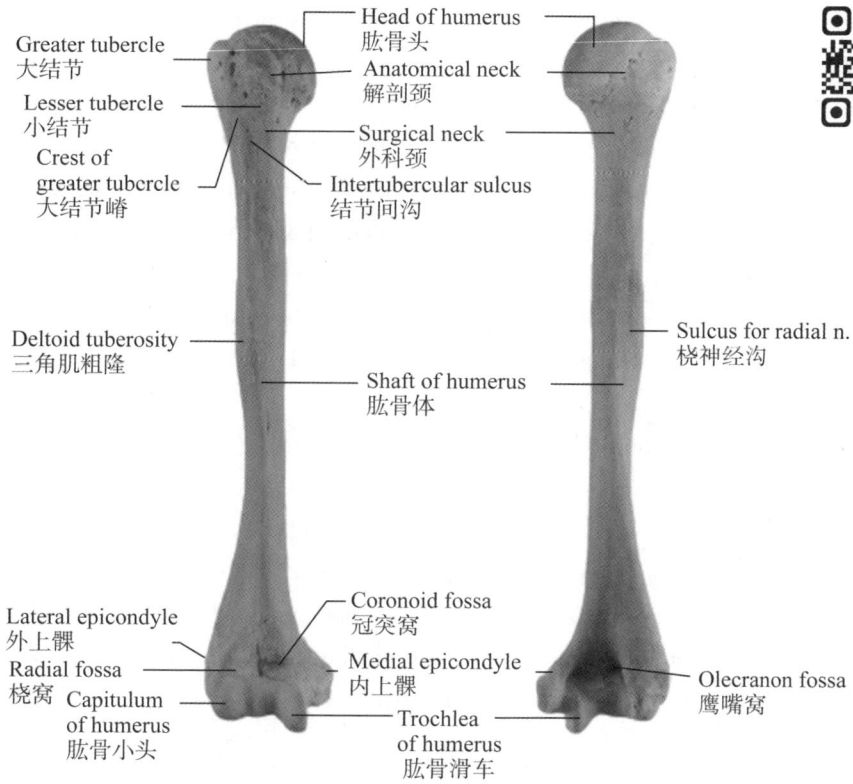

Fig.1-19   The humerus (n.: nerve)

3) The ulna (尺骨) (Fig.1-21). It refers to another long bone of the forearm, medial to

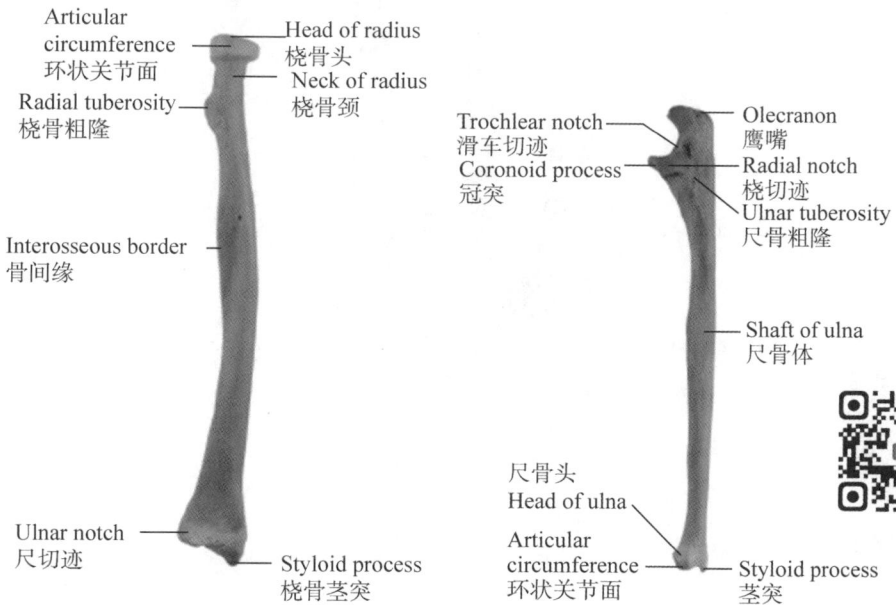

Articular
circumference
环状关节面

Radial tuberosity
桡骨粗隆

Head of radius
桡骨头

Neck of radius
桡骨颈

Trochlear notch
滑车切迹

Coronoid process
冠突

Olecranon
鹰嘴

Radial notch
桡切迹

Ulnar tuberosity
尺骨粗隆

Interosseous border
骨间缘

Shaft of ulna
尺骨体

尺骨头
Head of ulna

Articular
circumference
环状关节面

Ulnar notch
尺切迹

Styloid process
桡骨茎突

Styloid process
茎突

Fig.1-20   The radius

Fig.1-21   The ulna

the radius. The upper extremity of the ulna is connected to the trochlea of the humerus, the olecranon process that fits into the olecranon fossa of the humerus. There is also a radial notch for the head of the radius, and the ulnar tuberosity to which muscles attach. At the distal end of the ulna is a head and medial styloid process.

4) The bones of the hand (Fig.1-22). They can be subdivided into three segments: the carpus or wrist bones, the metacarpus and the phalanges or bones of the digits.

5) The carpal bones (腕骨). The carpal bones include eight short bones and are arranged into two rows to form the carpal tunnel. The proximal row consists of the scaphoid, lunate, triquetrum, pisiform, while the distal row consists of the trapezium, trapezoid, capitate, hamate.

6) The metacarpal bones (掌骨). They refer to the five long bones located between the phalanges and the carpus, conventionally numbered in a radio-ulnar order. Each metacarpal bone consists of a body and two extremities (head and base).

7) Phalanges (指骨). They refer to the digital bones in the hands. The thumbs have two phalanges while the other digits have three phalanges (the proximal phalange, the middle phalange and the distal phalange). The phalanges are classed as long bones. Each phalanx consists of a head, shaft and proximal base.

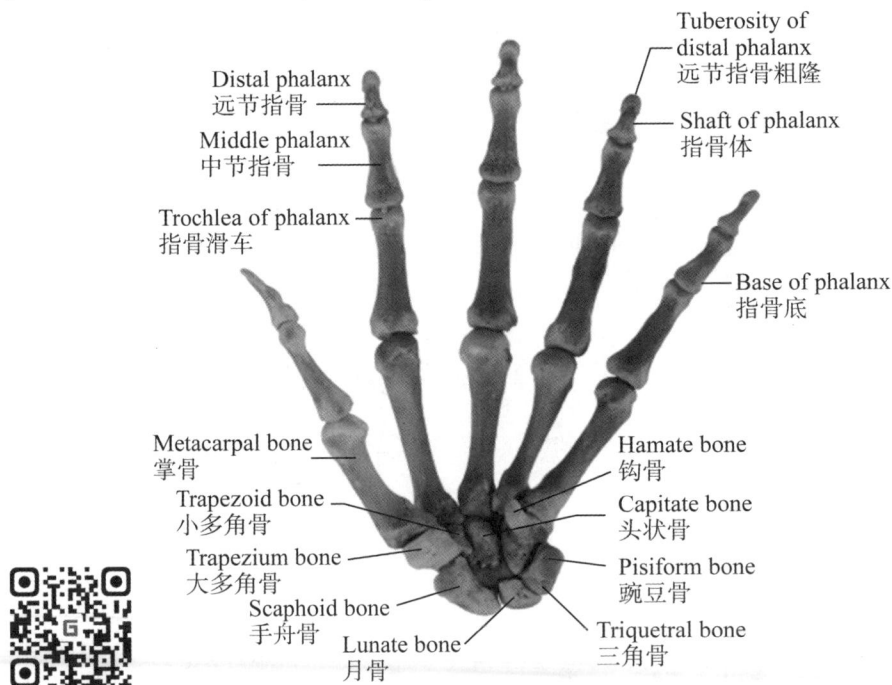

Distal phalanx
远节指骨

Middle phalanx
中节指骨

Trochlea of phalanx
指骨滑车

Tuberosity of distal phalanx
远节指骨粗隆

Shaft of phalanx
指骨体

Base of phalanx
指骨底

Metacarpal bone
掌骨

Trapezoid bone
小多角骨

Trapezium bone
大多角骨

Scaphoid bone
手舟骨

Lunate bone
月骨

Hamate bone
钩骨

Capitate bone
头状骨

Pisiform bone
豌豆骨

Triquetral bone
三角骨

Fig.1-22   Bones of the hand

2. Bones of the Lower Limbs

The bones of the lower limbs are the three fused components of the pelvic girdle; the femur and patella, the tibia and fibula, and the tarsus, metatarsus, phalanges and sesamoid bones. The pelvic girdle is formed by the hip bones, which articulate with each other in front, at the symphysis pubis. It is imperfect behind, but the gap is filled in by the upper part of the sacrum. The pelvic girdle, with the sacrum, is a complete ring, massive and comparatively rigid, in marked contrast to the lightness and mobility of the shoulder girdle.

(1) **The pelvic girdle**

1) The hip bone (髋骨) (Fig.1-23). The pelvic bone or coxal bone is a large flat bone, constricted in the center and expanding above and below. It is composed of three bones: the ilium, the ischium, and the pubis. At birth, these three component bones are separated by hyaline cartilage. They join each other in a Y-shaped portion of cartilage in the acetabulum. The two hip bones join at the pubic symphysis and together with the sacrum and coccyx (the pelvic part of the spine) comprise the skeletal component of the pelvis. Each hip bone is connected to the corresponding femur through the large ball and socket joint of the hip.

2) The ilium (髂骨) is the uppermost and largest bone of the pelvis, three surfaces and two parts: the body and the ala; the separation is indicated on the top surface by a curved line, the arcuate line, and on the external surface by the margin of the acetabulum. The superior border is the prominent iliac crest which is a site of attachment for a number of muscles and fascia of the abdominal wall, the back and the lower limb. It ends anteriorly at the anterior superior iliac spine and posteriorly at the posterior superior iliac spine.

3) The ischium (坐骨) forms the lower and back part of the hip bone, two main parts: the body and the inferior ramus. The body has upper and lower ends and femoral, posterior and pelvic surfaces. The body contains a prominent spine. The indentation inferior to the spine is the lesser sciatic notch. Continuing downward the posterior side, the ischial tuberosity is a thick, rough surfaced prominence below the lesser sciatic notch. The ramus extends inferiorly from the body and unites with the inferior ramus of the pubis. The ramus participates in the formation of the obturator foramen.

4) The pubis (耻骨) is the ventral and anterior part of the hip bone with three parts: the body, the superior ramus and the inferior ramus. The superior ramus passes up and back to the acetabulum and the inferior ramus passes back, down and laterally to join the ischial ramus inferomedial to the obturator foramen. The rounded upper border is known as the pubic crest. This crest ends laterally as the pubic tubercle which provides attachment to the medial end of the inguinal ligament. The left and right hip bones join at

the pubic symphysis.

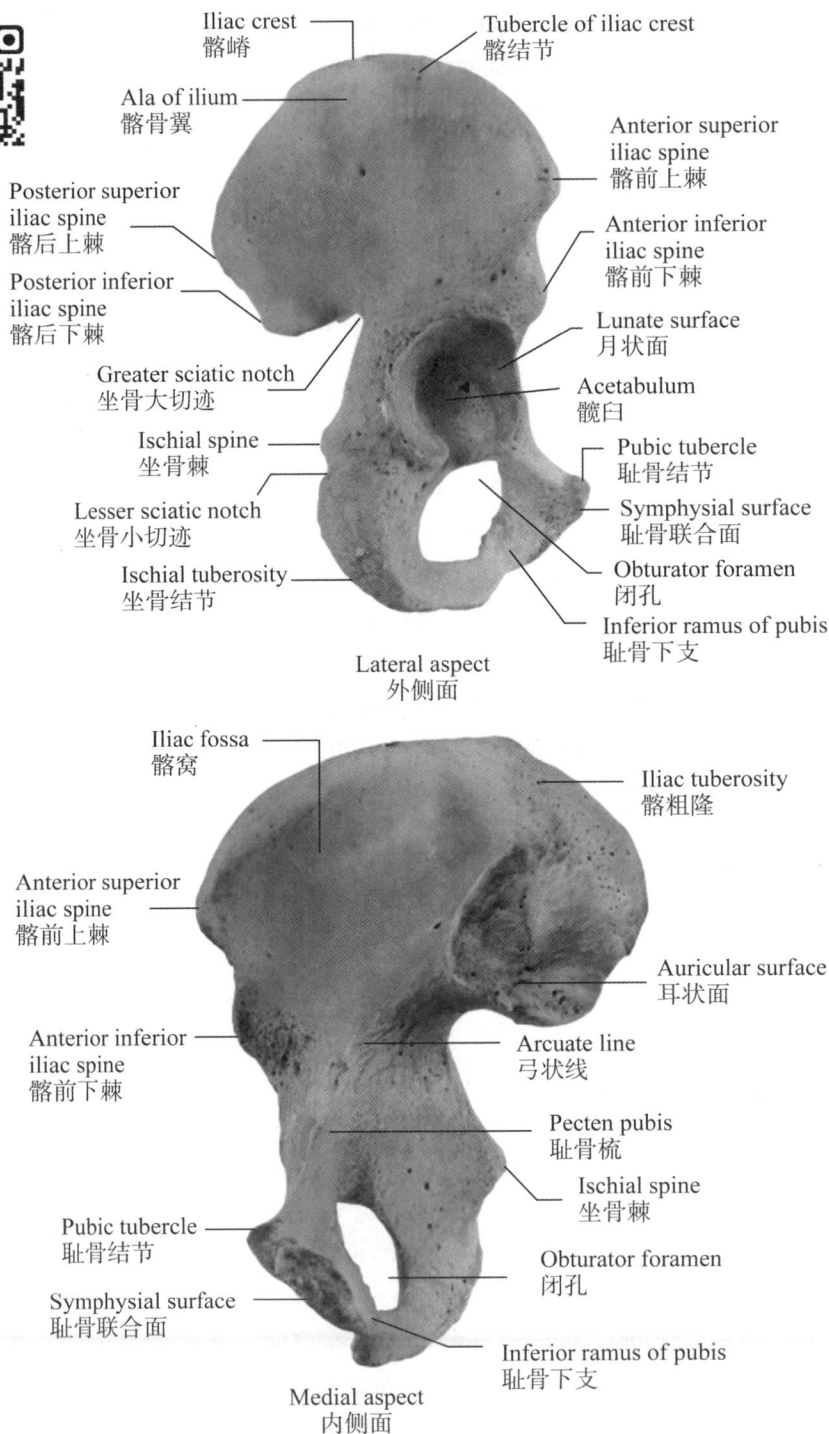

Iliac crest
髂嵴

Tubercle of iliac crest
髂结节

Ala of ilium
髂骨翼

Anterior superior
iliac spine
髂前上棘

Posterior superior
iliac spine
髂后上棘

Anterior inferior
iliac spine
髂前下棘

Posterior inferior
iliac spine
髂后下棘

Lunate surface
月状面

Greater sciatic notch
坐骨大切迹

Acetabulum
髋臼

Ischial spine
坐骨棘

Pubic tubercle
耻骨结节

Lesser sciatic notch
坐骨小切迹

Symphysial surface
耻骨联合面

Obturator foramen
闭孔

Ischial tuberosity
坐骨结节

Inferior ramus of pubis
耻骨下支

Lateral aspect
外侧面

Iliac fossa
髂窝

Iliac tuberosity
髂粗隆

Anterior superior
iliac spine
髂前上棘

Auricular surface
耳状面

Anterior inferior
iliac spine
髂前下棘

Arcuate line
弓状线

Pecten pubis
耻骨梳

Ischial spine
坐骨棘

Pubic tubercle
耻骨结节

Obturator foramen
闭孔

Symphysial surface
耻骨联合面

Inferior ramus of pubis
耻骨下支

Medial aspect
内侧面

Fig.1-23   The hip bone

(2) Free bones of the lower limbs

1) The femur (股骨) (Fig.1-24). As the longest and strongest bone in the skeleton, its length on average is 1/4 of a person's height. The femur is categorised as a long bone and comprises a diaphysis, the shaft (or body) and two epiphyses or extremities that articulate with adjacent bones in the hip and the knee. The femoral head faces anterosuperomedially to articulate with the acetabulum. The upper extremity of the right femur viewed from behind and above show the head, the neck, and the greater and lesser trochanter. The head of femur has a small groove, or fovea. The lower extremity of the femur (or distal extremity) has two oblong eminences known as the condyles. Anteriorly, the condyles are separated by a smooth shallow articular depression called the patellar surface. Posteriorly, a deep notch is the intercondylar fossa of femur. The popliteal surface of the femur is a triangular space found at the distal posterior surface of the femur.

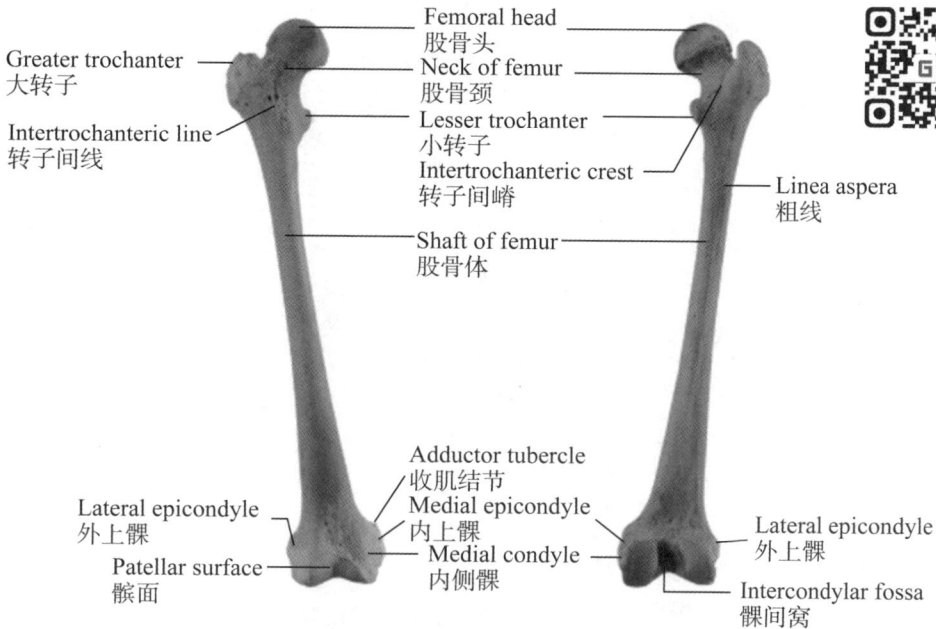

Fig.1-24　The femur

2) The tibia (胫骨) (Fig.1-25). The tibia is one of two bones in the lower leg(medial side), the other being the fibula(lateral side), and is a component of the knee and ankle joints. The tibia is composed of a body and two epiphyses, and the tibial shaft is triangular in section. The proximal extremity of the tibia is expanded in the transverse plane with a medial and lateral condyle. The upper surfaces of the condyles articulate with the femur to form the tibiofemoral joint. Here the medial and lateral intercondylar tubercles form the intercondylar eminence. The lower extremity of the tibia is much smaller than the upper extremity; it is prolonged downward on its medial side as a strong process, the medial

malleolus. The lower extremity of the tibia forms the ankle joint together with the fibula and the talus.

3) The fibula (腓骨) (Fig.1-25). The fibula is a leg bone located on the lateral side of the tibia and is much more slender than the tibia. Its upper extremity is small, placed toward the back of the head of the tibia, below the knee joint, and excluded from the formation of this joint. Its lower extremity inclines a little forward, so as to be on a plane anterior to that of the upper end, and forms the lateral part of the ankle joint.

4) The tarsal bones (跗骨). The tarsal bones are seven articulating short bones in each foot situated among the lower end of tibia, the fibula of the lower leg and the metatarsus. The joint between the tibia and the fibula above and the tarsus below is referred to as the ankle joint. The tarsal bones, seven in number, consist of the talus, the calcaneus (hindfoot), the cuboid, the navicular, and three cuneiform bones which form the arches of the foot serving as a shock absorber.

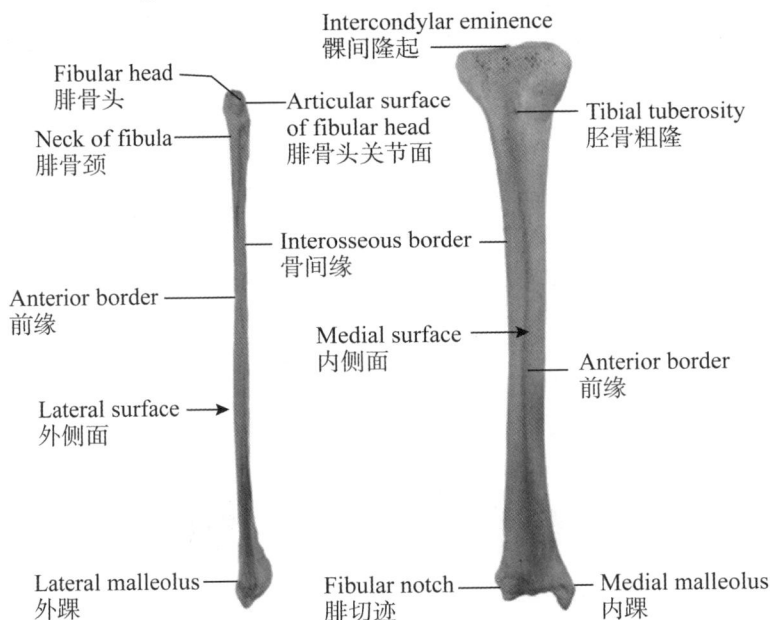

Fig.1-25　The tibia and fibula

5) The metatarsal bone (跖骨). The metatarsal bone consists of five bones which are numbered from the medial side (ossa metatarsalia I－V). Like the metacarpals, they are miniature long bones and have a shaft, proximal base and distal head.

6) The phalange of toe (趾骨). In number and general arrangement, they are comparable to those of the hand; the great toe has two phalanges, while each of the other toes has three. However, they vary in size, with the bodies notably shorter, especially those in the first row (Fig.1-26).

Distal phalanx
远节趾骨

Middle phalanx
中节趾骨

Proximal phalanx
近节趾骨

Intermediate
cuneiform bone
中间楔骨

Metatarsal bone
跖骨

Medial
cuneiform bone
内侧楔骨

Lateral
cuneiform bone
外侧楔骨

Navicular bone
足舟骨

Cuboid bone
骰骨

Talus
距骨

Trochlea of talus
距骨滑车

Calcaneus
跟骨

Superior view of right foot
右足上面观

Distal phalanx
远节趾骨

Middle phalanx
中节趾骨

Proximal phalanx
近节趾骨

Metatarsal bone
跖骨

Lateral
cuneiform bone
外侧楔骨

Intermediate
cuneiform bone
中间楔骨

Medial
cuneiform bone
内侧楔骨

Cuboid bone
骰骨

Navicular bone
足舟骨

Calcaneus
跟骨

Talus
距骨

Calcaneal tuberosity
跟骨结节

Inferior view of right foot
右足底面观

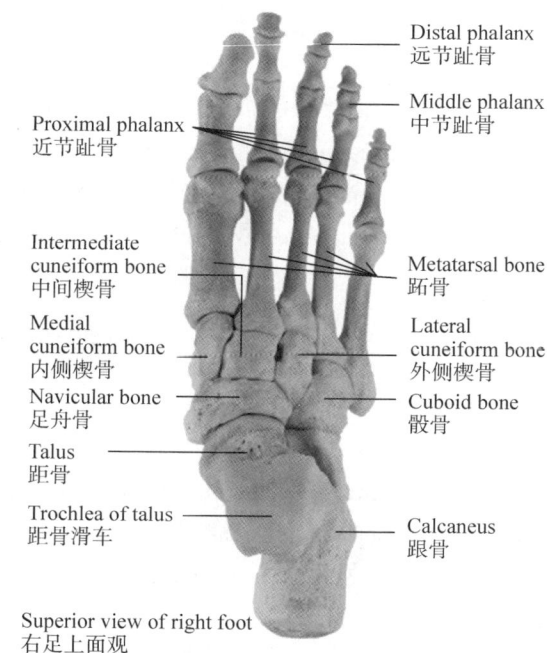

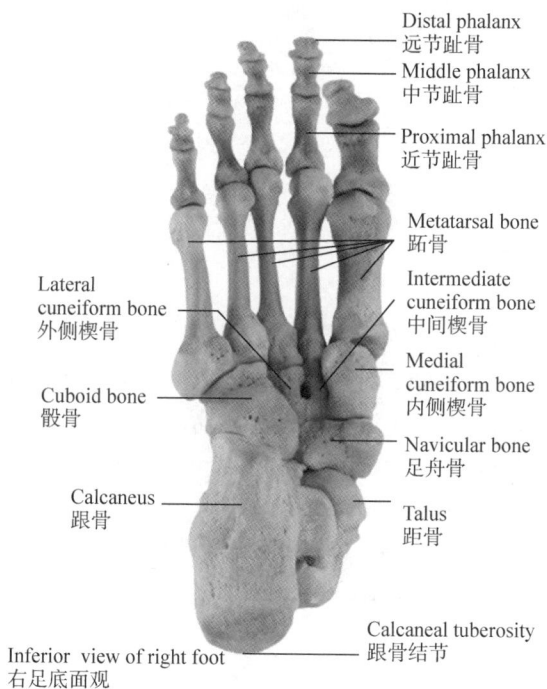

Fig.1-26 Bones of the foot

（吉林大学　刘海岩）

Exercise

1. A 46-year-old man was admitted to ICU due to an accident half of an hour before the admission. However, he had already died upon arrival. Autopsy revealed that one cervical vertebra was broken and a small piece of bony fragments was driven into his spinal cord. From which of the following bones was this fragment most likely derived?

(A) The atlas.

(B) The axis.

(C) The seventh cervical vertebra.

(D) The sixth cervical vertebra.

(E) The fifth cervical vertebra.

2. A 60-year-old woman was admitted to the emergency department due to a fall. The physical examination showed that her left leg was shortened with external rotation. The patient had a history of osteoporosis. Which part of the femur was most likely fractured according to these findings?

(A) The greater trochanter.

(B) The lateral epicondyle.

(C) The medical epicondyle.

(D) The neck.

(E) The shaft.

Answer

1. The correct answer is B.

The atlas (Choice A) is the first cervical vertebra, and it receives the odontoid process of axis (Choice B) which is the part of the second cervical vertebra. Odontoid process is susceptible to traumatic fracture, and bony fragments can injure the spinal cord. Because the first to the fourth sections of the spinal cord are closely related to respiratory activity, the damage in these sections will cause sudden death. Bone fragments from the cervical vertebrae in other choices (Choices C, D and E) do not usually cause sudden death.

2. The correct answer is D.

This is the typical presentation of a fracture of the neck of the femur. Dislocation of the head of the femur results in the leg rotation externally. Fracture of the femur at the greater trochanter (Choice A), the epicondyles (Choices B and C) or the shaft (Choice E) do not produce outward rotation of the entire limb.

1.2 Arthrology

1.2.1 General Description

1. Definition of the Arthrology (关节学)

Arthrology treats a connection between two or more bones or between the bone and the cartilage. The bones are connected together by the fibrous, cartilaginous, osseous tissues or joint.

2. Classification of Articulation

There are two main types: *synarthroses* (不动关节) and *diarthroses* (活动关节).

(1) **Synarthroses (immovable articulation)** (Fig. 1-27). They only have a little or have no movement, consisting of *fibrous joints* (纤维连结) (sutures, syndesmoses), *cartilaginous joints* (软骨连结) (synchondroses-hyaline cartilages, symphyses-fibrous cartilages) and *synostosis* (骨性结合).

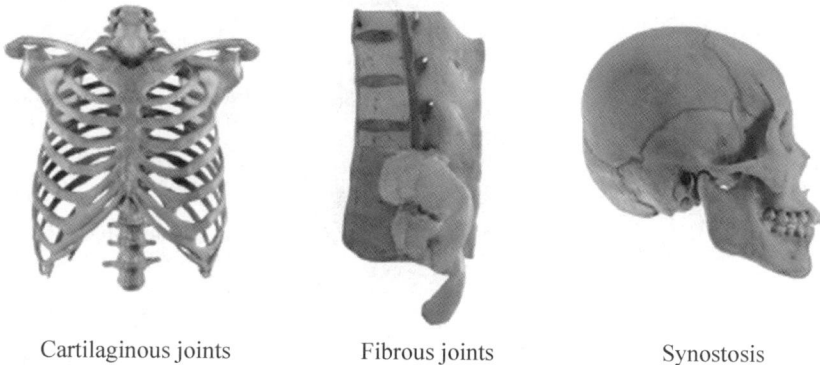

Cartilaginous joints   Fibrous joints   Synostosis

Fig.1-27   Synarthroses

(2) **Diarthroses (synovial joints or movable articulations).** They provide free movement.

1) Essential structures of a *synovial joint* (滑膜关节) (Fig.1-28)

Articular surface (关节面) is the portions of the bone that come into contact with one another within a joint. They have a layer of smooth hyaline cartilage.

Articular (joint) capsule (关节囊) is found in the space where two or more adjacent bones meet to form a synovial joint. There are two layers: *fibrous membrane* (纤维膜) (superficial, thickness) and *synovial membrane* (滑膜)(deep, thin, slippery, can pro-duce synovia that lubricates the joint).

Joint cavity (关节腔) is a closed cavity and contains the synovial fluid. It is negative to the atmosphere pressure.

2) Accessory structures of the synovial joints

Ligaments (韧带): Some fibrous membranes are arranged in parallel bundles of dense regular connective tissue. There are two kinds: intracapsular and extracapsular ligaments.

Articular disc (关节盘): It refers to the fibrocartilage pads between opposing surfaces in a joint, articular meniscus (半月板).

Articular labrum (关节唇) (lip): It is the fibrocartilage ring attached to the periphery of the joint cavity, and has the effect of deepening the joint cavity and enhancing joint stability.

Synovial folds and synovial bursa (滑膜襞和滑膜囊): It is the synovial layer protruding into the joint cavity. The synovial folds increase the surface area of the synovial membrane, which is conducive to the secretion and absorption of synovial fluid, and helps to alleviate collisions.

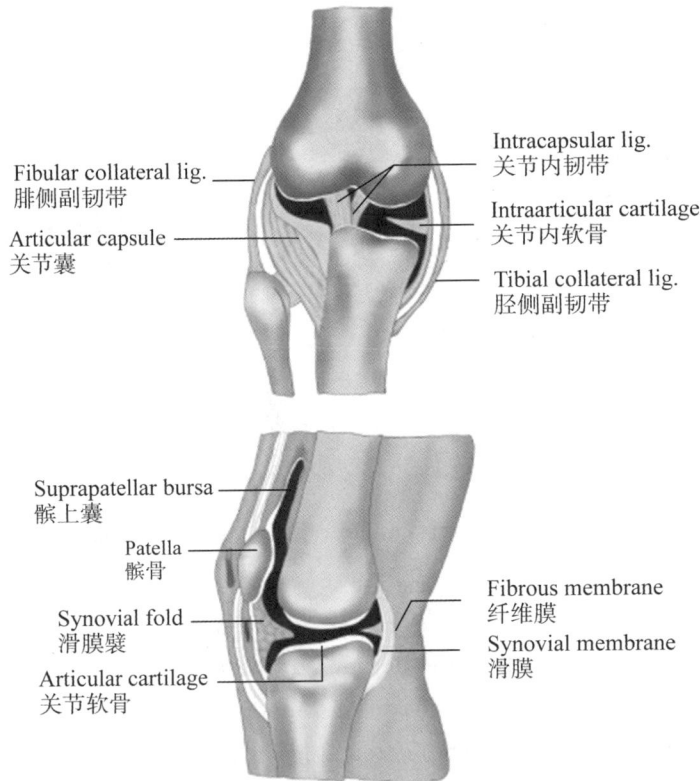

Fibular collateral lig. 腓侧副韧带

Articular capsule 关节囊

Intracapsular lig. 关节内韧带

Intraarticular cartilage 关节内软骨

Tibial collateral lig. 胫侧副韧带

Suprapatellar bursa 髌上囊

Patella 髌骨

Synovial fold 滑膜襞

Articular cartilage 关节软骨

Fibrous membrane 纤维膜

Synovial membrane 滑膜

Fig.1-28　Structure of the synovial joint

3) Movements of the joint (diarthroses)

Flexion (屈) and *extension* (伸) (in the coronal axis): Flexion means decreasing the angle of the joint relative to its anatomical position. Extension means increasing the angle of the joint relative to its anatomical position.

Adduction (收) and *abduction* (展) (in the sagittal axis): Abduction means away from the midline of the body. Adduction moving toward the midline of the body.

Rotation (旋转) (in the vertical axis or around its own long axis): It refers to a circular movement around a fixed point.

Pronation (旋前) and *supination* (旋后) (only for forearm): They include medial rotation and external rotation, and refer to rotation of the forearm so that in the anatomical position, turn your palm anteriorly(front) or posteriorly (back).

Inversion (内翻) and *eversion* (外翻): They refer to movements that tilt the sole of the foot away from (eversion) or towards (inversion) the midline of the body.

Circumduction (环转) (around 2 or 3 axises): It refers to the circular movement of a limb, which a combination of flexion, extension, adduction and abduction.

Gliding or *slipping* (滑动): It refers to movements in the plane joint)

4) Classification of synovial joints (according to the axis) (Fig.1-29).

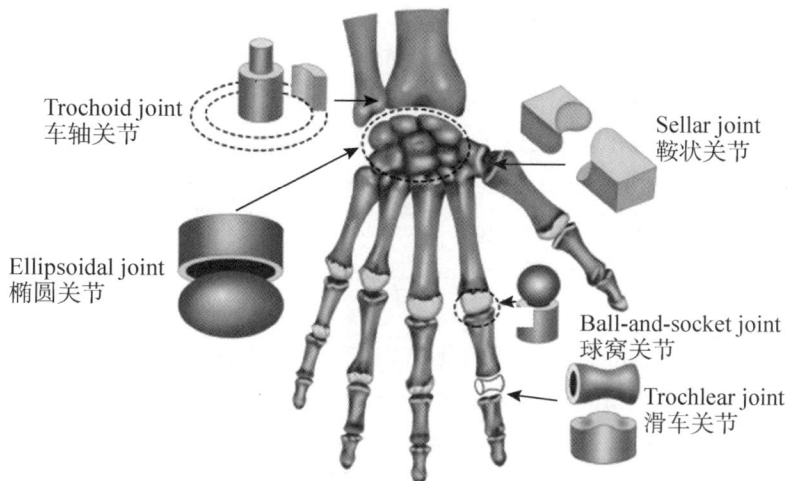

Fig.1-29 Classification of synovial joints

• The polyaxial joints

Plane joint (平面关节) (gliding joint): It is only a little glide.

Ball-and-socket joint (球窝关节): flexion and extension, adduction and abduction, medial and lateral rotation, circumduction.

• The biaxial joints

Ellipsoidal joint (椭圆关节) (condyloid joint): flexion and extension, adduction and abduction, circumduction.

Saddle joints (鞍状关节) (sellar joint): flexion and extension, adduction and abduction, circumduction are included.

• The uniaxial joints

Hinge joint (屈戍关节) (trochlear joint): only flexion and extension.

Pivot joint (车轴关节): trochoid joint rotation around a long axis.

1.2.2 Joints of the Trunk

Bones of the trunk include the vertebra (椎骨), the sternum (胸骨) and the costal bone (肋骨). It is formed by the vertebral column (脊柱) and the rib cage.

1. Vertebral Column

The vertebral column is a flexuous and flexible column, formed of 32 or 33 vertebrae, which are grouped under the names cervical (7), thoracic (12), lumbar (5), sacral (5), and coccygeal (3—4), according to the regions they occupy. The articulations of the vertebral column consist of i) a series of amphiarthrodial joints between the vertebral bodies, and ii) a series of diarthrodial joints between the vertebral arches.

(1) **Joints of the vertebral bodies** (Fig.1-30)

1) Intervertebral discs (椎间盘). They are between the bodies of adjacent vertebrae, composed of nucleus pulposus (髓核) and annulus fibrosus (纤维环). Nucleus pulposus is an inner soft, pulpy, highly elastic structure (gelatinous core). Annulus fibrosus is an outer fibrous ring, consisting of fibrocartilage. They adhere to thin layers of cartilage on the superior and inferior vertebral surfaces, the vertebral end-plates. There are 23 in number in adults (no intervertebral disc between the atlas and the axis) and the total thickness of all intervertebral discs accounts for approximately 1/4 of the total length of the spine above the sacrum.

2) Anterior longitudinal ligament (前纵韧带). The anterior longitudinal ligament is a broad and strong band of fibers, which extends along the anterior surfaces of the bodies of the vertebrae, from the axis to the sacrum. Strong band covering the anterior part of the vertebral bodies and intervertebral discs running from the anterior margin of foramen magnum to the S1—S2. Maintains stability of the intervertebral disc and prevents hyper extension of the vertebral column. The ligament fills the anterior concavities of the bodies at intermediate levels.

3) Posterior longitudinal ligament (后纵韧带). The posterior longitudinal ligament is situated within the vertebral canal, and extends along the posterior surfaces of the vertebrae bodies, from the body of the axis, where it is continuous with the membrana tectoria, to the sacrum. It is broader above than below, and thicker in the thoracic than in the cervical and lumbar regions. It is attached to the posterior aspect of the intervertebral discs and posterior edges of the vertebral bodies from the C2 vertebra to the sacrum. It prevents hyperflexion of the vertebral column and posterior protrusion of the discs.

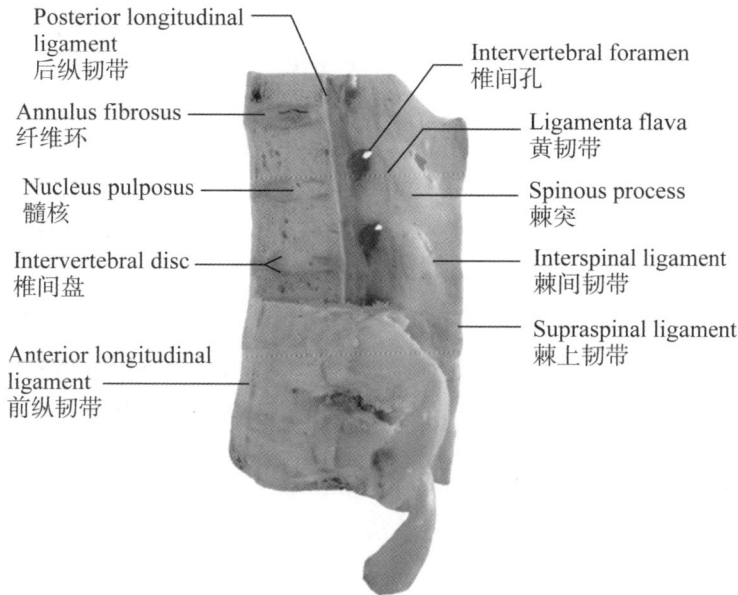

Posterior longitudinal ligament
后纵韧带

Annulus fibrosus
纤维环

Nucleus pulposus
髓核

Intervertebral disc
椎间盘

Anterior longitudinal ligament
前纵韧带

Intervertebral foramen
椎间孔

Ligamenta flava
黄韧带

Spinous process
棘突

Interspinal ligament
棘间韧带

Supraspinal ligament
棘上韧带

Fig.1-30   Joints of the vertebral bodies

(2) **Joints of the vertebral arches** (椎弓间的连结)

The vertebral arches are connected by synovial joints between superior and inferior articular processes and by accessory ligaments that connect the laminae and all processes.

1) Zygapophysial joints (关节突关节). They are formed by opposing articular processes of the adjacent vertebrae. They are mostly of the gliding type and move only slightly.

2) Ligamenta flava (黄韧带). It is thick, yellow and elastic plates, which are attached to the inferior or anterior surface of lamina. It is contributed to part of the posterior boundary of the vertebral canal and tends to prevent hyperflexion of the vertebral column.

3) Interspinal ligaments (棘间韧带). They are thin and membranous, which connect adjoining spinous processes and extend from the root to the apex of each process. They meet the ligamenta flava in front and the supraspinal ligament behind.

4) Intertransverse ligaments (横突间韧带). It connect adjoining transverse processes.

5) Supraspinal ligament (棘上韧带). It is a strong fibrous cord, which connects together the apices of the spinous processes from the seventh cervical vertebra to the sacrum. It continued with the ligamentum nuchae.

6) Ligamentum nuchae (项韧带). It is a fibrous membrane, which extends from the external occipital protuberance and median nuchal line to the spinous process of the seventh cervical vertebra, and forms a septum between the muscles on either side of the neck.

7) Atlantooccipital joint (寰枕关节). It lies between superior articulating surfaces of atlas and occipital condyles, consisting of two articular capsules. The posterior atlantoaxial, the anterior atlantoaxial and the transverse is supported by membrance and ligaments that join occipital bone and atlas. Atlantooccipital joint takes part in the action, including the nodding of head and the lateral tilting of head.

8) Atlantoaxial joint (寰枢关节). Three synovial joints are between the atlas and the axis. Laterally, paired joints are between articulating facets. Median joint is between dens of axis and anterior arch of atlas. They are supported by ligaments which are *apical ligament of dens* (齿突尖韧带), *alar ligament* (翼状韧带) and *transverse ligament of atlas* (寰椎横韧带). Action allows the atlas (and head) pivot on the axis and the vertebral column.

(3) Normal curvature of the vertebral column

The cervical curvature is convex forward, and the thoracic curve is convex backward, while the lumbar curve is convex forward and the sacral curve is convex backward (Fig.1-31). The movement of the vertebral column covers flexion, extension, lateral flexion and rotation.

2. Thoracic Cage (胸廓)

(1) **Composition**. Bones consist of twelve thoracic vertebrae, twelve pairs of ribs and

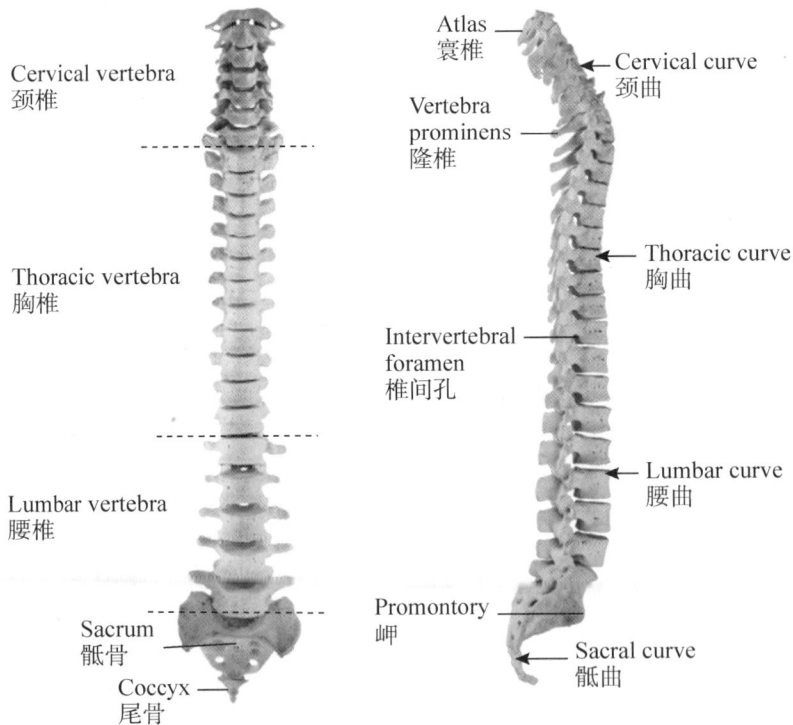

Fig.1-31　The vertebral column

costal cartilages, and sternum. Costovertebral joints (肋椎关节) consists of joints of costal head (肋头关节), costotransverse joints (肋横突关节), sternocostal joints (胸肋关节), sternocostal synchondrosis of the first rib, sternocostal joints, interchondral joints which are between costal cartilages 8, 9, and 10 to form the costal arch (肋弓). To increase the volume during inspiration, the ribs swing outward and upward, the second to the tenth ribs are elevated and their lower borders everted. The contrary movement decreases the volume during expiration.

(2) **General features of thoracic cage**. It is roughly cone-shape, narrow above and broad below, flattened from before-backwards, longer behind than in front. The superior thoracic aperture or superior aperture of thorax (胸廓上口) is bounded by the upper border of the manubrium, the first rib, and the vertebra T1. The inferior thoracic aperture or inferior aperture of thorax (胸廓下口) is bounded by the vertebra T12, the twelvth and the eleventh ribs, the costal arch and the xiphoid process. The infrasternal angle (胸骨下角) is formed by the costal arch of both sides. The intercostal space lies between the ribs.

(3) **Function**. The thoracic cage (Fig.1-32) protects the organs in the thoracic cavity and the upper abdominal cavity. It plays a vital role in the process of breathing.

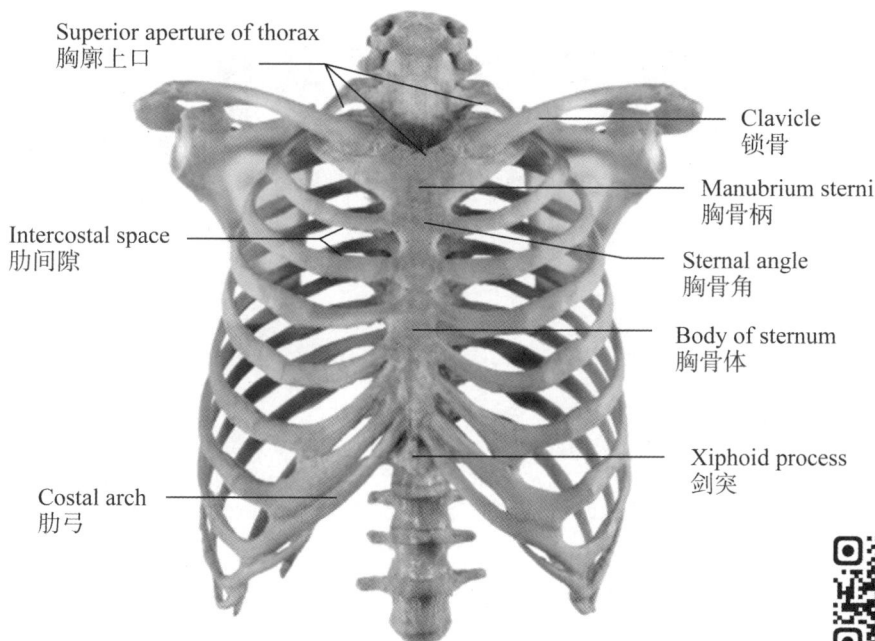

Fig.1-32   The thoracic cage

1.2.3   Joints of the Skull

Most bones of the skull are connected together by suture, synchodrosis, or synostosis. The suture is a type of fibrous joint which only occurs in the skull.

Coronal suture (冠状缝) lies between the frontal and two parietal bones. *Lambdoid suture* (人字缝) lies between the parietal and occipital bones and is continuous with the occipitomastoid suture. *Occipitomastoid suture* (枕乳突缝) lies between the occipital and temporal bones and is continuous with the lambdoid suture.

The temporomandibular joint (颞下颌关节) (Fig. 1-33) is a bilateral synovial articulation between the mandible (下颌骨) and the temporal bone (颞骨), formed by the mandibular fossa (下颌窝), the articular tubercle and the head of mandibule. Capsule is thin and lax in front and behind, strengthened by the ligaments as the temporomandibular (颞下颌韧带) (lateral), sphenomandibular (蝶下颌韧带) and stylomandibular ligaments (茎突下颌韧带). Articular disk separates surfaces, forming upper and lower compartments the joint. Movement is elevated or depressed, protruded or retracted; rotation may also occur as in chewing (a slight amount of side to side movement is also permitted).

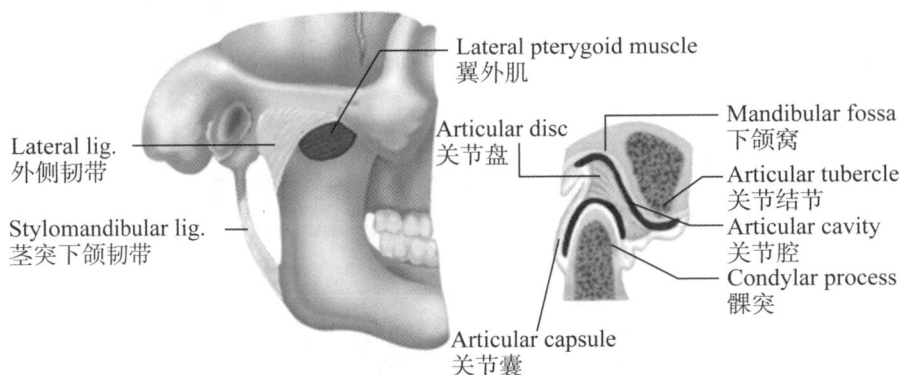

Fig.1-33　The temporomandibular joint

1.2.4　Joints of the Limbs

The joints of the upper limb and joints of the lower limb are included.

1. Joints of the Upper Limb

The articulations of the upper extremity are arranged as follows: sternoclavicular joint (胸锁关节), acromioclavicular joint (肩锁关节), shoulder joint (肩关节), elbow joint (肘关节), wrist joint (腕关节), radioulnar joint (桡尺关节), intercarpal joint (腕骨间关节), carpometacarpal joint (腕掌关节), intermetacarpal joint (掌骨间关节), metacarpophalangeal joint (掌指关节), interphalangeal joint of hand (指骨间关节).

(1) Joints of the girdle of the upper limb

1)Sternoclavicular joint (胸锁关节) (Fig.1-34). It is a synovial sellar joint of sternal end of clavicle, clavicular notch of sternum and the first costal cartilage. It is the only articulation between the upper limb and the axial skeleton.The ligaments of this joint are: the intrinsic ligaments (the anterior and posterior sternoclavicular ligaments); the extrinsic ligaments (the midline interclavicular ligament and the costoclavicular ligaments on each side). An articular disk is attached to the capsule, dividing the joint into two cavities between the sternal and clavicular surfaces. The movements are of the following kinds. This articulation admits of a limited amount of motion in nearly every direction—elevation and depression, forward and backward, rotation and circumduction of the acromial end of the clavicle.

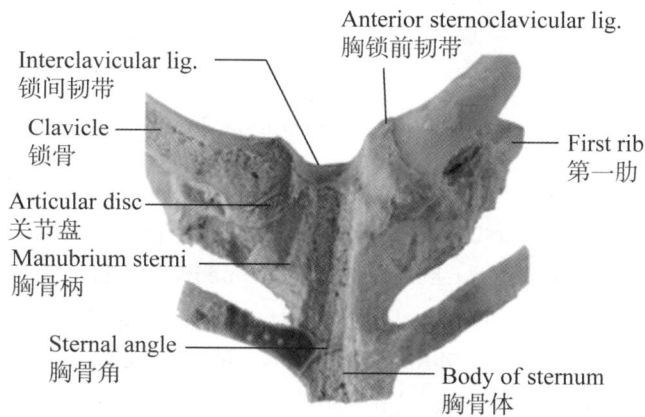

Fig.1-34　The sternoclavicular joint

2) Acromioclavicular joint (肩锁关节). The acromioclavicular articulation is a synovial plane joint between the acromial end of the clavicle and the acromion of the scapula. The movements of this articulation are of two kinds: a gliding motion of the articular end of the clavicle on the acromion; rotation of the scapula forward and backward upon the clavicle. Coraco-acromial arch (喙肩弓) formed by coraco-acromial ligament (喙肩韧带), coracoid process (喙突), and acromion (肩峰) that prevents the shoulder joint from superior dislocation.

(2) **Joints of free upper limb**

1) Glenohumeral (shoulder) joint (肩关节)(Fig.1-35). The shoulder joint is ball-and-socket joint. The joint is protected by an arch, formed by the coracoid process, the acromion, and the coracoacromial ligament. The bones entering into its formation are the hemispherical head of the humerus (肱骨) and the shallow glenoid cavity of the scapula.

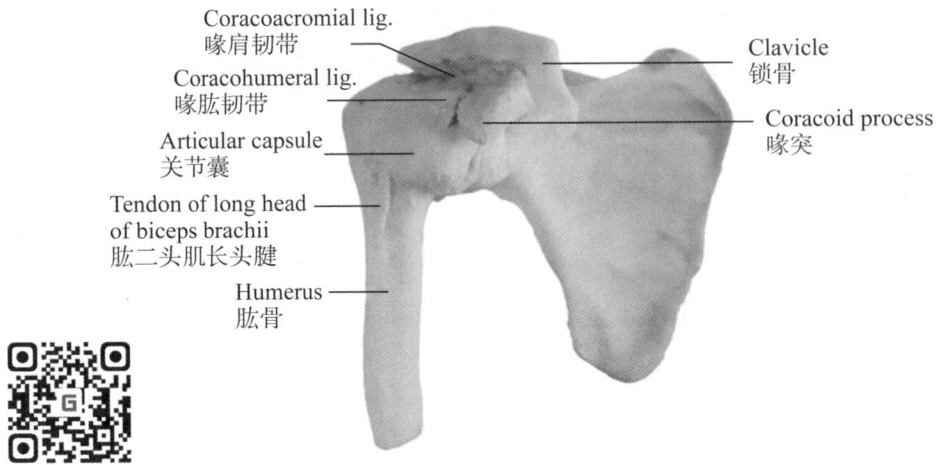

Fig.1-35　The shoulder joint

The capsule is thicker above and below than that elsewhere, and is so remarkably loose and lax, especially at the lower part. Attachments are proximal to glenoid labrum (盂唇), distal to anatomical neck of humerus, except medially where it is slightly distal to surgical neck. The tendon of long head of biceps brachii passes (肱二头肌长头腱) though the cavity. Glenoid labrum is a fibrocartilaginous rim attached around the margin of the glenoid cavity. Coracohumeral ligament (喙肱韧带) is a broad band which strengthens the upper part of the capsule, runs from the coracoid process to greater tubercle.

The shoulder joint is capable of every variety of movement, flexion, extension, adduction, abduction, medial and lateral rotation, circumduction.

2) The elbow joint (肘关节)(Fig. 1-36). The elbow joint is a ginglymus or hinge-joint, acting as a platform for the forearm and hand. Bones: lower end of humerus, upper ends of radius (桡骨) and ulna (尺骨). It consists of humeroulnar joint (肱尺关节) that is formed by trochlea of humerus (肱骨滑车) and troclear noch (hinge) (尺骨滑车切迹),

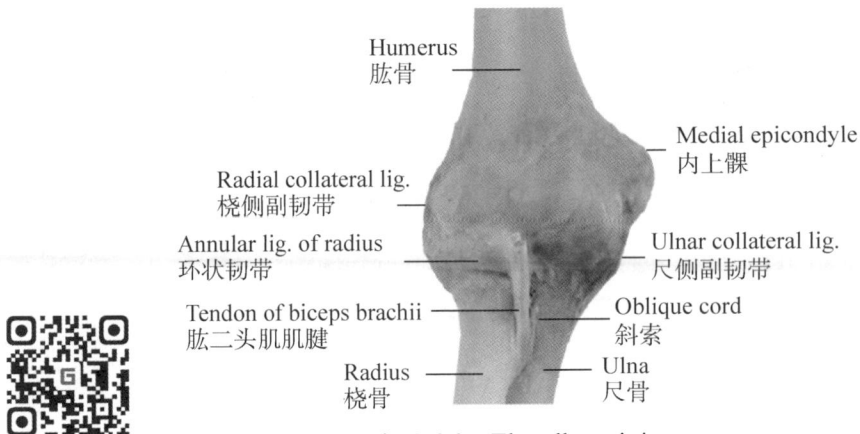

Fig.1-36　The elbow joint

humeroradial joint (肱桡关节) that is formed by capitulum of humerus (肱骨小头) and articular fovea of radius (桡骨头关节凹), and proximal radioulnar joint (桡尺近侧关节) that is formed by articular circumference of radius (桡骨环状关节面) and radial notch of ulna (尺骨桡切迹).

The capsule is thin and lax anteriorly and posteriorly, strongly thickened on either side by collateral ligaments. Radial collateral ligament (桡侧副韧带) is a short and narrow fibrous band, less distinct than the ulnar collateral, attached, above, to a depression below the lateral epicondyle of the humerus. Ulnar collateral ligament (尺侧副韧带) is a thick triangular band consisting of two portions, an anterior one and a posterior one united by a thinner intermediate portion. It is attached to medial epicondyle to medial border of trochlear notch. Annular ligament of radius (桡骨环状韧带) attached to anterior and posterior margins of radial notch of the ulna surrounds the head of radius. The movements are flexion and extension, pronation and supination.

The elbow joint allows for flexion and extension. The head of the radius can rotate and carry the hand to pronate and supinate.

3) Joints of the hand (Fig.1-37). They consist of the theradiocarpal joint (the wrist joint), the intercarpal joint, the carpometacarpal joints, the intermetacarpal joints, the metacarpophalangeal joints and the interphalangeal joints.

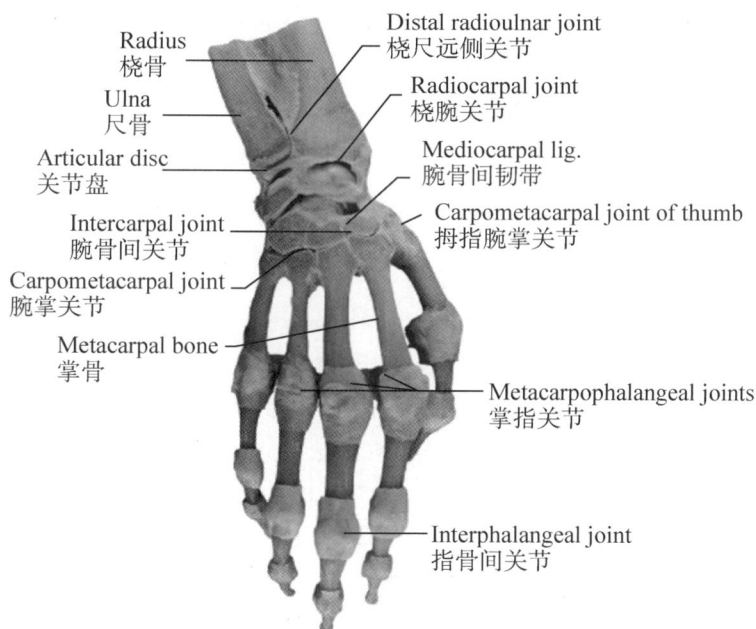

Fig.1-37 Joints of the hand

4) The radiocarpal joint (the wrist joint) (桡腕关节，腕关节). The wrist joint is a synovial, biaxial and ellipsoid joint. Bones refer to carpal articular surface of radius and articular disc below the ulna. including proximal row of carpal are scaphoid (手舟骨), lunate (月骨), and triquetral bones (三角骨), but not pisiform (豌豆骨).

5) The capsule. It is lax and strengthened by surrounding ligament. The movements permitted in this joint are flexion, extension, abduction, adduction, and circumduction.

6) The intercarpal joints (腕骨间关节). They are plane joints between the neighboring carpal bones. The movements of these joints are limited and considered as a part of all movements of the wrist joint.

7) The carpometacarpal joints. They are formed by the distal row of the carpal bones and the bases of the metacarpals. They share a common capsule with the intercarpal joints and the movements of them are slight except the carpometacarpal joint of the thumb. Carpometacarpal joint of thumb (拇指腕掌关节) is saddle-shaped by the trapezium (大多角骨) and the base of the first metacarpal (第 1 掌骨底). The capsule of the joint is thick but loose. The movements are flexion, extension, adduction, abduction, and opposition.

8) The intermetacarpal joints. They are plane joints, formed by the articulations between the opposed sides of the bases of the second, third, fourth and fifth metacarpal bones.

9) The metacarpophalangeal joints. They are the condyloid kind formed by the head of the metacarpal bones and the bases of the proximal phalanges. The movements are flexion, extension, abduction, adduction and circumduction.

10) The interphalangeal joints. They are typical hinge joints, formed by the heads of the phalanx proximally and the base of the phalanx distally. The movements are flexion and extension.

2. Joints of the Lower Limb

(1) Joints of the pelvic girdle of the lower limb

The pubic symphysis (耻骨联合), the sacroiliac joint (骶髂关节), the sacrotuberous (骶结节韧带) and sacrospinous ligaments (骶棘韧带)，the obturator membrane (闭孔膜), the obturator canal (闭膜管), the pelvis (骨盆).

1) Pubic symphysis (耻骨联合) (Fig.1-38). It is formed by symphysial surface and interpubic disc (fibrocartilage) (耻骨间盘). Ligaments include the superior pubic ligament (耻骨上韧带) and the arcuate pubic ligament (耻骨弓状韧带).

Superior pubic lig.
耻骨上韧带

Interpubic disc
耻骨间盘

Arcuate pubic lig.
耻骨弓状韧带

Superior ramus of pubis
耻骨上支

Obturator foramen
闭孔

Inferior ramus of pubis
耻骨下支

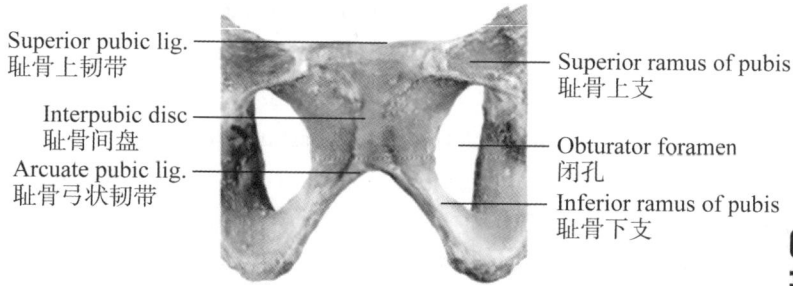

Fig.1-38　The pubic symphysis

2) Sacroiliac joint（骶髂关节）(Fig. 1-39). It refers to a stress-relieving joint consisting of syndesmotic and synovial parts, formed by auricular surface of sacrum （骶骨）and ilium（髂骨）. The sacral surface is covered by hyaline cartilage, and the thinner cartilage on the iliac surface is also hyaline in type. The ligaments of the sacroiliac joint are the anterior sacroiliac ligament, the posterior sacroiliac ligament and the interosseous sacroiliac ligament. The capsule is very tight and strengthened by ligaments. The movements are very limited because the joints are adapted to supporting the weight of the body.

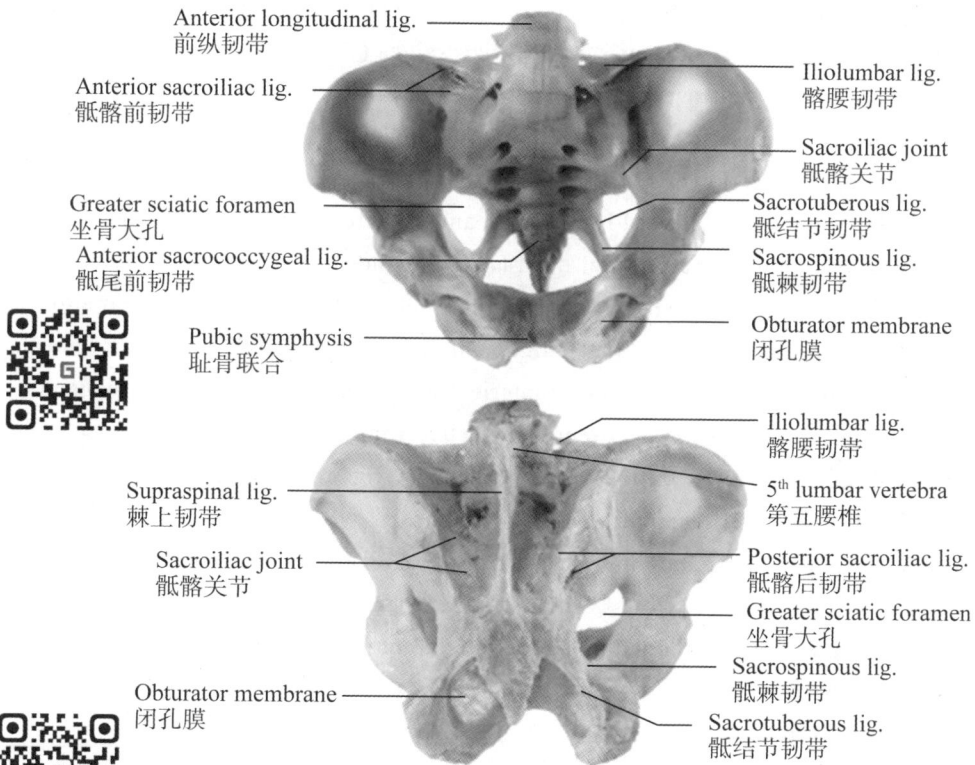

Anterior longitudinal lig.
前纵韧带

Anterior sacroiliac lig.
骶髂前韧带

Greater sciatic foramen
坐骨大孔

Anterior sacrococcygeal lig.
骶尾前韧带

Pubic symphysis
耻骨联合

Iliolumbar lig.
髂腰韧带

Sacroiliac joint
骶髂关节

Sacrotuberous lig.
骶结节韧带

Sacrospinous lig.
骶棘韧带

Obturator membrane
闭孔膜

Supraspinal lig.
棘上韧带

Sacroiliac joint
骶髂关节

Obturator membrane
闭孔膜

Iliolumbar lig.
髂腰韧带

5th lumbar vertebra
第五腰椎

Posterior sacroiliac lig.
骶髂后韧带

Greater sciatic foramen
坐骨大孔

Sacrospinous lig.
骶棘韧带

Sacrotuberous lig.
骶结节韧带

Fig.1-39　Ligaments of the pelvis

Iliolumbal ligament runs from transverse process of L5 to the posterosuperior part of the iliac crest. Sacrotuberous ligament (骶结节韧带) runs from lateral margins of sacrum and coccyx to the inner margin of ischial tuberosity (坐骨结节). Sacrospinous ligament (骶棘韧带) runs from ischial spine (坐骨棘) to lateral margins of sacrum and coccyx (尾骨). These two ligaments convert the sciatic notches (坐骨切迹) the greater and lesser sciatic foramina (坐骨大孔和坐骨小孔).

• The *obturator membrane* (闭孔膜) is fibrous in nature and spans the inner margin of the obturator foramen. It acts as a point of origin for both the obturator externus and obturator internus muscles. Superior and lateral is the obturator canal that passes through obturator vessels and nerves.

• The *pelvis* (骨盆) is formed by paired hip bones, sacrum, coccyx, and their articulations. The terminal line (界线) is a circular line formed by the promontory of the sacrum (骶骨岬), arcuate line (弓状线), pecten of pubis (耻骨梳), pubic tubercle (耻骨结节), upper border of pubic symphysis. The pelvis is divided into a greater (大骨盆)(or false) pelvis and a lesser (or true) pelvis (小骨盆) by the terminal line. The pelvic inlet (superior) of the lesser pelvis is the terminal line. The pelvic outlet (inferior) of the lesser pelvis is bounded by the apex of the coccyx, the sacrotuberous and sacrospinous ligaments, the ischial tuberosities, pubic arch and the lower border of the pubic symphysis.

In anatomical position, anterior superior iliac spines (髂前上棘) and pubic tubercle (耻骨结节) are on the same vertical plane, while the tip of the coccyx and the superior border of pubic symphyses are on the same horizontal plane.

(2) **Joints of the free lower limb**

1) The hip joint (髋关节) (Fig. 1-40) is an enarthrodial or ball-and-socket joint, formed by the reception of the femoral head (股骨头) into the cup-shaped cavity of the acetabulum (髋臼). Articular capsule is strong and dense. It is attached to the margin of the acetabulum and transverse acetabular ligament (髋臼横韧带), down to surround the neck of the femur intertrochanteric line (anterior) and 1 cm above the intertrochanteric crest (posterior). The capsule is strengthened by a number of ligaments including acetabular labrum (髋臼唇), transverse acetebular ligament, ligaments, iliofemoral ligament (髂股韧带), the ligament of head of femur (股骨头韧带) (runs an artery that supplies the femoral head), pubofemoral ligament (耻股韧带), ischiofemoral ligament (坐股韧带), zona orbicularis (轮匝带). The movements of the hip are very extensive, and consist of flexion, extension, adduction, abduction, circumduction, and rotation.

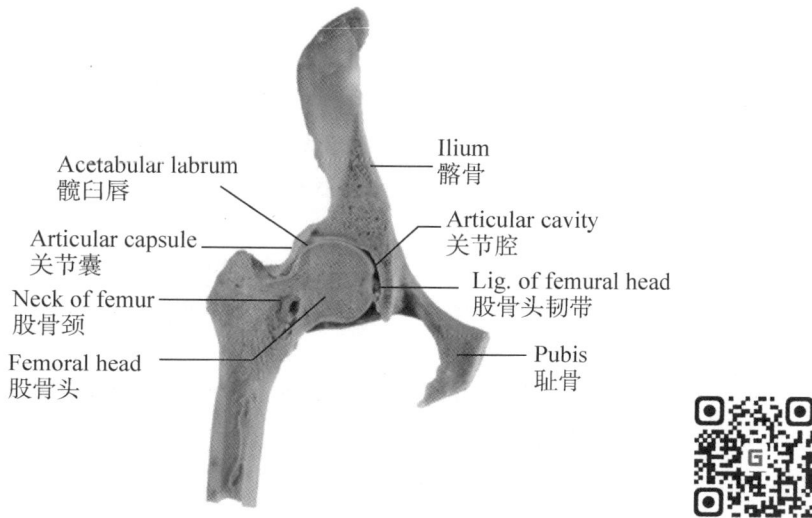

Acetabular labrum
髋臼唇

Articular capsule
关节囊

Neck of femur
股骨颈

Femoral head
股骨头

Ilium
髂骨

Articular cavity
关节腔

Lig. of femoral head
股骨头韧带

Pubis
耻骨

Fig.1-40　The hip joint

2) The knee joint (膝关节)(Fig.1-41). It is a ginglymus or hinge-joint, but is really of a much more complicated joint, formed by lower end of femur, upper end of tibia (胫骨) and patella (髌骨). It consists of the tibiofemoral (胫股关节) and patellofemoral articulations (髌股关节).

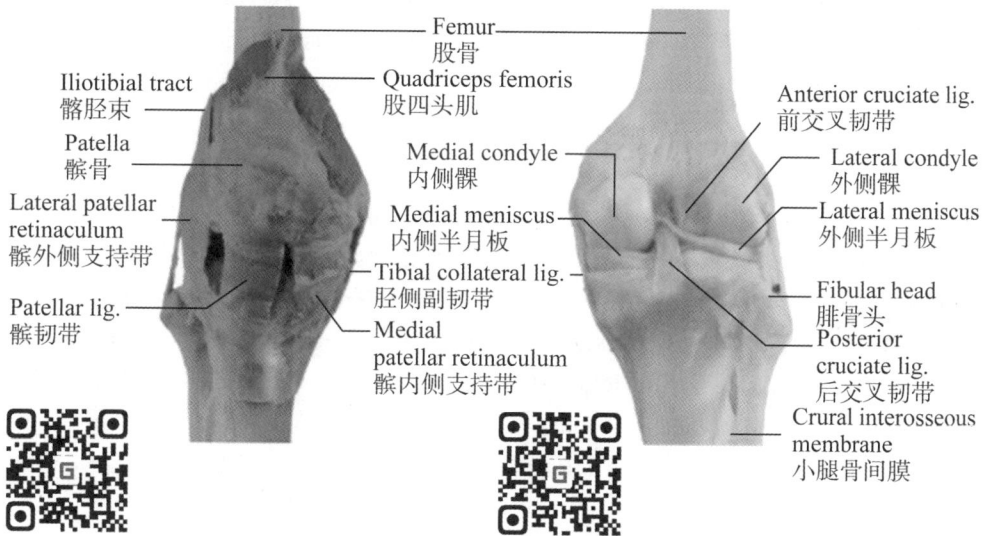

Iliotibial tract
髂胫束

Patella
髌骨

Lateral patellar
retinaculum
髌外侧支持带

Patellar lig.
髌韧带

Femur
股骨

Quadriceps femoris
股四头肌

Medial condyle
内侧髁

Medial meniscus
内侧半月板

Tibial collateral lig.
胫侧副韧带

Medial
patellar retinaculum
髌内侧支持带

Anterior cruciate lig.
前交叉韧带

Lateral condyle
外侧髁

Lateral meniscus
外侧半月板

Fibular head
腓骨头

Posterior
cruciate lig.
后交叉韧带

Crural interosseous
membrane
小腿骨间膜

Fig.1-41　The knee joint

The articular capsule is attached to the borders of the articular surfaces of these bones and the menisci. It is strengthened by ligaments, including the follows: the patellar ligament (髌韧带), the continuation of the tendon of the quadriceps femoris; the fibular collateral ligament (腓侧副韧带) from the lateral condyle of the femur and below to the lateral side of the head of the fibula; the tibial collateral ligament (胫侧副韧带) from the tubercle on the medial condyle of the femur to the medial condyle and the medial surface of the body of the tibia; the oblique popliteal ligament (腘斜韧带) from the medial condyle of the tibia to the lateral condyle of the femur; the anterior cruciate ligament (前交叉韧带) from the front of the intercondylar eminence of the tibia to the medial aspect of the lateral condyle of the femur that prevents anterior displacement of the tibia; the posterior cruciate ligament (后交叉韧带) from the posterior intercondylar eminence of the tibia to the lateral side of the medial condyle of the femur that prevents posterior displacement of the tibia.

The medial meniscus (内侧半月板) is larger and nearly semicircular C-shaped. The lateral meniscus (外侧半月板) is nearly circular and covers a somewhat greater proportion of the tibial surface as O-shaped.

The knee joint is primarily a hinge joint and the movements are flexion and extension. In a semi-flexed position, the joint allows slight abduction and adduction, and little rotation of the leg.

3) The tibiofibular syndesmosis (胫腓连结). The superior (proximal) tibiofibular joint (胫腓关节) is a synovial joint between the lateral tibial condyle and the head of the fibula. The inferior tibiofibular joint is usually considered a syndesmosis, consisting of the anterior and posterior tibiofibular and interosseous ligaments. The interosseous membrane of the leg (小腿骨间膜) is between the interosseous crests of the tibia and fibula, and separates the front and back muscles of the leg. There is almost no movement between the tibia and the fibula.

4) Joints of the foot (足关节)(Fig.1-42).

Ankle-joint (踝关节): It is a ginglymus, or hinge-joint, formed by the lower ends of tibia and fibula, trochlea of talus (距骨滑车). Articular capsule is a broad, thin, membranous layer, attached from the anterior margin of the lower end of the tibia to the superior articular surface of talus, and supported on each side by strong collateral ligaments. The strong medial or deltoid ligament is from medial malleolus of the tibia to the navicular bone, talus and calcaneus as posterior talotibial ligament, calcaneo-tibial ligament, tibialscaphoid ligament, anterior talotibial ligament. The lateral collateral ligaments extend from the lateral melleolus to the talus and the calcaneus as the anterior talofibular ligament (距腓前韧带), the shortest of the three, passes from the anterior margin of the lateral malleolus (外踝) to the talus. The calcaneofibular ligament (跟腓韧带), the longest of the three, running from the apex of the fibular malleolus downward and slightly backward to the calcaneus. The posterior talofibular ligament (距腓后韧带) runs from the fibular malleolus to a prominent tubercle on the posterior surface of the talus.

The movements are dorsiflexion (背屈) and plantar flexion(跖屈) (extension). Little abduction and adduction are possible.

Intertarsal joints (跗骨间关节): The articulations between the tarsal bones, including the subtalar joint, the talocalcaneonavicular joint and the calcaneocuboid joint. The Chopart joint is composed of the talonavicular joint medially and the calcaneocuboid joint laterally.

Tarsometatarsal joints (跗跖关节): These are approximately plane synovial joints. The bones entering into their formation are the first, second, and third cuneiforms (楔骨), and the cuboid (骰骨), which articulate with the bases of the metatarsal bones. The bones are connected by dorsal and plantar tarsometatarsal (跗跖韧带) and cuneometatarsal interosseous ligaments (楔跖骨间韧带).

Intermetatarsal joints (跖骨间关节): The base of the first metatarsal is not connected with that of the second by any ligaments, in this respect the great toe. The bases of the other four metatarsals are connected by the dorsal and plantar intermetatarsal ligaments (跖骨间韧带).

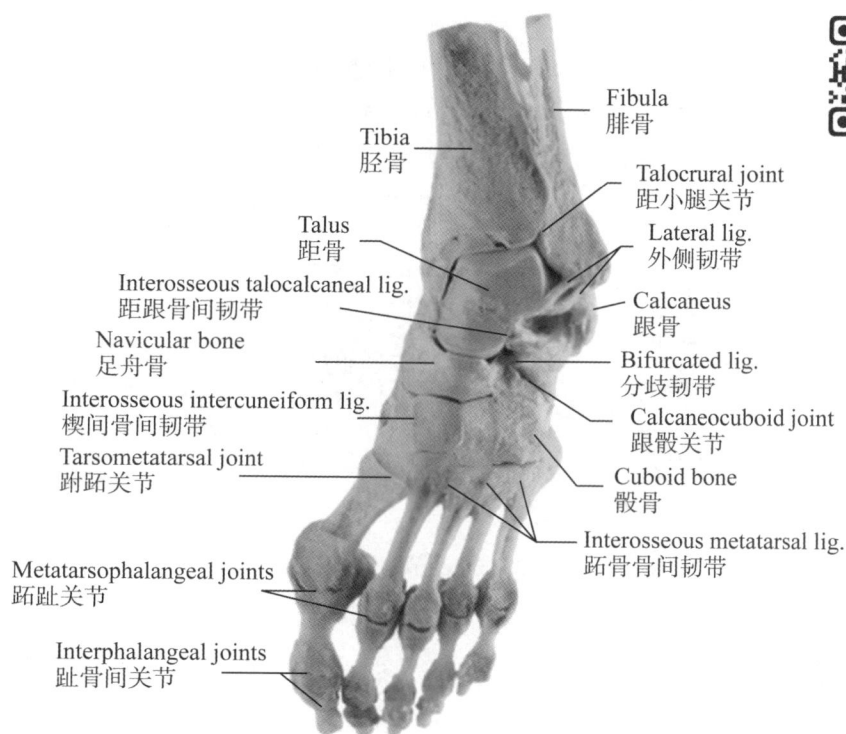

Fig.1-42　Coronal section through the joints of the foot

Metatarsophalangeal joints (跖趾关节): The metatarsophalangeal articulations are of the condyloid kind, formed by the reception of the rounded heads of the metatarsal bones in shallow cavities on the ends of the first phalanges.

Interphalangeal joints (趾骨间关节): The interphalangeal articulations are almost pure hinge joints, and each has a plantar and two collateral ligaments. The arrange-ment of these ligaments is similar to that in the metatarsophalangeal articulations: the Extensor tendons supply the places of dorsal ligaments.

The arch of the foot (足弓) (Fig.1-43) supports the weight of the body in the erect posture with the least expenditure of material (the heads of Ⅰ & Ⅴ metatarsal bone, calcaneal tuberosity). The foot is constructed of a series of arches formed by the tarsal (跗骨) and metatarsal bones (跖骨), and strengthened by the ligaments and tendons of the foot as medial longitudinal arch, lateral longitudinal arch and transverse arches.

The medial part of the longitudinal arch of the foot (内侧纵弓) is formed by the calcaneus, the talus, the navicular, the three cuneiforms, and the first, the second, and the third metatarsals.

The lateral part of the longitudinal arch of the foot (外侧纵弓) is formed by the calcaneus, the cuboid, and the fourth and the fifth metatarsals.

The transverse arch (横弓) is formed by the cuboid, three cuneiforms and all metatarsals; the intermediate cuneiform is the keystone of this arch. It gives the foot stability and resilience and protects plantar vessels and nerves.

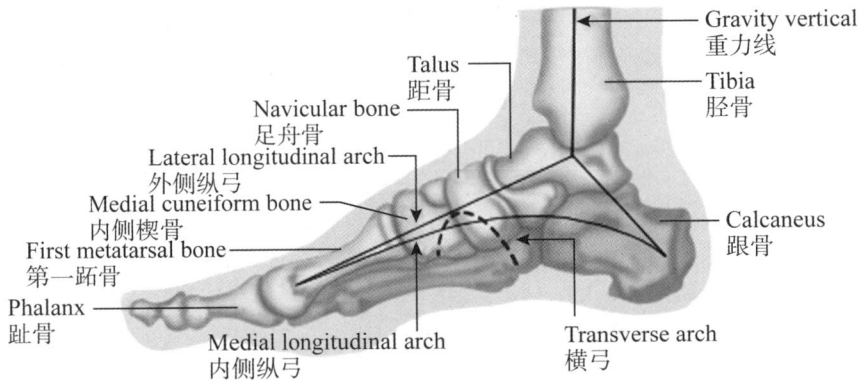

Fig.1-43   The arch of the foot

(浙江大学医学院   张晓明)

Exercise

1. A rugby player suffers a powerful blow to the outside of the weight-bearing leg when the knee joint is in semi flexion position. He immediately falls and cannot speak due to knee pain. Three structures in the knee joint most vulnerable to be injure are _____.

(A) the anterior cruciate ligament, the lateral meniscus, the lateral collateral ligament

(B) the posterior cruciate ligament, the lateral meniscus, the medial collateral ligament

(C) the anterior cruciate ligament, the medial meniscus, the medial collateral ligament

(D) the posterior cruciate ligament, the medial meniscus, the medial collateral ligament

(E) the anterior cruciate ligament, the posterior cruciate ligament, the lateral meniscus

2. A 44-year-old man was admitted to hospital after a car accident. He suffered severe neck pain when his car was struck from behind. Radiologic examination revealed that the ligament on the anterior surface of the cervical vertebral bodies were damaged. Which ligament was most likely to break?

(A) The anterior longitudinal ligament.

(B) The ligamentum flavum.

(C) The nuchal ligament.

(D) The posterior longitudinal ligament.

(E) The transverse cervical ligament.

Answer

1. The correct answer is C.

The anterior cruciate ligament starts from the anterior medial side of the intercondylar eminence of the tibia, and stops to the anterior angle of the lateral meniscus. The anterior cruciate ligament is the axis of rotation of the knee joint. It is easily damaged since it is relatively thin. The medial collateral ligament starts from the adductor tubercle at the top of the medial epicondylar of the femur and ends at the medial surface of the tibia. The medial collateral ligament is also easily broken when the outside of the leg suffers a powerful blow. The medial meniscus is connected to the medial collateral ligament which suffers more pressure than the lateral meniscus; therefore, they are commonly injured in lateral blows to the knees.

The lateral collateral ligament is located at the lateral side of the knee joint, starting from the external epicondylar of the femur and ending at the capitulum of the fibula, the main function of the lateral collateral ligament is to prevent knee varus which is easily damaged when the inner side of the knees or legs are subjected to violent blows. The lateral meniscus is located on the medial and lateral articular surfaces of the tibial plateau and it suffers less pressure. The upper end of the posterior cruciate ligament is attached to the lateral side of the medial condyle of the femur, and to the posterior intercondylar fossa of the tibia which is relatively thick. These three structures are very uncommon to injure.

2. The correct answer is A.

The anterior longitudinal ligament (Choice A) lies in front of the vertebral bodies along vertebral column. The ligamentum flavum (Choice B) connects the lamina of two adjacent vertebrae. The nuchal ligament (Choice C) is an elastic membrane that extends from the spinous processes of cervical vertebrae. The posterior longitudinal ligament (Choice D) is located at the posterior edge of the vertebral body. The transverse cervical ligament (Choice E) is associated with the pelvic region of the body.

1.3　Myology

1.3.1　General Description

The muscles are connected with the bones, cartilages, ligaments, and skin, either directly, or through the intervention of fibrous structures called tendons or aponeuroses. The muscles vary extremely in their form. In the limbs, they are of considerable length, especially the more superficial ones; they surround the bones, and constitute an important protection for the various joints. In the trunk, they are broad, flattened, and expanded, and assist in forming the walls of the trunk cavities. Hence the terms, long, broad, short, etc., are used in the description of a muscle.

1. Three Variations of Muscular Tissue

1) According to the gross structure, there are skeletal muscle, smooth muscle and cardiac muscle.

2) According to the microscopic structure, there are striped (striated) muscle (skeletal muscle and cardiac muscle) and unstriated muscle (smooth muscle).

3) According to the function, there are voluntary muscle (skeletal muscle) and involuntary muscle (smooth and cardiac muscles).

2. Morphology of Skeletal Muscles

There are kinds of skeletal muscles: long, short, broad, orbicular, bibelly muscles (Fig.1-44).

According to the direction of muscular fibers, the skeletal muscles divides into bipennate muscles, unipennate muscles, multipennate muscles.

According to the tendinous number, the skeletal muscles divides into digastric muscles, biceps muscles, triceps muscles, quadriceps muscles.

Long muscle
长肌

Multibelly muscle
多腹肌

Tendinous
intersection
腱划

Flat muscle
扁肌

Orbicular muscle
轮匝肌

Bibelly muscle
二腹肌

Biceps muscle
二头肌

Triceps muscle
三头肌

Unipennate muscle
半羽肌

Bipennate muscle
羽肌

Multipennate muscle
多羽肌

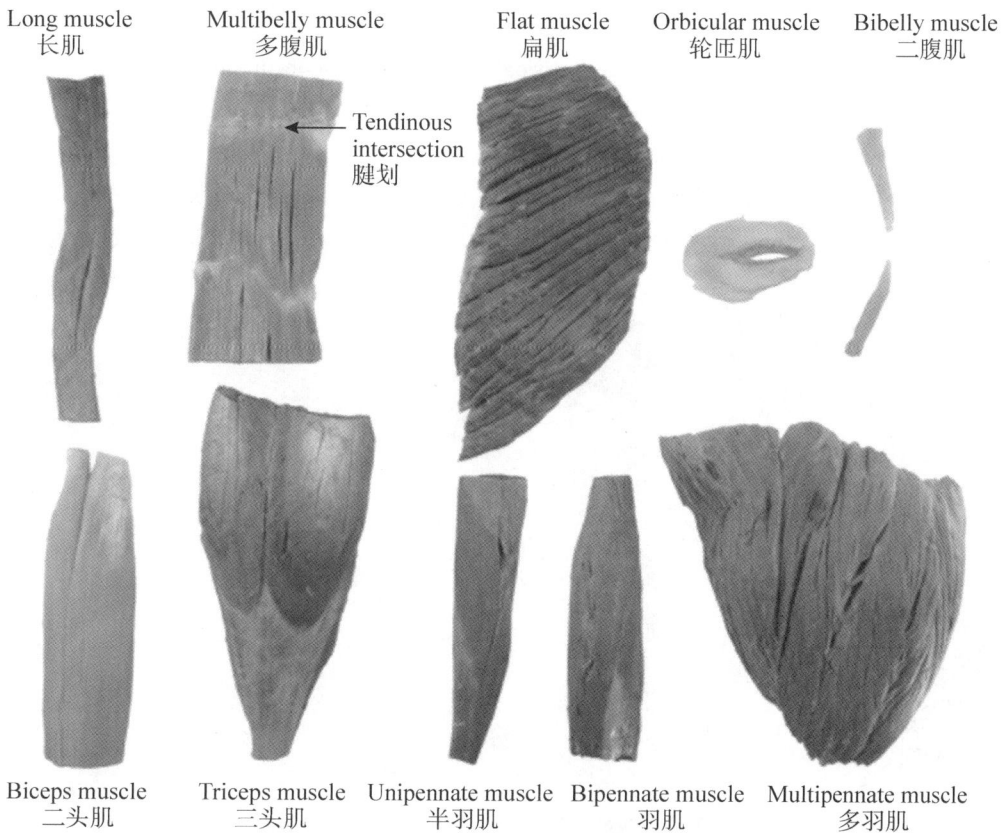

Fig.1-44　Classification of skeletal muscles

3. Gross Structure of Skeletal Muscles

Forces developed by skeletal muscles are transferred to bone by tendons, aponeuroses and fasciae, whereas ligaments prevent excessive separation of adjacent bones. Belly and tendon (肌腹和肌腱): aponeurosis, tendinous intersection, intermediate tendon. For example, digastric muscle, triceps muscle, biceps muscle, quadriceps muscle.

4. Origin, Insertion of Skeletal Muscles

1) The fixation of muscles. Most muscles are attached to bones, cartilages, ligaments, fasciae or combination of them, some are attached to organs, skin or mucous membrane.

2) Origin and insertion. In general, when a muscle contracts or shortens, fixed attachment is origin, the moveable one is insertion, so in limbs, the distal parts of muscles usually are insertion. Sometimes, the flexion and movement parts of the muscle may be exchanged for each other.

5. Action of the Muscles

In studying the mechanical action of muscles, the individual muscle cannot always be treated as a single unit, since different parts of the same muscle may have entirely different actions, as with the Pectoralis major, the Deltoid, and the Trapezius where the nerve impulses control and stimulate different portions of the muscle in succession or at different times. Most muscles are, however, in a mechanical sense unit. But in either case, the muscle fibers constitute the elementary motor elements.

Prime movers or agonists are from contract actively. Antagonists oppose the action of a prime mover. Synergist cooperates in performing an action. The last one is fixators (Fig.1-45).

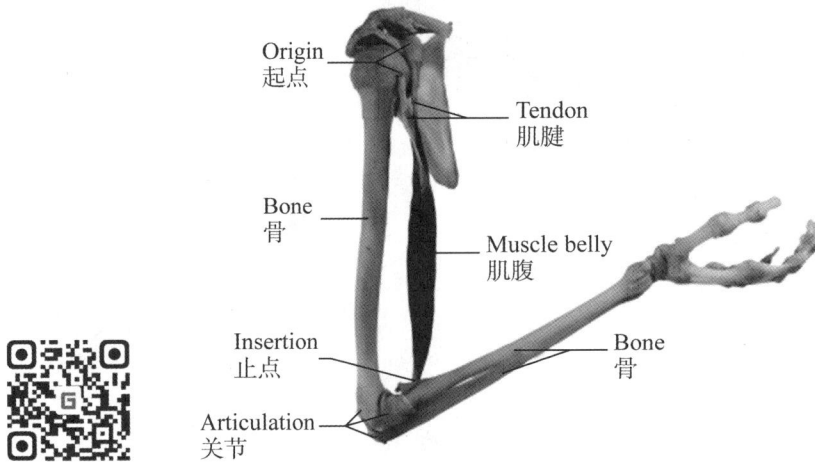

Fig.1-45　The starting and ending points of muscles

6. Nomenclature of Muscles

The names of muscles indicate the shape, location, actions or their combination of muscles.

7. Accessory Structures of Muscles

(1) The fascia (筋膜)

It refers to a band or sheet of connective tissue fibers, primarily collagen that forms beneath the skin to attach, stabilize, enclose, and separate muscles and other internal organs. Fasciae are classified according to their distinct layers as in superficial fascia, deep (or muscle) fascia. The superficial fascia (浅筋膜) consists of fat, the trunks of subcutaneous vessels and nerves, the superficial lymph notes and the mammary gland and cutaneous muscles, covering almost the entire body. It is composed of loose connective tissue and contains fat in varying quantities. It varies in thickness in different individuals and different parts of the body. Deep fascia (proper fascia) (深筋膜) forms some sheaths for each or group of muscles and for vessels and nerves. The intermuscular septa separate the groups of muscles. There is retinaculum for its underlying tendons (Fig.1-46).

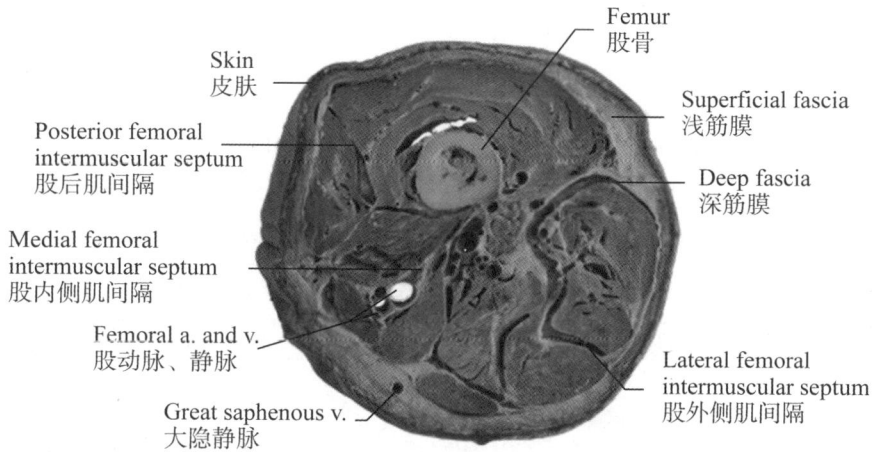

Skin
皮肤

Posterior femoral
intermuscular septum
股后肌间隔

Medial femoral
intermuscular septum
股内侧肌间隔

Femoral a. and v.
股动脉、静脉

Great saphenous v.
大隐静脉

Femur
股骨

Superficial fascia
浅筋膜

Deep fascia
深筋膜

Lateral femoral
intermuscular septum
股外侧肌间隔

Fig.1-46　Horizontal section of mid-thigh (fascia)

(2) The synovial tendon sheath (or tendinous sheath)(腱鞘)

It refers to a layer of membrane around a tendon. It permits the tendon to stretch and not adhere to the surrounding fascia. It has two layers: One is fibrous layer (or fibrous sheath of tendon), and the other is synovial layer (or synovial sheath of tendon) which can be divided into the parietal layer and the visceral layer (synovial fluid).

(3) The synovial bursa (滑膜囊)

It refers to a small fluid-filled sac lined by a synovial membrane with an inner capillary layer of viscous fluid (similar in consistency to that of a raw egg white). It provides a cushion between bones and tendons and/or muscles around a joint.

(4) The sesamoid bones (籽骨)

The sesamoid bones refer to the bones embedded within a tendon or a muscle, providing a smooth surface for tendons to slide over, increasing the tendon's ability to transmit muscular forces (Fig.1-47).

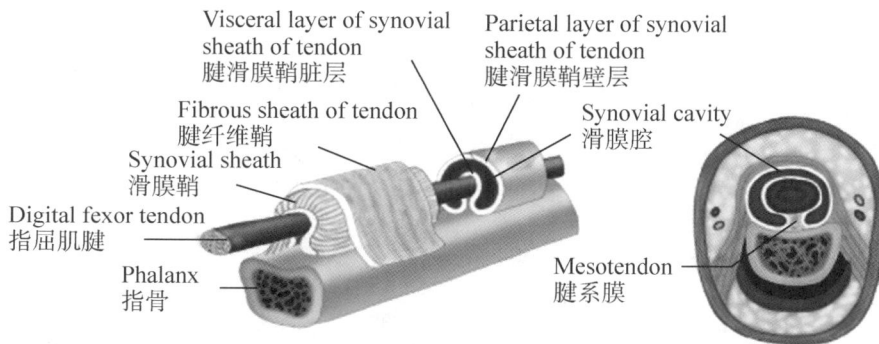

Visceral layer of synovial
sheath of tendon
腱滑膜鞘脏层

Fibrous sheath of tendon
腱纤维鞘

Synovial sheath
滑膜鞘

Digital fexor tendon
指屈肌腱

Phalanx
指骨

Parietal layer of synovial
sheath of tendon
腱滑膜鞘壁层

Synovial cavity
滑膜腔

Mesotendon
腱系膜

Fig.1-47　Schematic diagram of sheath of tendon

1.3.2   Muscles of the Human Body

The muscles of the human body (Table 1-1) can be divided into four parts: the muscles of the head (Figs. 1-48 & 1-49), the muscles of the trunk(Figs. 1-52—1-56), the muscles of the neck (Figs. 1-50 & 1-51) and the muscles of the limbs (Figs. 1-57—1-65).

Table 1-1   Name, origin, insertion, innervation and main action of

major muscles of the human body

Name	Origin	Insertion	Innervation	Main Actions
Sternocleido mastoid	Anterior surface of manubrium, medial of clavicle	Mastoid process	Accessory nerve	Bilaterally: flexes head; Unilaterally: turns face toward opposite side
Trapezius	Superior nuchal line, external occipital protuberance, nuchal ligament, spinous processes of C7—T12	Lateral third of clavicle, acromion, spine of scapula	Accessory nerve	Elevates, retracts, and rotates scapula; lower fibers depress scapula
Levator scapulae	Transverse processes of C1—C4 vertebrae	Medial border of the scapula from the superior angle to the spine	Dorsal scapular nerve (C5)	Elevates scapula
Scalene anterior	Anterior tubercles of the transverse processes of vertebrae C3—C6	Scalene tubercle of the first rib	Brachial plexus, C5—C7	Elevates the first rib; flexes and laterally bends the neck
Scalene middle	Posterior tubercles of the transverse processes of vertebrae C2—C7	Upper surface of the first rib behind the subclavian artery	Brachial plexus, C3—C8	Elevates the first rib; flexes and laterally bends the neck
Scalene posterior	Posterior tubercles of the transverse processes of vertebrae C5—C7	Lateral surface of the second rib	Brachial plexus, C7—C8	Elevates the second rib; flexes and laterally bends the neck
Latissimus dorsi	Spinous processes of T7—L5, iliac crest, and last three ribs	Intertubercular sulcus of humerus	Thoracodorsal nerve	Extends, adducts, and medially rotates humerus
Pectoralis major	Sternal half of clavicle, sternum to the seventh rib, cartilages of true ribs	Intertubercular sulcus of humerus	Medial and lateral pectoral nerves	Flexes, adducts, and medially rotates arm

(To be continued)

Table 1-1

Name	Origin	Insertion	Innervation	Main Actions
External intercostal	The lower border of a rib within an intercostal space	The upper border of the rib below, coursing, downward and medially	Intercostal nerves (T1—T11)	Keeps the intercostal space from blowing out or sucking in during respiration
Diaphragm	Xiphoid process, costal margin, fascia over the quadratus lumborum and psoas major muscle (lateral & medial arcuate ligaments), vertebral bodies L1—L3	Central tendon of the diaphragm	Phrenic nerve (C3—C5)	Pushes the abdominal viscera inferiorly, increasing the volume of the thoracic cavity (inspiration)
Transversus thoracis	Posterior surface of the sternum	Inner surfaces of costal cartilages 2—6	Intercostal nerves 2—6	Compresses the thorax for forced expiration
Deltoid	Lateral third of clavicle, acromion, spine of scapula	Deltoid tuberosity of humerus	Axillary nerve	Flexes, medially rotates, abducts, extends and laterally rotates arm
Biceps brachii	Supraglenoid tubercle and coracoid process of scapula	Radial tuberosity, fascia of forearm	Musculocutaneous nerve	Flexes and supinates forearm at elbow
Triceps brachii	Long head: infraglenoid tubercle of the scapula; lateral head: posterolateral humerus & lateral intermuscular septum; medial head: posteromedial surface of the inferior 1/2 of the humerus	Olecranon process of the ulna	Radial nerve	Extends the forearm; the long head extends and adducts arm
Brachialis	Anterior surface of the lower one-half of the humerus and the associated intermuscular septa	Coronoid process of the ulna	Musculocutaneous nerve	Flexes the forearm
Coracobrachi-alis	Coracoid process of the scapula	Medial side of the humerus at mid-shaft	Musculocutaneous nerve (C5, C6)	Flexes and adducts the arm

(To be continued)

Table 1-1

Name	Origin	Insertion	Innervation	Main Actions
Brachioradialis	Upper two-thirds of the lateral supracondylar ridge of the humerus	Lateral side of the base of the styloid process of the radius	Radial nerve	Flexes the elbow, assists in pronation & supination
External abdominal oblique	External surfaces of ribs 5—12	Linea alba, pubic tubercle, anterior half of iliac crest	Anterior rami of six thoracic nerves	Compresses and supports abdominal viscera, flexes and rotates trunk
Internal abdominal oblique	Thoracolumbar fascia, anterior 2/3 of the iliac crest, lateral 2/3 of the inguinal ligament	Lower 3 or 4 ribs, linea alba, pubic crest	Intercostal nerves 7—11, subcostal, iliohypogastric and ilioinguinal nerves	Flexes and laterally bends the trunk
Transversus abdominis	Lower 6 ribs, thoraolumbar fascia, anterior 3/4 of the iliac crest, lateral 1/3 of inguinal ligament	Linea alba, pubic crest and pecten of the pubis	Intercostal nerves 7—11, subcostal, iliohypogastric and ilioinguinal nerves	Flexes and laterally bends trunk
Rectus abdominis	Pubic symphysis, pubic crest	Xiphoid process, costal cartilages 5—7	Anterior rami of six thoracic nerves	Flexes trunk, compresses abdominal viscera
Psoas major	Bodies and transverse processes of lumbar vertebrae	Lesser trochanter of femur (with iliacus) via iliopsoas tendon	Branches of the ventral primary rami of spinal nerves L2—L4	Flexes the thigh; flexes & laterally bends the lumbar vertebral column
Quadratus lumborum	Posterior part of the iliac crest and the iliolumbar ligament	Transverse processes of lumbar vertebrae 1—4 and the 12th rib	Subcostal nerve and ventral primary rami of spinal nerves L1—L4	Laterally bends the trunk, fixes the 12th rib
Quadriceps	Anterior inferior iliac spine, greater trochanter, anterior and lateral surfaces of femur	Base of patella	Femoral nerve	Extends leg at knee joint and flexes thigh at hip joint

(To be continued)

Table 1-1

Name	Origin	Insertion	Innervation	Main Actions
Sartorius	Anterior superior iliac spine	Medial surface of the tibia (pes anserinus)	Femoral nerve	Flexes, abducts and laterally rotates the thigh; flexes leg
Adductor longus	Medial portion of the superior pubic ramus	Linea aspera of the femur	Anterior division of the obturator nerve	Adducts, flexes, and medially rotates the femur
Adductor magnus	Ischiopubic ramus and ischial tuberosity	Linea aspera of the femur; the ischiocondylar part inserts on the adductor tubercle of the femur	Posterior division of the obturator nerve; tibial nerve (ischiocondylar part)	Adducts, flexes, and medially rotates the femur; extends the femur (ischiocondylar part)
Iliopsoas	Iliac fossa; bodies and transverse processes of lumbar vertebrae	Lesser trochanter of the femur	Branches of the ventral primary rami of spinal nerves L2—L4; branches of the femoral nerve	Flexes the thigh; flexes and laterally bends the lumbar vertebral column
Biceps femoris	Long head: ischial tuberosity; short head: lateral lip of the linea aspera	Head of fibula and lateral condyle of the tibia	Long head: tibial nerve; short head: common fibular (peroneal) nerve	Extends the thigh, flexes the leg
Gluteus maximus	Ilium posterior to posterior gluteal line, dorsal surface of sacrum	Lateral condyle of tibia, gluteal tuberosity of femur	Inferior gluteal nerve	Extends flexed thigh, assists in lateral rotation, and abducts thigh
Gluteus medius	External surface of the ilium between the posterior and anterior gluteal lines	Greater trochanter of the femur	Superior gluteal nerve	Abducts the femur; medially rotates the thigh
Gluteus minimus	External surface of the ilium between the anterior and inferior gluteal lines	Greater trochanter of the femur	Superior gluteal nerve	Abducts the femur; medially rotates the thigh

(To be continued)

Table 1-1

Name	Origin	Insertion	Innervation	Main Actions
Piriformis	Anterior surface of sacrum	Upper border of greater trochanter of femur	Ventral rami of S1—S2	Laterally rotates and abducts thigh
Tibialis anterior	Lateral tibial condyle and the upper lateral surface of the tibia	Medial surface of the medial cuneiform and the 1st metatarsal	Deep fibular (peroneal) nerve	Dorsi flexes and inverts the foot
Tibialis posterior	Interosseous membrane, posteromedial surface of the fibula, posterolateral surface of the tibia	Tuberosity of the navicular and medial cuneiform, metatarsals 2—4	Tibial nerve	Plantar flexes the foot; inverts the foot
Gastrocnemius	Lateral and medial condyle of femur	Posterior aspect of calcaneus	Tibial nerve	Plantar flexes foot at ankle joint
Soleus	Posterior surface of head and upper shaft of the fibula, soleal line of the tibia	Dorsum of the calcaneus via the calcaneal (Achilles') tendon	Tibial nerve	Plantar flexes the foot

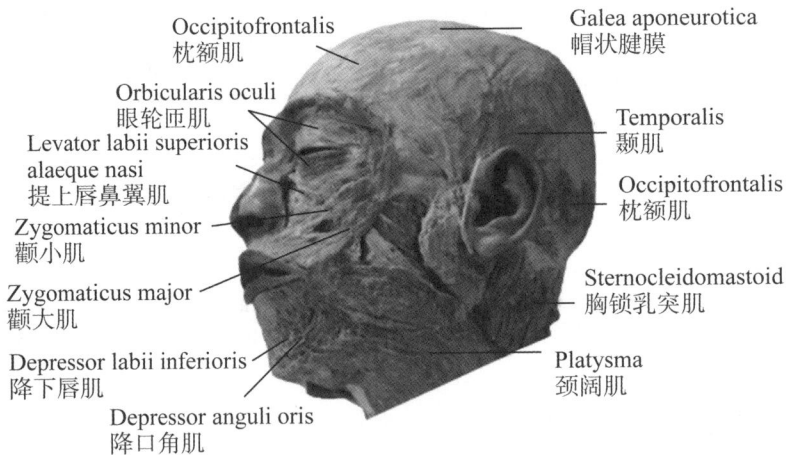

Fig.1-48　Head muscle

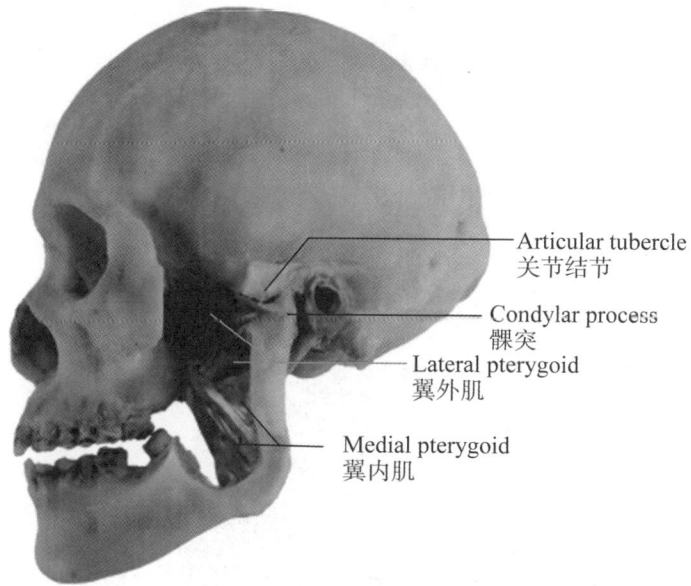

Articular tubercle
关节结节

Condylar process
髁突

Lateral pterygoid
翼外肌

Medial pterygoid
翼内肌

Fig.1-49   The lateral pterygoid and medial pterygoid muscle

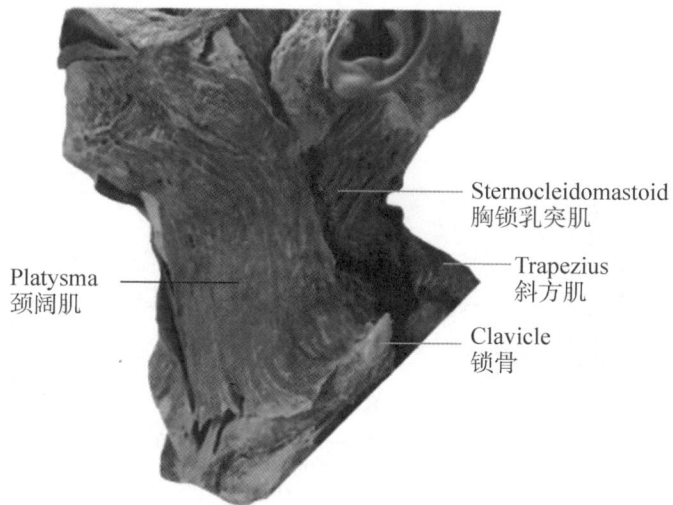

Sternocleidomastoid
胸锁乳突肌

Trapezius
斜方肌

Platysma
颈阔肌

Clavicle
锁骨

Fig.1-50   Superficial and lateral cervical muscles (front)

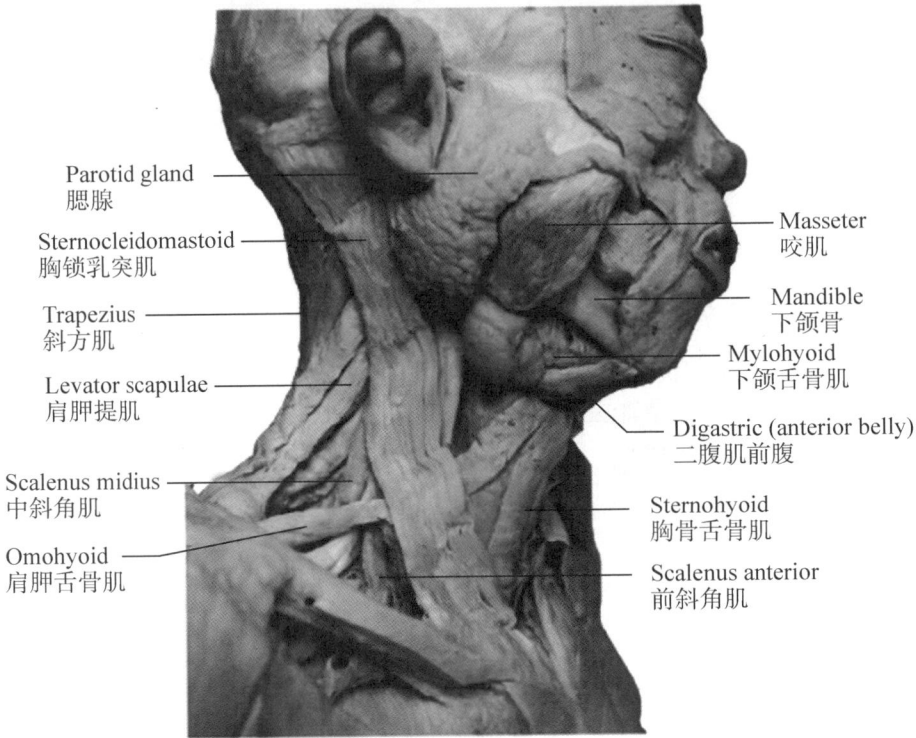

Parotid gland
腮腺

Sternocleidomastoid
胸锁乳突肌

Trapezius
斜方肌

Levator scapulae
肩胛提肌

Scalenus midius
中斜角肌

Omohyoid
肩胛舌骨肌

Masseter
咬肌

Mandible
下颌骨

Mylohyoid
下颌舌骨肌

Digastric (anterior belly)
二腹肌前腹

Sternohyoid
胸骨舌骨肌

Scalenus anterior
前斜角肌

Fig.1-51   Cervical muscle (side)

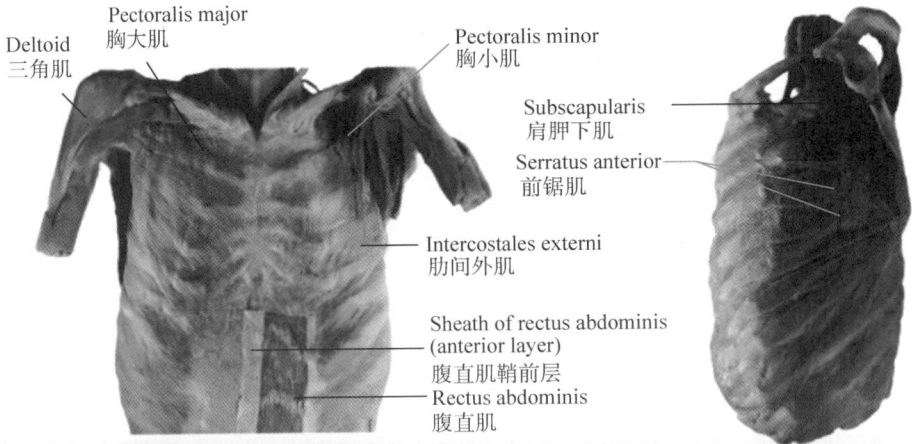

Deltoid
三角肌

Pectoralis major
胸大肌

Pectoralis minor
胸小肌

Subscapularis
肩胛下肌

Serratus anterior
前锯肌

Intercostales externi
肋间外肌

Sheath of rectus abdominis
(anterior layer)
腹直肌鞘前层

Rectus abdominis
腹直肌

Fig.1-52   Muscles of the thorax and abdomen

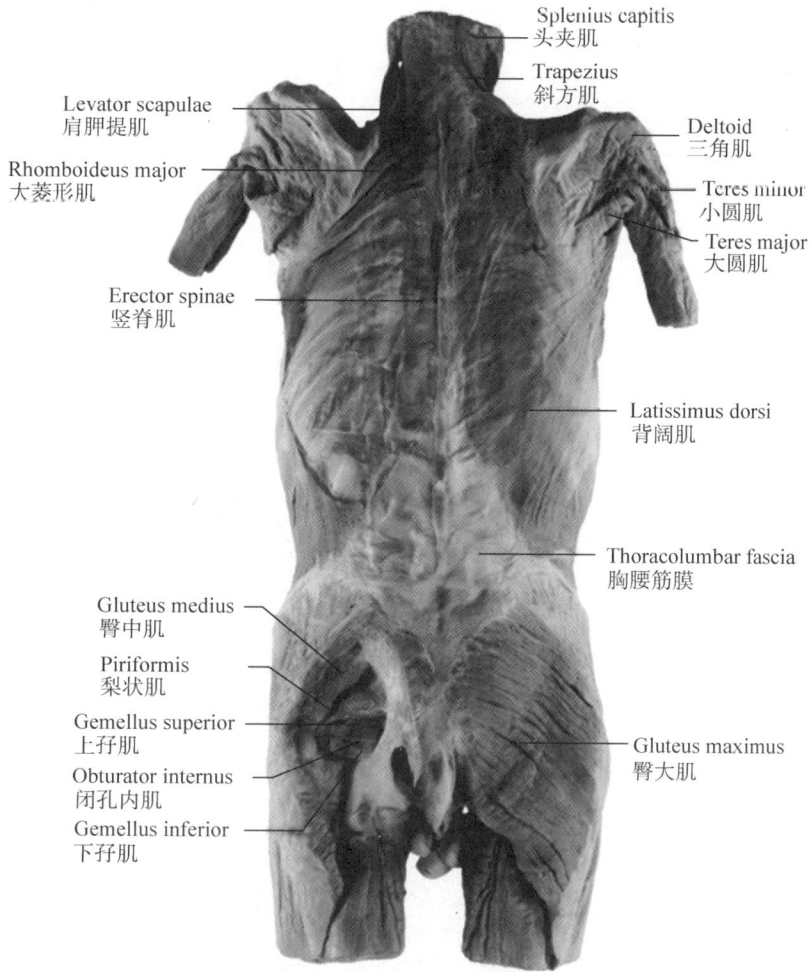

Splenius capitis
头夹肌

Trapezius
斜方肌

Levator scapulae
肩胛提肌

Deltoid
三角肌

Rhomboideus major
大菱形肌

Teres minor
小圆肌

Teres major
大圆肌

Erector spinae
竖脊肌

Latissimus dorsi
背阔肌

Thoracolumbar fascia
胸腰筋膜

Gluteus medius
臀中肌

Piriformis
梨状肌

Gemellus superior
上孖肌

Obturator internus
闭孔内肌

Gluteus maximus
臀大肌

Gemellus inferior
下孖肌

Fig.1-53   Muscles of the back

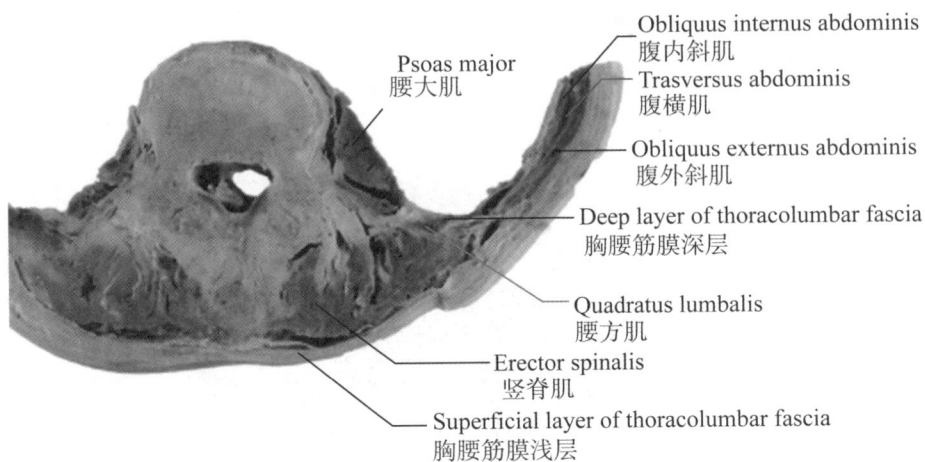

Psoas major
腰大肌

Obliquus internus abdominis
腹内斜肌

Trasversus abdominis
腹横肌

Obliquus externus abdominis
腹外斜肌

Deep layer of thoracolumbar fascia
胸腰筋膜深层

Quadratus lumbalis
腰方肌

Erector spinalis
竖脊肌

Superficial layer of thoracolumbar fascia
胸腰筋膜浅层

Fig.1-54   Thoracolumbar fascia

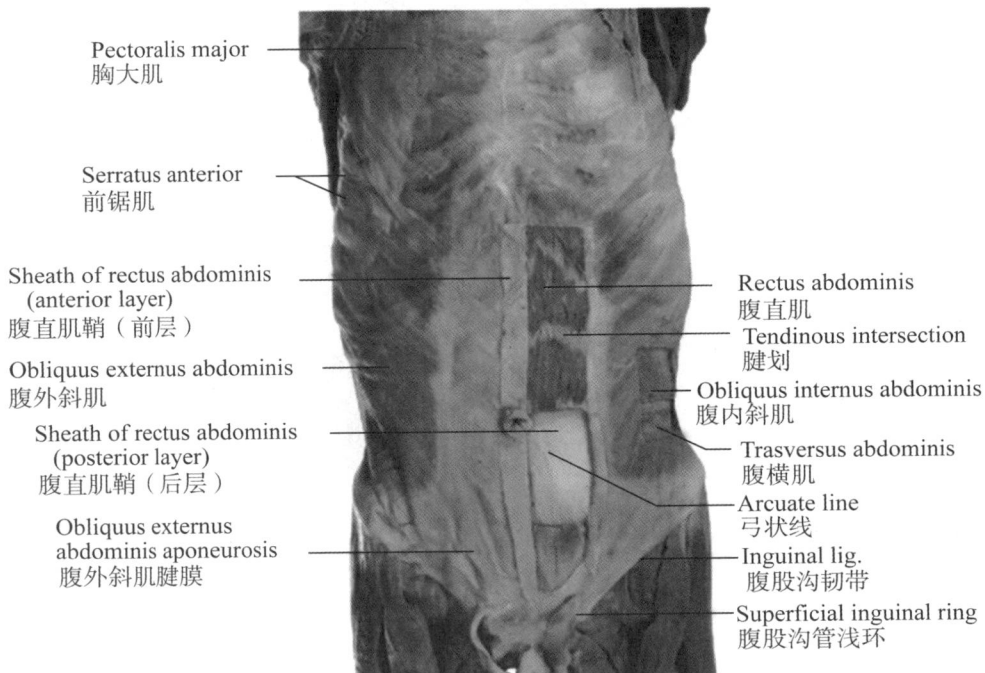

Pectoralis major
胸大肌

Serratus anterior
前锯肌

Sheath of rectus abdominis
(anterior layer)
腹直肌鞘（前层）

Obliquus externus abdominis
腹外斜肌

Sheath of rectus abdominis
(posterior layer)
腹直肌鞘（后层）

Obliquus externus
abdominis aponeurosis
腹外斜肌腱膜

Rectus abdominis
腹直肌

Tendinous intersection
腱划

Obliquus internus abdominis
腹内斜肌

Trasversus abdominis
腹横肌

Arcuate line
弓状线

Inguinal lig.
腹股沟韧带

Superficial inguinal ring
腹股沟管浅环

Fig.1-55   Anterior lateral wall muscles of the abdomen

Rectus abdominis
腹直肌

Transversus abdominis aponeurosis
腹横肌腱膜

Obliquus externus abdominis aponeurosis
腹外斜肌腱膜

Obliquus internus abdomins aponeurosis
腹内斜肌腱膜

Transversus abdominis
腹横肌

Obliquus externus abdominis
腹外斜肌

Linea alba
白线

Above the umbilicus
脐以上

Obliquus internus abdominis
腹内斜肌

Rectus abdominis
腹直肌

Transversus abdominis aponcurosis
腹横肌腱膜

Obliquus externus abdominis aponeurosis
腹外斜肌腱膜

Obliquus internus abdominis aponeurosis
腹内斜肌腱膜

Transversus abdominis
腹横肌

Obliquus externus abdominis
腹外斜肌

Linea alba
白线

Below the arcuate line
弓状线以下

Obliquus internus abdominis
腹内斜肌

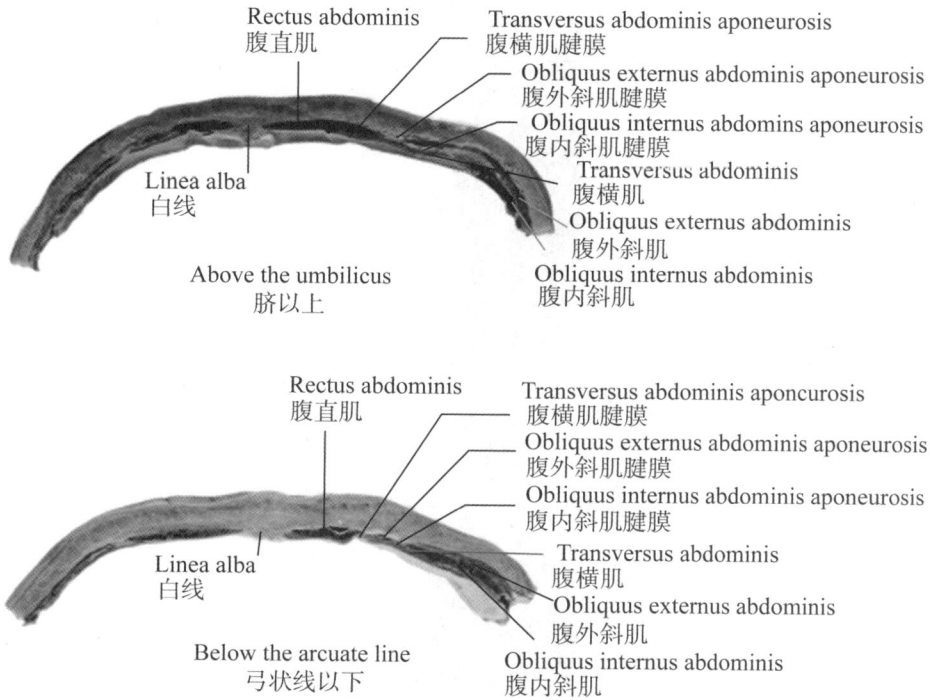

Fig.1-56   Transverse section of the anterior abdominal wall

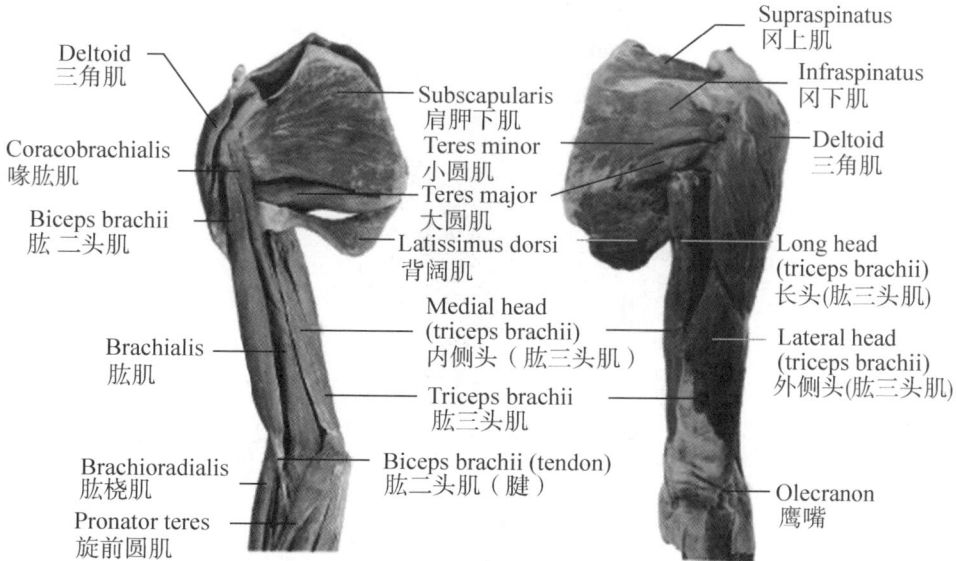

Deltoid
三角肌

Coracobrachialis
喙肱肌

Biceps brachii
肱二头肌

Brachialis
肱肌

Brachioradialis
肱桡肌

Pronator teres
旋前圆肌

Subscapularis
肩胛下肌

Teres minor
小圆肌

Teres major
大圆肌

Latissimus dorsi
背阔肌

Medial head
(triceps brachii)
内侧头（肱三头肌）

Triceps brachii
肱三头肌

Biceps brachii (tendon)
肱二头肌（腱）

Supraspinatus
冈上肌

Infraspinatus
冈下肌

Deltoid
三角肌

Long head
(triceps brachii)
长头(肱三头肌)

Lateral head
(triceps brachii)
外侧头(肱三头肌)

Olecranon
鹰嘴

Fig.1-57   Muscles of the shoulder and the arm

Biceps brachii muscle
肱二头肌

Brachioradialis
肱桡肌

Pronator teres
旋前圆肌

Flexor digitorum
profundus
指深屈肌

Flexor pollicis longus
拇长屈肌

Flexor carpi radialis (tendon)
桡侧腕屈肌腱

Flexor carpi
ulnaris (tendon)
尺侧腕屈肌腱

Abductor pollicis brevis
拇短展肌

Lumbricalis
蚓状肌

Flexor pollicis longus
拇长屈肌

Adductor pollicis
拇收肌

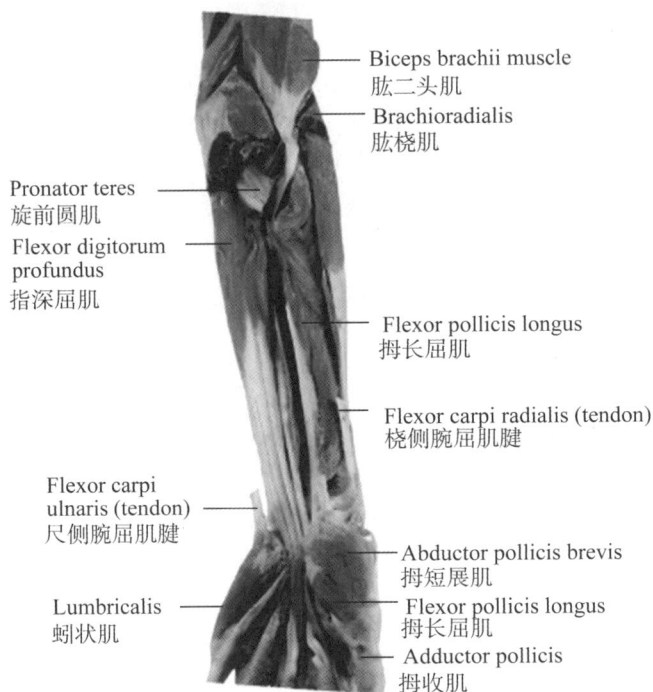

Fig.1-58　Muscles of the anterior aspect of the forearm

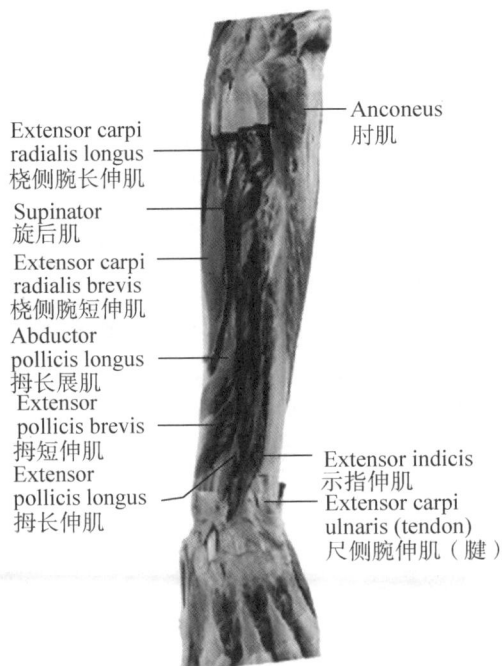

Anconeus
肘肌

Extensor carpi
radialis longus
桡侧腕长伸肌

Supinator
旋后肌

Extensor carpi
radialis brevis
桡侧腕短伸肌

Abductor
pollicis longus
拇长展肌

Extensor
pollicis brevis
拇短伸肌

Extensor
pollicis longus
拇长伸肌

Extensor indicis
示指伸肌

Extensor carpi
ulnaris (tendon)
尺侧腕伸肌（腱）

Fig.1-59　Muscles of the posterior aspect of the forearm

68

Fibrous sheath
纤维鞘

Lumbricalis
蚓状肌

Flexor digitorum
superficialis (tendon)
指浅屈肌（腱）

Flexor digiti
minimi brevis
小指短屈肌

Abductor
digiti minimi
小指展肌

Flexor carpi ulnaris
尺侧腕屈肌

Adductor pollicis
拇收肌

Flexor pollicis brevis
拇短屈肌

Abductor pollicis brevis
拇短展肌

Flexor retinaculum
屈肌支持带

Palmaris longus (tendon)
掌长肌（腱）

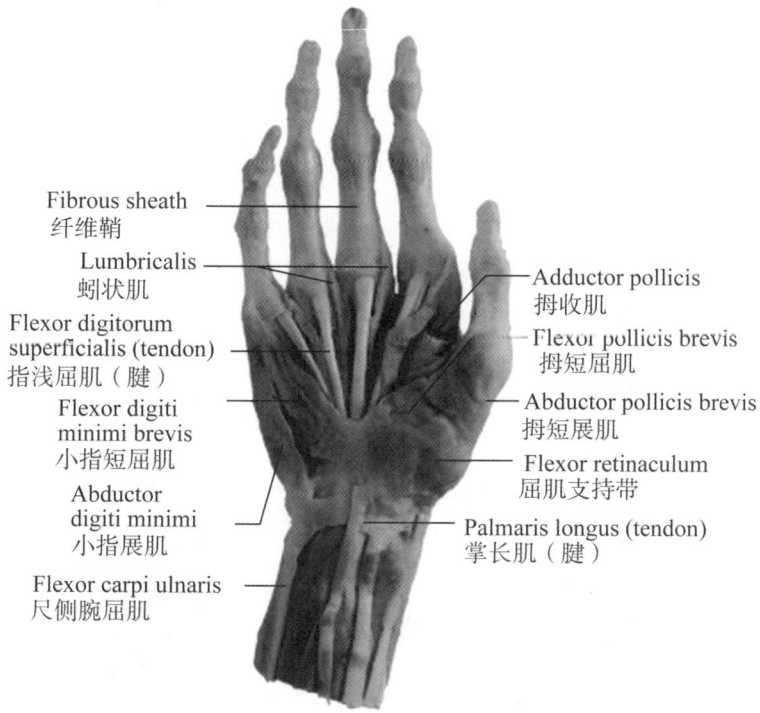

Fig.1-60   Muscles of the palm of the hand

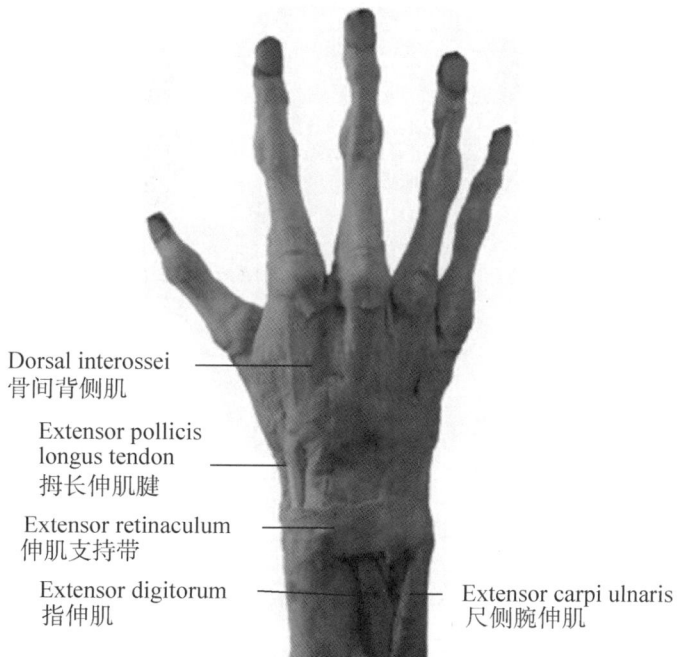

Dorsal interossei
骨间背侧肌

Extensor pollicis
longus tendon
拇长伸肌腱

Extensor retinaculum
伸肌支持带

Extensor digitorum
指伸肌

Extensor carpi ulnaris
尺侧腕伸肌

Fig.1-61   Muscles of the dorsum of the hand

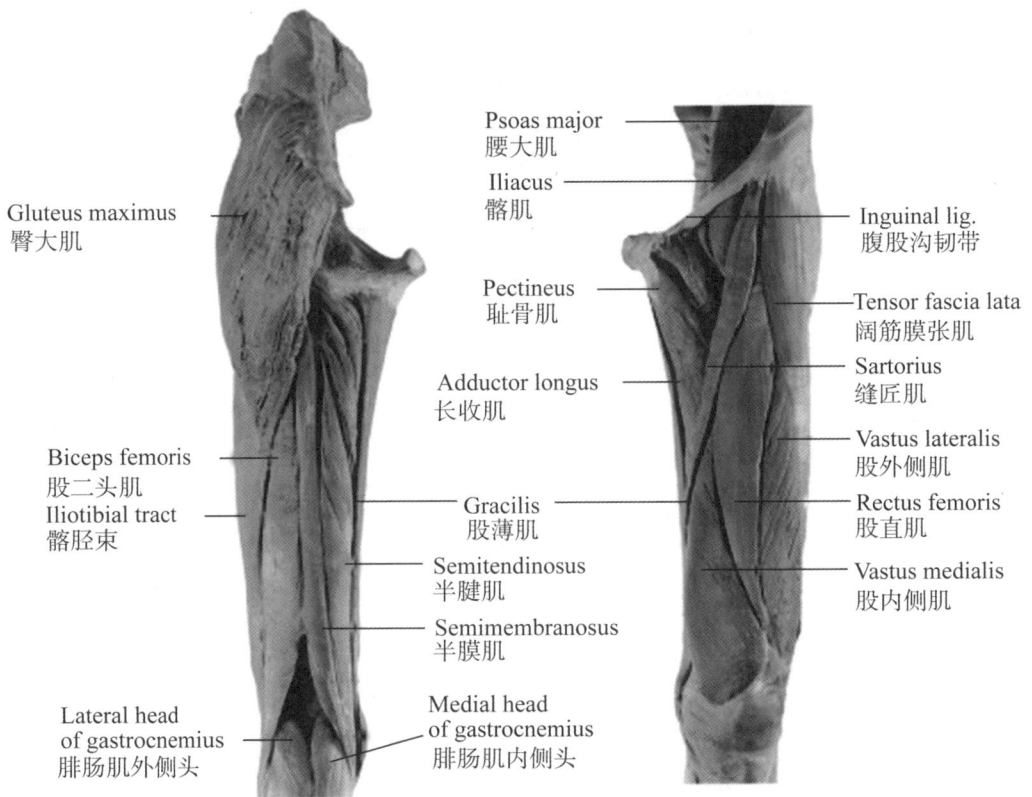

Gluteus maximus
臀大肌

Biceps femoris
股二头肌
Iliotibial tract
髂胫束

Lateral head
of gastrocnemius
腓肠肌外侧头

Psoas major
腰大肌

Iliacus
髂肌

Pectineus
耻骨肌

Adductor longus
长收肌

Gracilis
股薄肌

Semitendinosus
半腱肌

Semimembranosus
半膜肌

Medial head
of gastrocnemius
腓肠肌内侧头

Inguinal lig.
腹股沟韧带

Tensor fascia lata
阔筋膜张肌

Sartorius
缝匠肌

Vastus lateralis
股外侧肌

Rectus femoris
股直肌

Vastus medialis
股内侧肌

Fig.1-62　Gluteus and muscles of the thigh

Tibialis anterior
胫骨前肌

Peroneus longus
腓骨长肌

Peroneus brevis
腓骨短肌

Extensor digitorum longus
趾长伸肌

Inferior extensor retinaculum
伸肌下支持带

Superior extensor retinaculum
伸肌上支持带

Extensor digitorum longus
趾长伸肌

Extensor digitorum brevis
趾短伸肌

Extensor hallucis brevis
蹞短伸肌

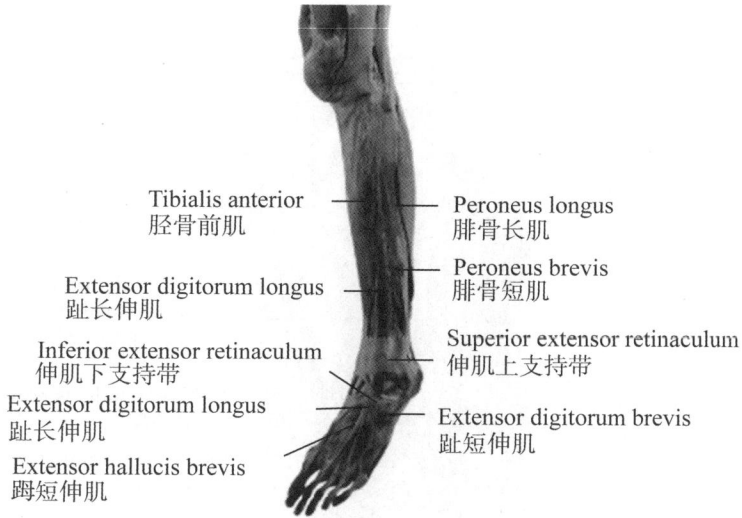

Fig.1-63   Muscles of antero-lateral aspect of the leg and dorsum of the foot

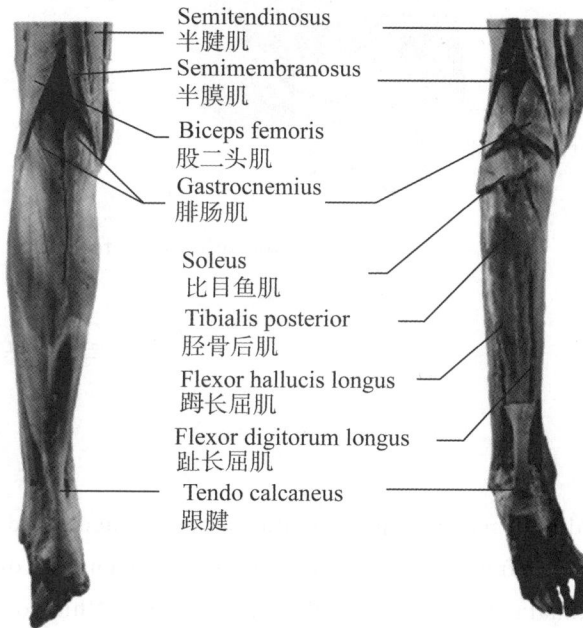

Semitendinosus
半腱肌

Semimembranosus
半膜肌

Biceps femoris
股二头肌

Gastrocnemius
腓肠肌

Soleus
比目鱼肌

Tibialis posterior
胫骨后肌

Flexor hallucis longus
蹞长屈肌

Flexor digitorum longus
趾长屈肌

Tendo calcaneus
跟腱

Fig.1-64   Muscles of posterior aspect of the leg

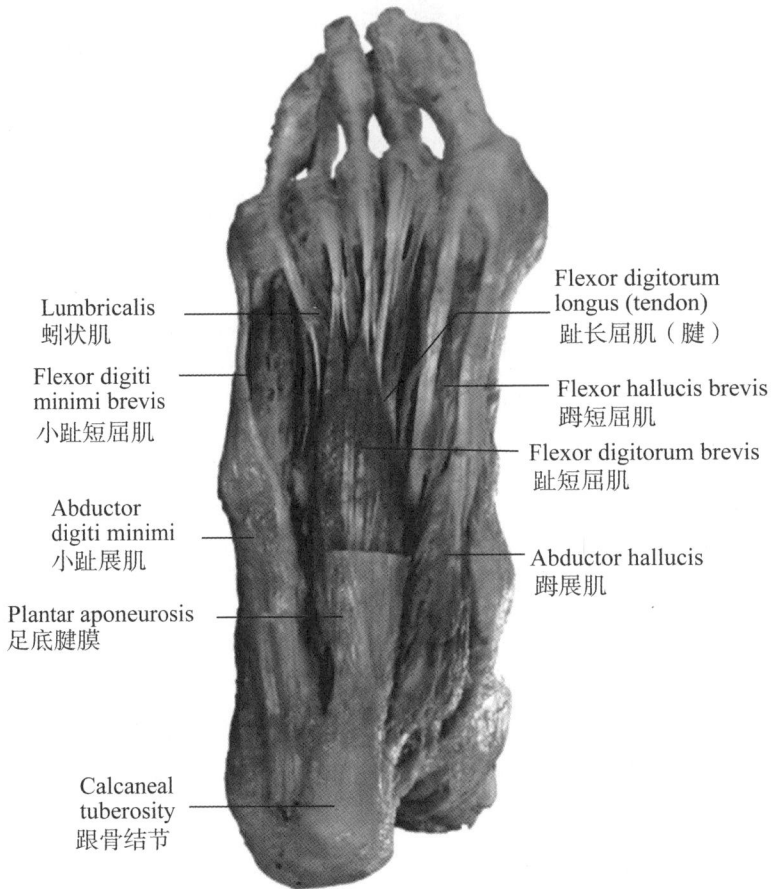

Lumbricalis
蚓状肌

Flexor digiti
minimi brevis
小趾短屈肌

Abductor
digiti minimi
小趾展肌

Plantar aponeurosis
足底腱膜

Calcaneal
tuberosity
跟骨结节

Flexor digitorum
longus (tendon)
趾长屈肌（腱）

Flexor hallucis brevis
踇短屈肌

Flexor digitorum brevis
趾短屈肌

Abductor hallucis
踇展肌

Fig.1-65　Muscles of the sole of the foot

（复旦大学基础医学院　高璐）

Exercise

1. A 49-year-old man was hospitalized after a car accident. Radiographic examination showed a transverse fracture of the radius near the attachment of the pronator teres muscle, and the proximal part of the radius deviated laterally. Which of the following muscles was most likely to cause this deviation?

(A) The pronator teres.

(B) The pronator quadratus.

(C) The brachialis.

(D) The supinator.

(E) The brachioradialis.

2. A 37-year-old woman falled down from her bicycle and the chest hit the stone. The physician found a superficial stab wound on the lateral aspect of the thoracic wall at the third rib. Although she had little bleeding nor breathing difficulty, the medial edge of the scapula was raised. Which of the following muscles was most likely to be damaged?

(A) The levator scapulae.

(B) The pectoralis minor.

(C) The rhomboid major.

(D) The supraspinatus.

(E) The serratus anterior.

Answer

1. The correct answer is D.

The pronator teres muscle (Choice A) starts from the forearm fascia of the medial epicondylar of the humerus and stops downward at the middle of the lateral side of the radius. The function of the pronator teres muscle is to rotate the forearm forward. The muscle fibers of the pronator anterior (Choice B) muscle originate from the anterior and medial side of the distal ulna and end at the anterior and medial side of the distal radius, pulling the radius medially. The brachioradialis muscle (Choice E) originates from the upper lateral epicondyle of the humerus, ends at the bottom of the styloid process of the radius, it is far below the fracture. The brachial (Choice C) muscle starts from the lower part of the front of the humerus and ends at the ulnar tuberosity and the coronoid process which do not act on the radius. The supinator muscle (Choice D) mainly starts from the upper part of the lateral epicondyle of the humerus and the lateral edge of the ulna, and ends in the front of the upper part of the radius which can cause a lateral deviation when fracture occurs.

2. The correct answer is E.

The levator scapula muscle (Choice A) starts from the transverse processes of the four uppermost cervical vertebrae (C1—C4) as well as ends at the upper corner of the scapula and the upper part of the spine edge of the scapula. The function of the levator scapulae is to lift the scapula and rotate the inferior angle of the scapula medially when the spine is fixed. Therefore, it is not damaged by an injury to the superolateral thoracic wall.

The pectoralis minor muscle (Choice B) starts from the front of the third to the fifth ribs and the fascia on the surface of the intercostal muscle, as well as ends at the coracoid process of the scapula. The pectoralis minor muscle can lift the ribs, but it can only move when inhaling. It is also not likely to be damaged by injury to the superolateral thoracic wall.

The rhomboid muscle (Choice C) starts from the spinous processes of the upper thoracic vertebrae (T1—T4) and ends at the medial border of the scapula. The function of the rhomboid muscle is to retract the scapula and make the scapula close to the spine which is not responsible for the arm abduction.

The supraspinatus muscle (Choice D) starts from the supraspinatus fossa of the scapula and ends at the greater tubercle of the humerus. This muscle plays a critical role in arm abduction and maintaining the stability of shoulder joint. It is also not damaged by an injury to the superolateral thoracic wall.

The serratus anterior muscle (Choice E) is attached to the surface of the lateral wall of the thorax, which starts from the external surface of the first to the ninth ribs, and ends at the medial border of the scapula. One function of the serratus anterior muscle is to press the scapula against the thorax. If the anterior serratus muscle is damaged, the medial border of the scapula is raised.

The Alimentary System

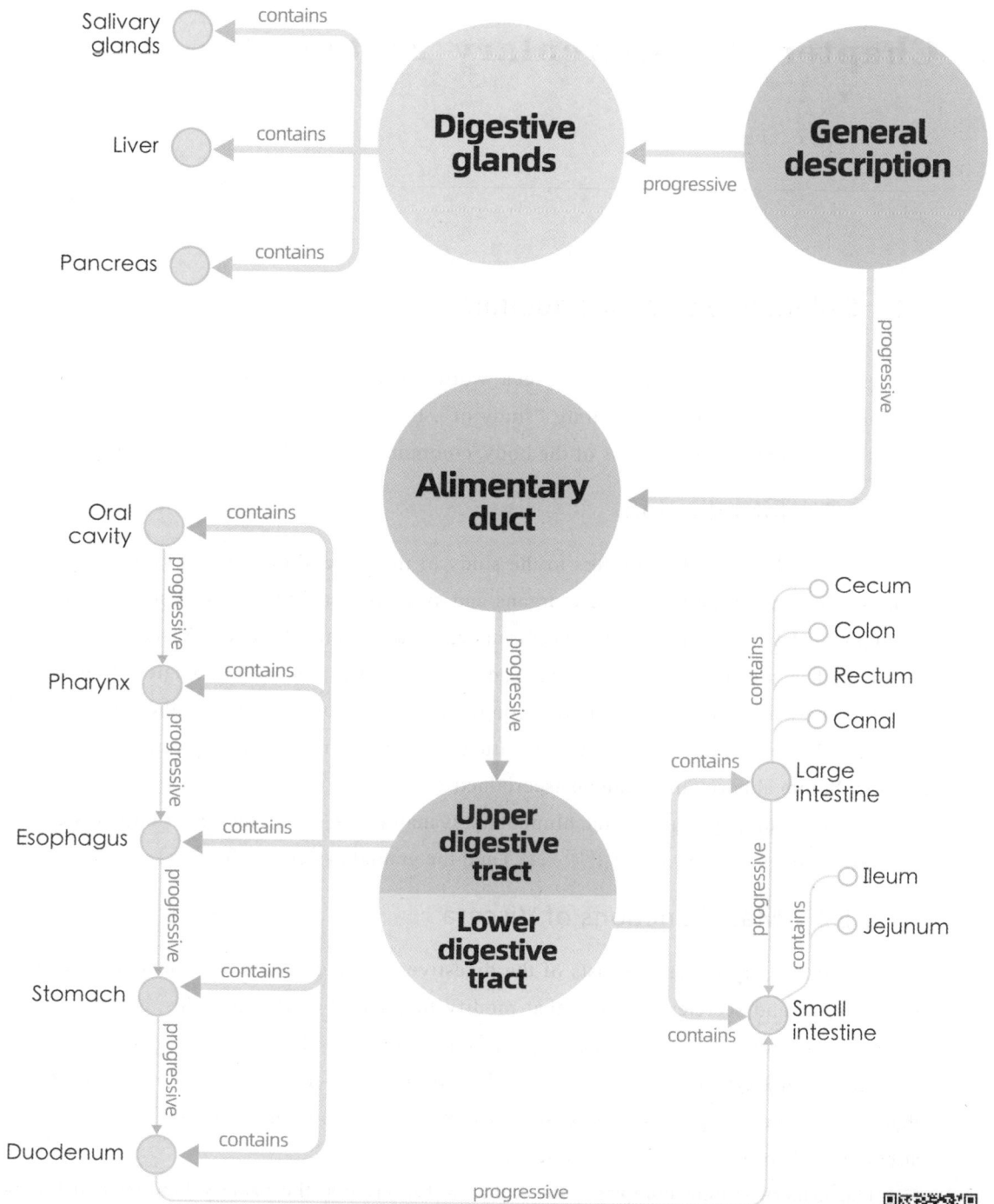

The Alimentary System

Chapter 2   Alimentary System

2.1   Splanchnology Introduction

Splanchnology comes from the Greek words "splanchno-", meaning "viscera" or internal organs, and "-logy", meaning "study of". It refers to the branch of anatomy that studies the viscera, the soft organs of the body, commonly referred to as visceral organs.

2.1.1   Introduction

Splanchnology (内脏学) refers to the study of the visceral organs and viscera refers to the soft organs of the body. These organs and systems of organs differ in structure and development but are united for the performance of a common function. Visceral organs are situated in the thoracic, abdominal, and pelvic cavities and are associated with the pleura or the peritoneum. They are also connected directly or indirectly to the outside of the body. Understanding the normal position and function of each visceral organ is essential before abnormalities can be ascertained.

The splanchnology include the alimentary system (消化系统), the respiratory system (呼吸系统), the urinary system (泌尿系统) and the genital system (生殖系统).

2.1.2   Main Functions of Viscera

The alimentary system consists of the digestive tube and certain accessory organs. It ingests foods and secretes enzymes that modify the size of food molecules, absorbs the products of this digestive action and eliminates the unused residue.

The respiratory system consists of the larynx, trachea, bronchi, lungs, and the pleurae. It carries out gas exchanges, supplies oxygen for the living cells and removes the carbon dioxide produced by cell metabolism.

The urinary system comprises the kidneys, the ureters, the urinary bladder and the urethra. It keeps the body in homeostasis by removing and restoring a selected amount of water and solutes. It also excretes a selected amount of various wastes.

The genital system consists of an internal organ and an external organ. It produces germ cells.

2.1.3   Reference Lines of the Thorax

The chest wall, commonly referred to as "the thoracic wall", is the structure that surrounds the vital organs within the thoracic cavity. Anatomical landmarks that play an important role in clinical examination and thoracic surgery include anterior median line (前正中线), sternal line (胸骨线), midclavicular line (锁骨中线), parasternal line (胸骨旁线), anterior axillary line (腋前线), midaxillary line (腋中线), posterior axillary line (腋后线), scapular line (肩胛线), paravertebral line (脊柱旁线), posterior median line (后正中线) (Fig.2-1).

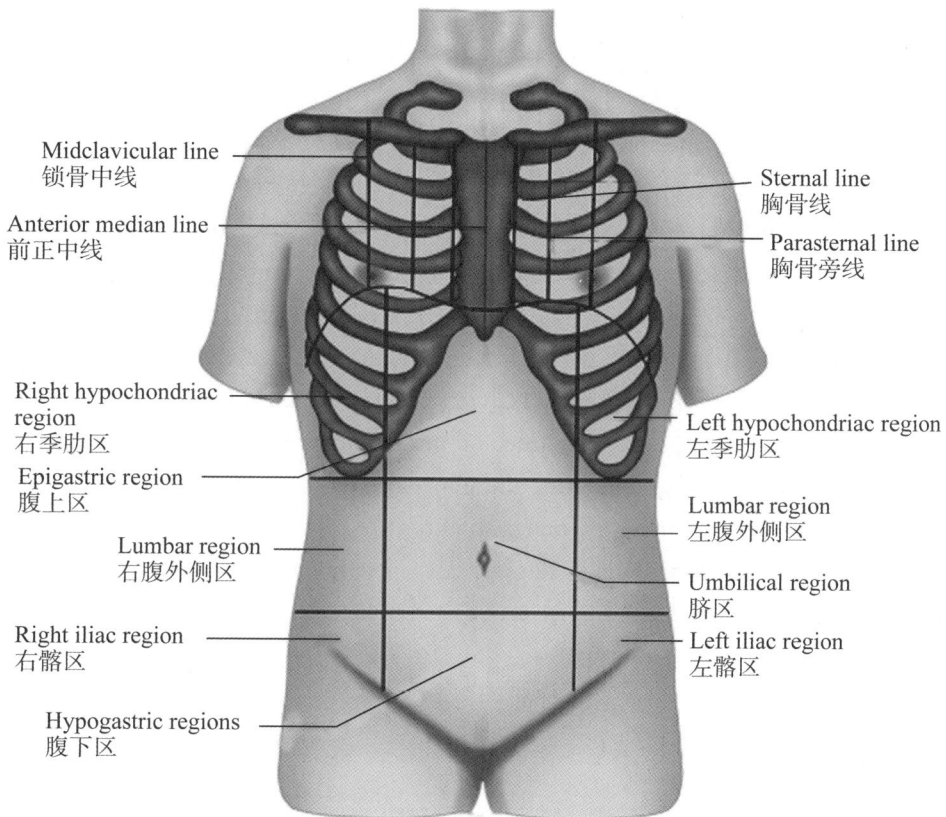

Fig.2-1   Reference line and abominal regions

2.1.4   Reference Lines of Abdomen and Abdominal Regions

Abdominal surface anatomy can be described when viewed from the front side of the abdomen in two ways: i) divided into nine regions by two vertical and two horizontal imaginary planes, and ii) divided into four quadrants by single vertical and horizontal imaginary planes.

Reference lines of the abdomen are a transverse line through the umbilicus (transumbilical line) and a vertical line in the midline of the body (median line). They divide the abdomen into four regions, including the right upper quadrant (RUQ) (右上腹), the left upper quadrant (LUQ) (左上腹), the right lower quadrant (RLQ) (右下腹) and the left lower quadrant (LLQ) (左下腹).

A more detailed regional approach subdivides the abdomen with one horizontal line immediately inferior to the ribs, one immediately superior to the pelvis, and two vertical lines drawn from the midpoint of the inguinal ligament into nine regions: the left hypochondriac region (左季肋区), containing the spleen; the right hypochondriac region (右季肋区), containing the liver; the epigastric region (腹上区), containing the bottom edge of the liver and the upper area of the stomach; the right lumbar region (右腰区), containing the ascending colon and the right edge of the small intestine; the umbilical region (脐区), containing the transverse colon and the upper region of the small intestine; the left lumbar region (左腰区), containing the left edge of the transverse colon and the left edge of the small intestine; the right iliac region (右腹股沟区), containing the ascending colon and vermiform appendix; the left iliac region (左腹股沟区), containing the lower left region of the small intestine and descending colon; the lower central square hypogastric region (腹下区), containing the upper region of the bladder, the lower region of the small intestine and female internal genital organs.

These nine regions or four quadrants are of clinical importance when physical examination and describing pathologies are related to the abdomen.

(福建医科大学　罗道枢)

2.2   Alimentary Canal & Gland

2.2.1   General Description

The alimentary system (消化系统)(Fig. 2-2) is responsible for several functions, including digestion, absorption, and immune response. It consists of the digestive tube (alimentary canal, 消化管) and certain accessory organs (alimentary glands, 消化腺).

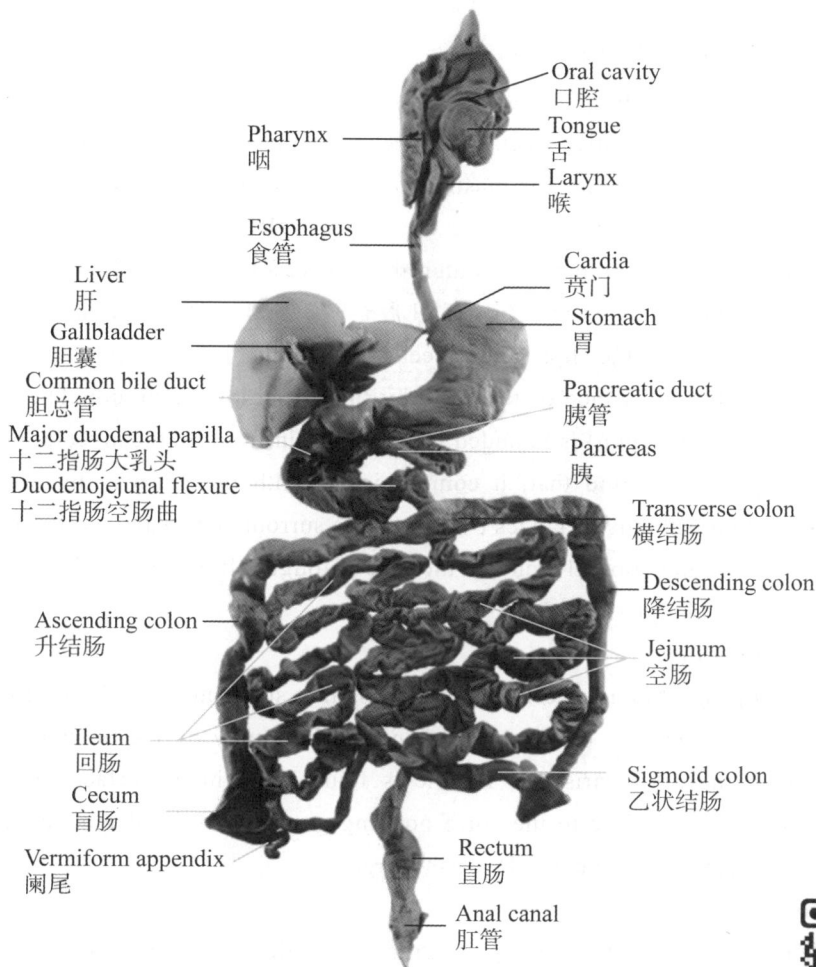

Fig.2-2   The alimentary system

Digestion begins in the upper gastrointestinal tract, consisting of the oral cavity (口腔), the pharynx (咽), the esophagus (食管), the stomach (胃) and the duodenum (十二指肠). This process starts with mastication in the mouth, which corresponds to the action of chewing food. Digestion then continues in the lower gastrointestinal tract consisting of the

jejunum (空肠), the ileum (回肠), the cecum (盲肠) and the appendix (阑尾), the colon (结肠), the rectum (直肠), and the anal canal (肛管).

The alimentary glands (消化腺) contain the salivary glands, including the parotid gland (腮腺), the submandibular gland (下颌下腺) and the sublingual gland (舌下腺), the liver (肝脏) and the pancreas (胰腺).

The functions of the alimentary system include ingesting foods, secreting enzymes, absorbing nutrients and eliminating unused residues.

2.2.2　Oral Cavity

The oral cavity (Figs. 2-3 & 2-4) is also known as mouth, located at the commencement of the digestive tract. The cheeks, tongue, and palate frame the mouth. It houses the structures necessary for mastication and speech, which include the teeth, the tongue and associated structures such as the salivary glands. It is a nearly oval-shaped cavity which consists of two parts: an outer, the oral vestibule (口腔前庭), and an inner, larger part, the oral cavity proper (固有口腔). The oral vestibule is a slit-like space, bounded externally by the lips and cheeks, internally by the gums and teeth. It communicates with the surface of the body by the orifice of the mouth. The oral cavity proper (cavum oris proprium) is bounded laterally and in front by the alveolar arches with their contained teeth; behind that, it communicates with the pharynx by a constricted aperture termed the isthmus of fauces (咽峡) that is surrounded by the uvula, free edge of the palatal velum, palatoglossal arch and the root of tongue. It is the boundary between the oral cavity and the pharynx.

1. The Oral Lips

The oral lips (口唇) are the two fleshy folds that surround the orifice of the mouth. They are formed externally by the integument and internally by the mucous membrane, between which the orbicularis oris muscle is found. The inner surface of each lip is connected in the middle line to the corresponding gum by a fold of mucous membrane, called the frenulum (with the upper being the larger).

2. The Cheeks

The cheeks (buccae)(颊) correspond to the two sides of the face, and are continuous with the lips at the front. They are composed externally of integument and internally of mucous membrane, which is tightly adherent to the buccinator. Between the two there is a muscular stratum, a large quantity of fat, areolar tissue, vessels, nerves and buccal glands.

3. The Roof of the Oral Cavity

The roof of the oral cavity is called the palate (腭). The anterior region of the palate serves as a wall (or septum) between the oral and nasal cavities. It is created by the maxillary and palatine bones of the skull (the hard palate) and the posterior region is the

Tooth
牙

Hard palate
硬腭

Soft palate
软腭

Uvula
腭垂

Epiglottis
会厌

Root of tongue
舌根

Terminal sulcus
界沟

Vallate papillae
轮廓乳头

Body of tongue
舌体

Apex of tongue
舌尖

Palatopharyngeal arch
腭咽弓

Palatoglossus arch
腭舌弓

Palatine tonsil
腭扁桃体

Lingual tonsil
舌扁桃体

Foliate papilla
叶状乳头

Median sulcus of tongue
舌正中沟

Fungiform papilla
菌状乳头

Filiform papilla
丝状乳头

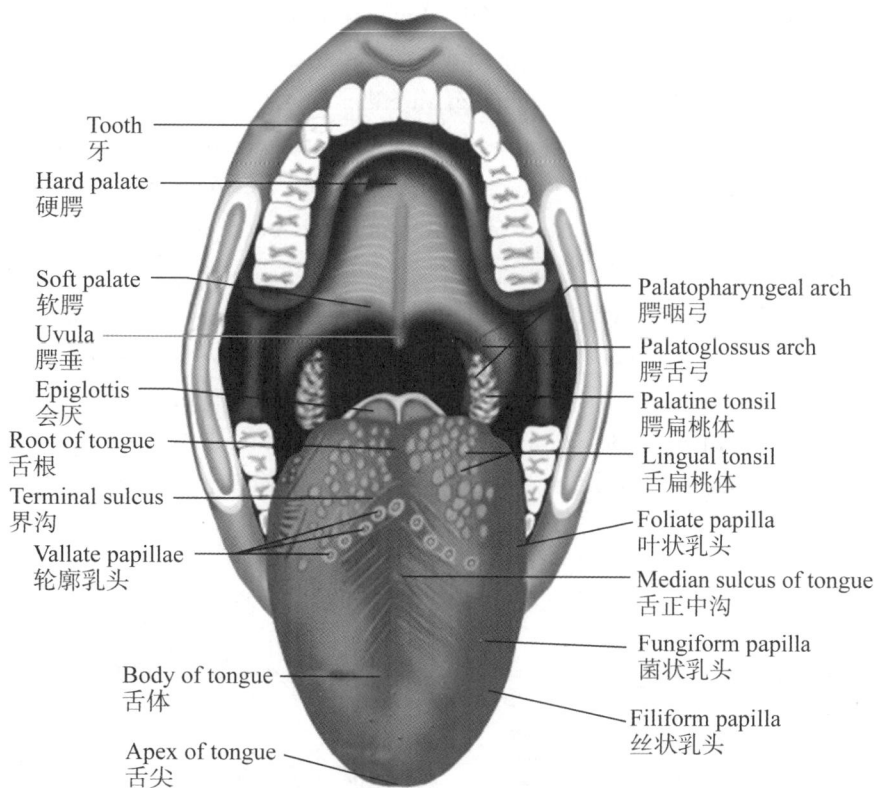

Fig.2-3   The cavity of the mouth (sagittal section)

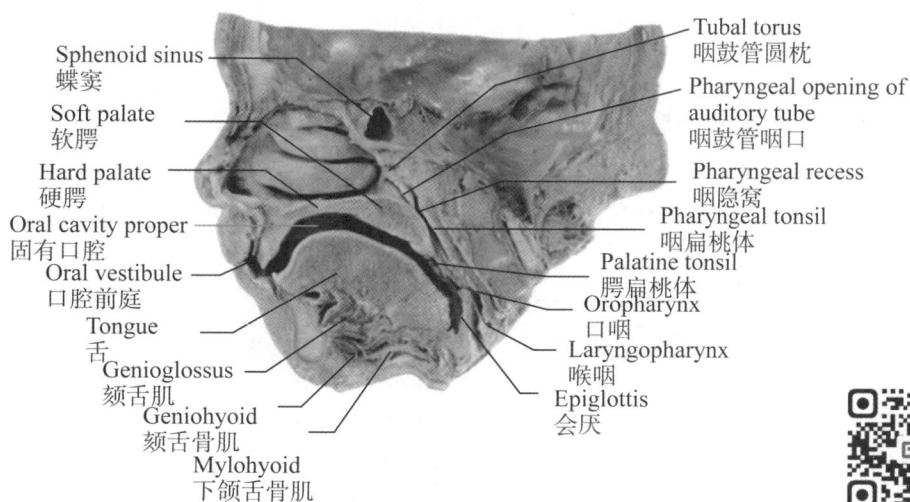

Sphenoid sinus
蝶窦

Soft palate
软腭

Hard palate
硬腭

Oral cavity proper
固有口腔

Oral vestibule
口腔前庭

Tongue
舌

Genioglossus
颏舌肌

Geniohyoid
颏舌骨肌

Mylohyoid
下颌舌骨肌

Tubal torus
咽鼓管圆枕

Pharyngeal opening of
auditory tube
咽鼓管咽口

Pharyngeal recess
咽隐窝

Pharyngeal tonsil
咽扁桃体

Palatine tonsil
腭扁桃体

Oropharynx
口咽

Laryngopharynx
喉咽

Epiglottis
会厌

Fig.2-4   The cavity of the mouth (sagittal aspect)

soft palate that is mainly composed of skeletal muscles. A fleshy bead of tissue called the uvula drops down from the center of the posterior edge of the soft palate. Two muscular folds extend downward from the soft palate, on either side of the uvula. Toward the front, the palatoglossal arch lies next to the base of the tongue; behind it, the palatopharyngeal arch forms the superior and lateral margins of the fauces. Between these two arches lies the palatine tonsil (腭扁桃体), clusters of lymphoid tissue that protect the pharynx.

4. The Teeth

The teeth (牙) are secured in the alveolar processes (sockets) of the maxilla and the mandible and mainly provided with two sets according to their appearance at different periods of life. The first set appear at about six months after birth and erupt before the age of three. They are called the deciduous tooth (乳牙) or milk teeth. The second set appears at an early period, around six years old, may continue until old age, around $18-21$ years old, named permanent tooth (恒牙) (Fig.2-5).

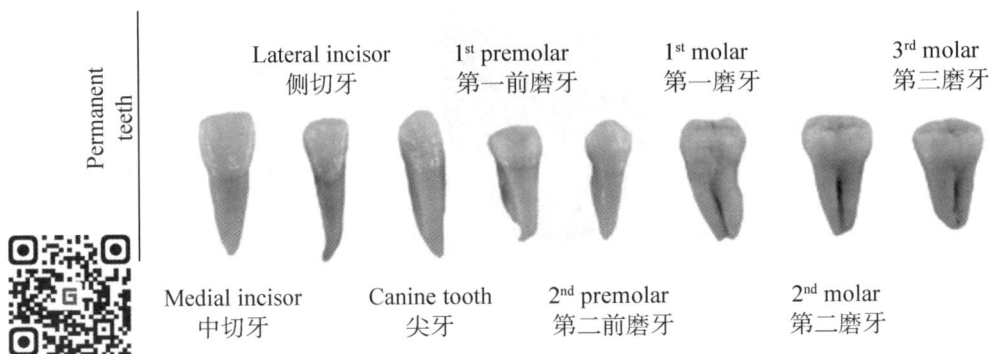

Fig.2-5　The teeth

Each tooth consists of three portions: the crown of tooth (牙冠), which is the portion projecting above the gum line; the root of tooth (牙根), which is embedded within the alveolus of maxilla and mandible; and the neck of tooth (牙颈), the constricted portion between the crown and the root.

The permanent teeth (恒牙) are 32 in number: four incisors (切牙), two canine teeth (尖牙), four premolars (前磨牙), and six molars (磨牙), in each jaw. The deciduous teeth (乳牙) are twenty in number: four incisors, two canines, and four molars, in each jaw.

The tooth includes a pulp cavity of tooth (牙髓腔), containing loose connective tissue through which run nerves and blood vessels called dental pulp (牙髓). The region of the pulp cavity that runs through the root of the tooth is called the root canal (牙根管) and apical foramen (根尖孔). Surrounding the dental cavity is dentine of tooth (牙质), a bone-like tissue. In the root of each tooth, the dentin is covered by an even harder bone-like layer called cementum (牙骨质) and periodontal membrane(牙周膜). In the crown of each tooth, the dentin is covered by an outer layer of enamel (牙釉质), the hardest substance in the body.

5. The Tongue

The tongue (舌) (Fig. 2-6) is the principal organ for the sense of taste, and an important organ of speech; it also assists in the mastication and deglutition of food. It is situated in the floor of the mouth, within the curve of the body of the mandible, partly oral and partly pharyngeal in position. It is composed of a root, an apex, a curved dorsum and an inferior surface.

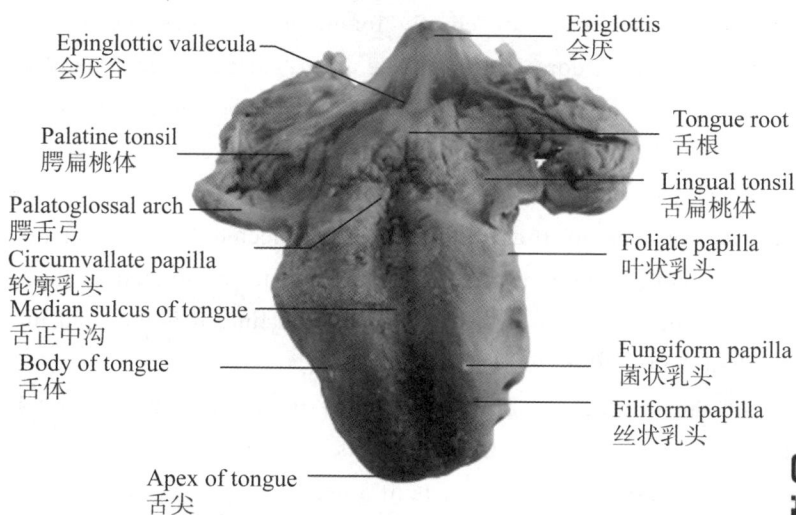

Fig.2-6   The tongue

The root of tongue (舌根) is directed backward, and connected with the hyoid bone by the hyoglossi and genioglossi muscles and the hyoglossal membrane; with the epiglottis by three folds (glossoepiglottic) of mucous membrane; with the soft palate by the glossopalatine arches; and with the pharynx by the constrictores pharyngis superiores and the mucous membrane. The two parts of the tongue (anterior and posterior) are divided by the terminal sulcus.

The apex of tongue (舌尖) is thin and narrow, and directed forward against the lingual surfaces of the lower incisor teeth.

Mucosa of the tongue (舌黏膜). The mucous membrane of the anterior 2/3 of the dorsum is thick, rough and is covered by numerous lingual papilla (舌乳头), a lots of small elevation formed by epithelium. They are thickly distributed over the anterior 2/3 of its dorsum, giving the surface a characteristic roughness. The varieties of papillae seen on the dorsal surface of the tongue are vallate papillae (轮廓乳头), fungiform papillae (菌状乳头), filiform papillae (丝状乳头) and foliate papillae (叶状乳头). The filiform papillae

(丝状乳头) covers the anterior two-thirds of the dorsum. They are very minute, filiform in shape and are arranged in diagonal lines parallel with the two rows of the papillae vallatae, except at the apex of the organ, where their direction is transverse. It has no tastebuds (味蕾). The vallate papillae (轮廓乳头) (circumvallate papillae) are large in size, varying from 8—12 in number and have dome-shaped structures. They are situated on the surface of the tongue immediately in front of the terminal sulcus. Each papilla is 1—2 mm in diameter, and is generally covered with nonkeratinized stratified squamous epithelium. The fungiform papillae (菌状乳头) are larger, rounded and deep red in color projections on the tongue. They are chiefly found on the sides and apex, and can be described as irregular on the dorsal surface. The apical surface of each papilla usually has one or more taste buds. The foliate papillae (叶状乳头) are similar to those of the skin, and are present on each side of the tongue. Each zone is covered by a series of red, leaf-like mucosal ridges, with numerous taste buds.

The inferior surface of the tongue. It is connected with the mandible by the genioglossi; the mucous membrane is reflected from it to the lingual surface of the gum and on to the floor of the mouth, where at the middle line, it is elevated into a distinct vertical fold called the frenulum linguae.

Muscles of the tongue (舌肌). The tongue divides into two lateral halves by a median fibrous septum that extends throughout its entire length and is fixed below to the hyoid bone. In either half, there are two sets of muscles, extrinsic and intrinsic; the former has its origins outside the tongue that control its movement; the latter is contained entirely within the tongue and alters its shape. The extrinsic muscles consists of genioglossus, hyoglossus, styloglossus (and chondroglossus) and palato-glossus. The intrinsic muscles consists of longitudinalis superior, transversus, longitudinalis inferior and verticalis.

2.2.3 Pharynx

The pharynx (Fig.2-7) is the part of the digestive tube which is located behind and communicates with the nasal cavities, mouth and larynx. It is a musculo-membranous tube, with the base upward and the apex downward, extending from the base of the skull to the level of the cricoid cartilage in front and the sixth cervical vertebra behind (level 1st—6th cervical vertebrae). The pharynx is 12—14 cm long and its width varies with muscle tension. It can be subdivided into the nasopharynx, the oropharynx and the laryngopharynx.

1. The Nasopharynx (鼻咽)

It lies behind the nose and above the level of the soft palate: it differs from the oral and laryngeal parts of the pharynx in that its cavity always remains patent. As an opening of auditory tube, the nasopharynx allows air to flow freely between the nasal cavities and the nasopharynx.

2. The Oropharynx (口咽)

It extends from the soft palate to the upper border of the epiglottis. It opens anteriorly through the isthmus faucium into the mouth, while at its lateral wall, between the two palatine arches, the palatine tonsil can be found.

3. The Laryngopharynx (喉咽)

It extends from the upper border of the epiglottis to the lower border of the cricoid cartilage, where it is continuous with the esophagus(lower level of C3 to the upper level of C6). While during deglutition, the laryngopharynx would be elevated together with the elevated hyoid. Anteriorly it presents the triangular entrance of the larynx, the base of which is directed forward and is formed by the epiglottis, while its lateral boundaries are constituted by the aryepiglottic folds. On either side of the laryngeal orifice is a recess, termed the sinus piriformis, which is bounded medially by the aryepiglottic fold, laterally by the thyroid cartilage and hyothyroid membrane.

2.2.4　Esophagus

The esophagus (Fig. 2-8) is a muscular canal, about $20-25$ cm long in adults, extending from the pharynx to the stomach. It begins in the neck at the lower border of the

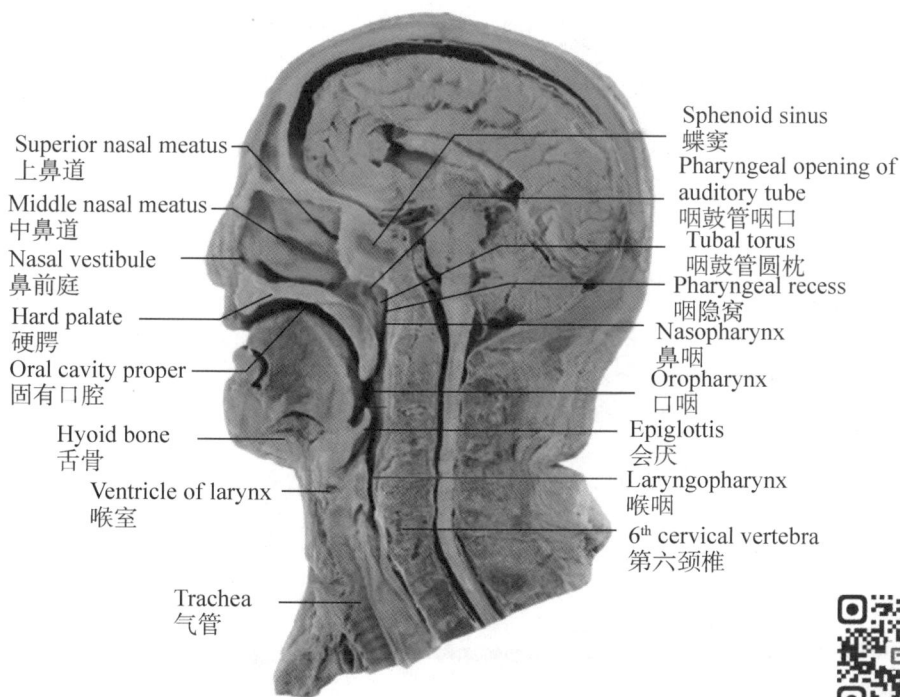

Fig.2-7　The pharynx

cricoid cartilage (C6), descends along the front of the vertebral column, through the superior and posterior mediastina, passes through the diaphragm to enter the abdomen, and ends at the cardiac orifice of the stomach (T11). It is subdivided into the cervical portion, the thoracic portion and the abdominal portion.

1. The Cervical Portion (颈部)

The cervical portion of the esophagus is in relation with the trachea in front; and at the lower part of the neck, where it projects to the left side with the thyroid gland; it rests upon the vertebral column and longus colli muscles; on either side it is in relation with the common carotid artery (especially the left, as it inclines to that side), and the posterior part of the thyroid gland; the recurrent nerves ascend between it and the trachea. The thoracic duct is located at the left of the cervical portion of the esophagus.

2. The Thoracic Portion

The thoracic portion (胸部) of the esophagus is at first situated in the superior mediastinum between the trachea and the vertebral column, a little to the left of the median line. It then passes behind and to the right of the aortic arch, descends through the posterior mediastinum along the right side of the descending aorta, and then runs in front and a little to the left of the aorta where it enters the abdomen through the diaphragm at

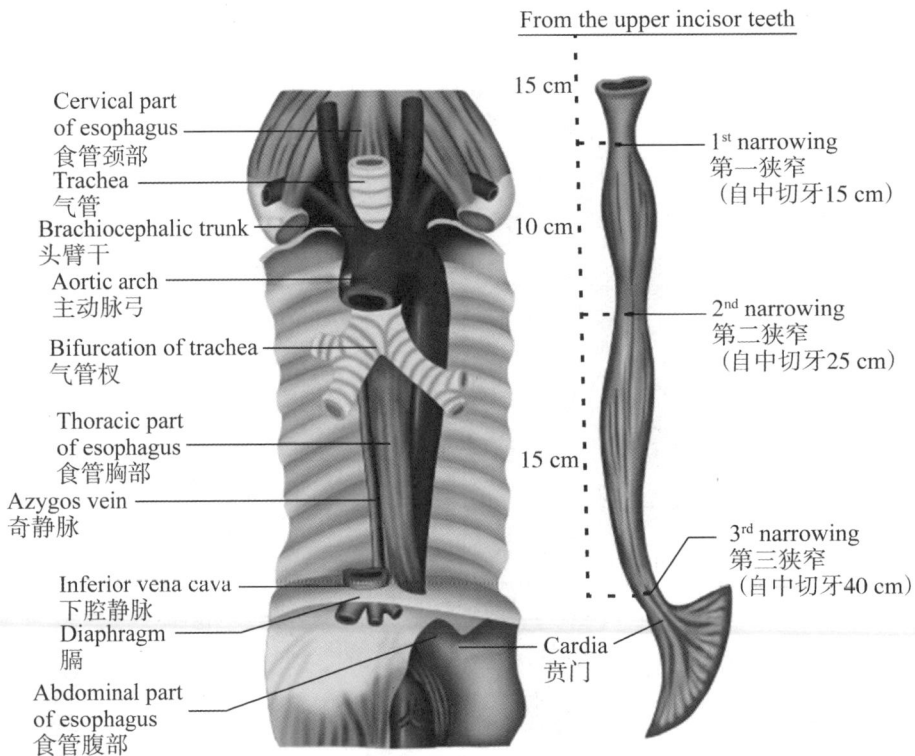

From the upper incisor teeth

15 cm
10 cm
15 cm

Cervical part of esophagus
食管颈部
Trachea
气管
Brachiocephalic trunk
头臂干
Aortic arch
主动脉弓
Bifurcation of trachea
气管杈
Thoracic part of esophagus
食管胸部
Azygos vein
奇静脉
Inferior vena cava
下腔静脉
Diaphragm
膈
Abdominal part of esophagus
食管腹部

1st narrowing
第一狭窄
(自中切牙15 cm)

2nd narrowing
第二狭窄
(自中切牙25 cm)

3rd narrowing
第三狭窄
(自中切牙40 cm)

Cardia
贲门

Fig.2-8　The esophagus

the level of T10.

3. The Abdominal Portion

The abdominal portion (腹部) of the esophagus lies in the esophageal groove on the posterior surface of the left lobe of the liver. It measures about 1.0—2.5 cm in length, and only its front and left aspects are covered by the peritoneum. It extends obliquely to the left and slightly to the back and ends at the gastro-esophageal junction.

4. Three Constrictions of the Esophagus

The first constriction is the commencement of the esophagus, surrounded by cricopharyngeal, about 15 cm from the incisor teeth.

The second constriction is crossed by the aortic arch and the left principal bronchus anteriorly, about 25 cm from the incisor teeth.

The third constriction is where the esophagus passes through the diaphragm, about 40 cm from the incisor teeth.

The esophageal glands (食管腺) are small compound racemose glands of the mucous type. They are lodged in the submucous tissue, and each opens upon the surface by a long excretory duct. The mucosal mucous glands located in the abdominal esophagus are called esophageal cardiac glands.

2.2.5   Stomach

1. Shape and Position

The shape and position of the stomach (Fig.2-9) are so greatly modified by changes within itself. It is located between the end of the esophagus and the beginning of the small intestine, and lies most in the epigastric regions, and umbilical & left hypochondriac regions of abdomen. Cardiac orifice is at the left side of the 11th thoracic vertebra. Pyloric orifice is at the right side of the 1st lumbar vertebra.

2. Components

The stomach presents two orifices, two borders(curvatures), two surfaces and four parts.

(1) Two orifices

They refer to the cardia and the pylorus. The orifice by which the esophagus communicates with the stomach is known as the cardia (贲门), and is situated on the left of the midline at the level of the 11th thoracic vertebra. The pylorus (幽门) communicates with the duodenum, and its position is usually indicated on the surface of the stomach by a circular groove known as the duodenopyloric constriction. This orifice lies 1—2 cm to the right of the middle line at the level of the lower border of the L1 vertebra.

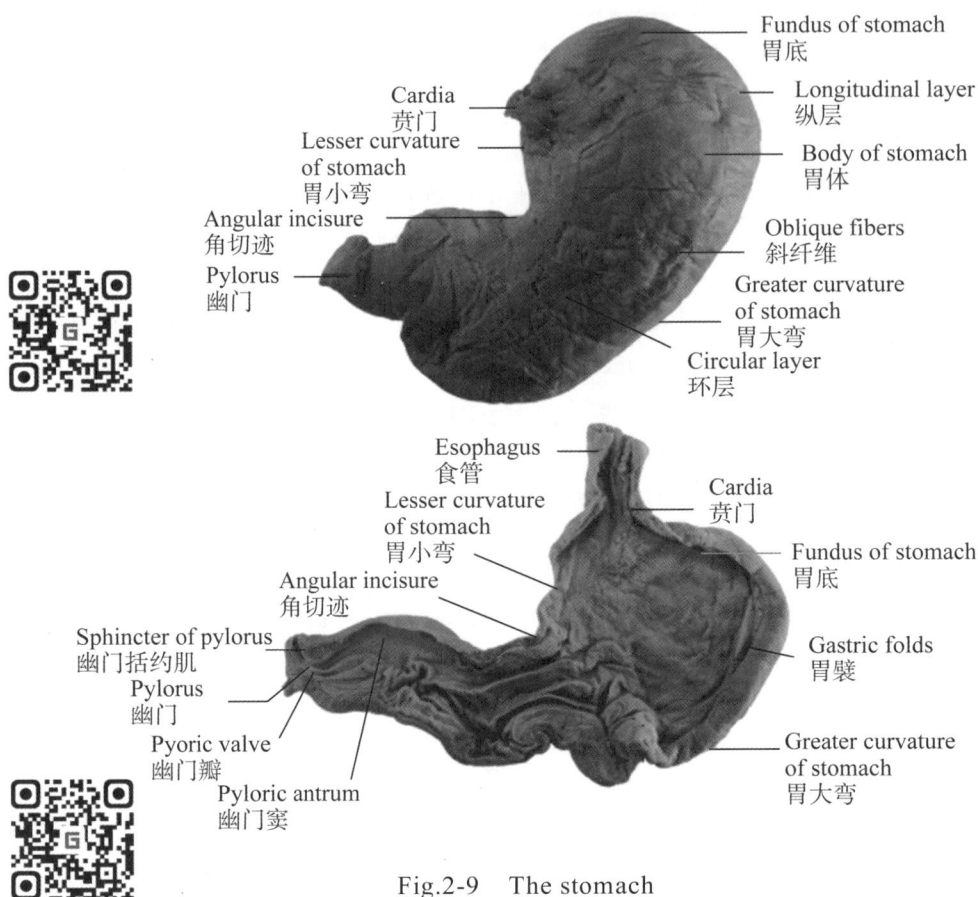

Fig.2-9 The stomach

(2) Two curvatures

They refer to the greater curvature (胃大弯) and the lesser curvature (胃小弯). The lesser curvature (curvatura ventriculi minor), extends between the cardiac and pyloric orifices where it forms the right or posterior border of the stomach. It descends as a continuation of the right margin of the esophagus in front of the fibers of the right crus of the diaphragm, turning right it crosses the first lumbar vertebra and ends at the pylorus. The lesser curvature ends at the pylorus, right to the midline. The greater curvature (curvatura ventriculi major) is directed mainly forward, and is two to three times as long as the lesser curvature. Starting from the cardiac orifice at the incisura cardiaca, it forms an arch backward, upward, and to the left; the highest point of the convexity is on a level with the sixth left costal cartilage. The greater curvature ends at the pylorus, the lower border of the first lumbar vertebra.

(3) Four parts

The fundus of stomach (胃底), the body of stomach (胃体), the cardiac part (贲门部) and the pyloric part (幽门部) are included. As the name implies, the cardia surrounds the cardiac orifice, which is the opening between the esophagus and the stomach. The fundus is the superior dilation of the stomach, which is located superiorly relative to the horizontal plane of the cardiac orifice. A plane passing through the angular incisure on the lesser curvature divides the stomach into a left portion (body) and a right portion (pyloric part). The pyloric part represents the outflow section of the stomach, passing partly digested food from the stomach into the duodenum via the pyloric orifice, the opening and closing of which are controlled by the pyloric sphincter (pylorus), a circular layer of the smooth muscle. The pylorus is further divided into two distinct areas: the pyloric antrum connected to the stomach and the pyloric canal connected to the duodenum.

(4) **Two surfaces**

The anterior surface (前面) and the posterior surface (后面) are included. The anterior surface is covered by the peritoneum and directly attached to the anterior abdominal wall. Its lateral part lies behind the left costal arch and its superior left part curves backwards and contacts with the visceral surface of the spleen.

3. Position and Relations

The stomach is the most dilated part of the digestive tube, and is situated between the end of the esophagus and the duodenum. It lies mostly in the epigastric region of the abdomen. The position is so greatly modified by changes within itself, but the cardiac orifice is at the left side of T11 and pyloric orifice is at the right side of L1. It is covered and connected to other organs by the peritoneum. The lesser omentum connects the stomach to the liver and then extends around the stomach. The greater omentum continues inferiorly from the stomach to greater curvature, and then turns back to the transverse colon. The stomach is located inside the abdominal cavity in a small area called the bed of the stomach [related to the omental bursa (the lesser sac), the pancreas, the left kidney and the adrenal gland, the spleen and the splenic artery].

2.2.6　Small Intestine

1.The Duodenum

The duodenum (十二指肠) (Fig. 2-10) is the first of the three parts of the small intestine that receives partially digested food from the stomach and its name is equal in length to the breadth of 12 fingers (25 cm). It is the shortest, the widest, and the most fixed part of the small intestine. It has a C-shape, and is closely related to the head of the pancreas (L1—L3 level), consisting of four sections: the superior part (上部), the descending part (降部), the horizontal part (水平部) and the ascending part (升部).

(1)**The superior part.** It lies intraperitoneally and is enlarged proximally (duodenal bulb). It is connected to the liver by the hepatoduodenal ligament. The superior part ends at the superior duodenal flexure and becomes the descending part.

(2)**The descending part.** It lies retroperitoneally. The common bile duct and the pancreatic duct unify to a conjoint duct at the hepatopancreatic ampulla (ampulla of Vater, 肝胰壶腹) and empties into the descending part of the duodenum at major duodenal papilla (papilla of Vater). Many people have an accessory pancreatic duct which empties into the minor duodenal papilla (papilla of Santorini). The transition from the descending to the horizontal part of the duodenum takes place at the inferior duodenal flexure.

(3)**The horizontal part.** It runs ventrally from the abdominal aorta and inferior vena cava, extending from right to left.

(4)**The ascending part.** It is the last part of the duodenum which joins the intraperitoneally lying jejunum at the duodenojejunal flexure. Here the duodenum is attached to the back of the abdominal wall through the suspensory ligament of the duodenum (the ligament of Treitz, 十二指肠悬韧带). Clinically, the ligament of Treitz serves as a landmark demarcating the boundary between the upper and the lower gastrointestinal tract.

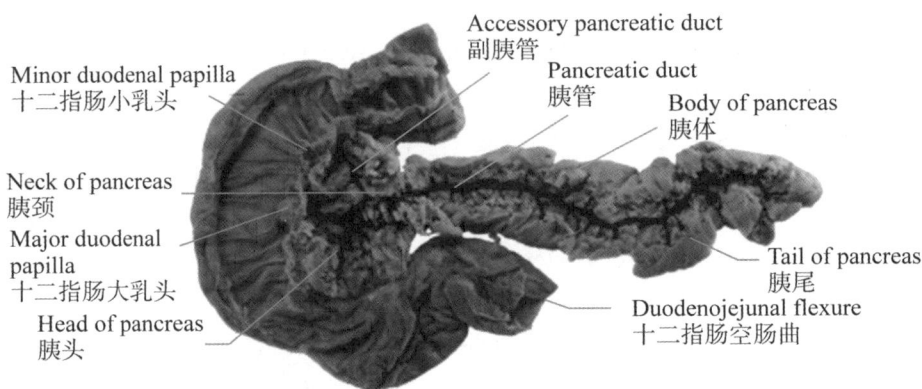

Fig.2-10　The duodenum and major duodenal papilla

2.The Jejunum and the Ileum

The remainders of the small intestine from the end of the duodenum is called the jejunum and the ileum. The term "jejunum" refers to the upper 2/5 part, while the term "ileum" refers to the lower 3/5 part (Table 2-1).

(1)**The jejunum**

The jejunum (空 肠) is the middle of the small intestine, situated between the duodenum and the ileum. It constitutes approximately 40% of the entire length of the small intestine and plays a significant role in digestion. Compared to the ileum, the jejunum is thicker, wider, more vascular, and has a deeper color, resulting in a greater weight per unit length. The proximal jejunum is characterized by prominent circular folds known as plicae circulares, which are formed by the mucous membrane.

(2)The ileum

The ileum (回肠) is the distal portion of the small intestine, succeeding the jejunum. It is narrower in diameter compared to the jejunum and has a thinner and less vascular coat. Unlike the jejunum, the ileum possesses fewer circular folds, which are small and diminish towards its lower end. However, it is characterized by larger and more numerous aggregated lymph nodules known as Peyer's patches.

Table 2-1   Comparison of the jejunum and the ileum

The jejunum	The ileum
Upper 2/5	Lower 3/5
Wider in diameter and the wall is thicker	Thinner in diameter and the wall is thinner
Red and more vascular	Less red and less vascular
The circular mucosal folds are larger and more in number	The circular mucosal folds are shorter and few in number
Only solitary lymphatic follicles	Solitary and aggregated lymphatic follicles

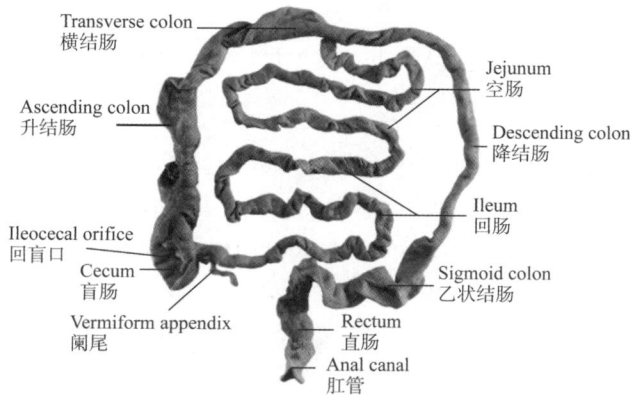

Fig.2-11   The Jejunum and the ileum

2.2.7   Large Intestine

The large intestine spans from the termination of the ileum to the anus, measuring approximately 1.0−1.5 meters in length. Its primary function involves the absorption of water from intestinal contents, leading to the formation of feces. Additionally, the large intestine serves as a storage site for feces before defecation and harbors a crucial microflora essential for our well-being. Its caliber is the largest at its commencement at the caecum (盲肠), and gradually diminishes as far as the sigmoid colon (乙状结肠), and then expands in the rectum (直肠), where there is a dilatation of considerable size at its lower third just above the anal canal, which iscalled rectal ampulla.

Three distinctive anatomical features characterize the large intestine (Fig. 2-12), including the epiploic appendices (肠脂垂, the fat attached externally to the walls), the colic band (also named the teniae coli, three longitudinal bands of the smooth muscle located underneath the peritoneum that extends along the large intestine, 结肠带), which forms the haustrum of the colon (结肠袋). Anatomically, the large intestine can be subdivided into the caecum (盲肠), the colon (结肠), the rectum (直肠), and the anal canal (肛管).

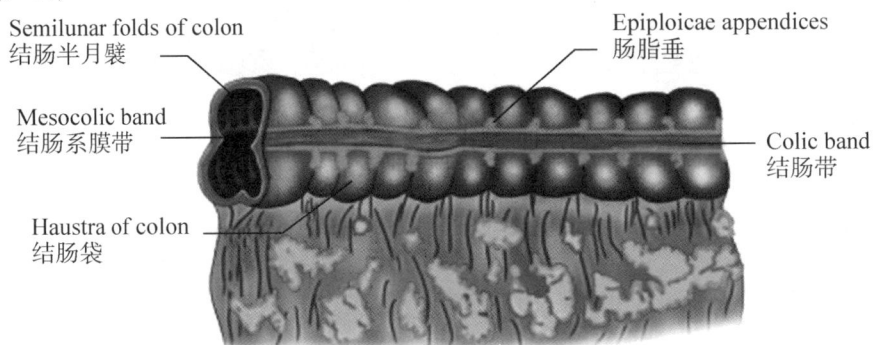

Semilunar folds of colon
结肠半月襞

Mesocolic band
结肠系膜带

Haustra of colon
结肠袋

Epiploicae appendices
肠脂垂

Colic band
结肠带

Fig.2-12　Anatomical features characterizing the large intestine

1. The Caecum

The caecum (盲肠), which marks the beginning of the large intestine, is approximately 6 cm in length and is positioned adjacent to the anterior abdominal wall. It receives chyme from the ileum and connects to the ascending colon of the large intestine. The boundary between the caecum and the ileum is demarcated by the ileocecal valve (ICV, 回盲瓣), also known as Bauhin's valve, while the separation from the colon is defined by the cecocolic junction. The vermiform appendix (阑尾) is attached to the caecum (Fig.2-13).

Although the caecum is typically intraperitoneal, the ascending colon is retroperitoneal. The vermiform appendix is a long, narrow, worm-shaped tube that originates from the apex of the caecum. It may extend in various directions, including upward behind the caecum, to the left behind the ileum and mesentery, or downward into the lesser pelvis. In adults, the length of the appendix typically ranges from 6 cm to 10 cm.

McBurney's point (麦氏点), which represents the surface projection of the root of the vermiform appendix, is located at the junction of the middle and the lateral thirds of a line drawn between the right anterior superior iliac spine and the umbilicus.

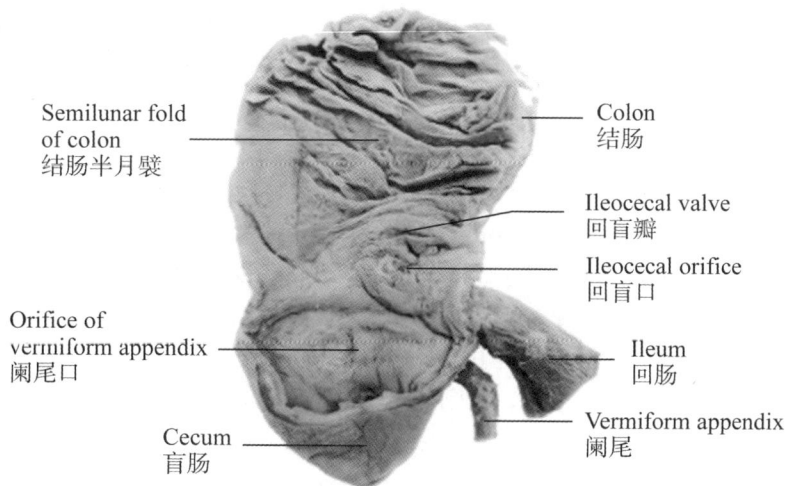

Fig.2-13   The caecum and appendix

2. The Colon

The colon, situated between the cecum and the rectum, constitutes a significant portion of the large intestine. It is comprised of four distinct regions: the ascending (升结肠), the transverse (横结肠), the descending (降结肠)and the sigmoid colon (乙状结肠). The primary functions of the colon encompass fluid and electrolyte reabsorption, essential for maintaining fluid balance within the body. Furthermore, the microflora inhabiting the colon play a crucial role in energy production via fermentation processes.

(1) Measuring approximately 15−20 cm in length, **the ascending colon** (升结肠) is located retroperitoneally and is anchored to the posterior abdominal wall by Toldt's fascia. Originating from the cecum, it ascends upwards, traversing along the under surface of the right lobe of the liver, adjacent to the gallbladder. At this juncture, it resides within a shallow indentation known as the colic impression. Subsequently, it sharply bends forward and to the left, and the right colic (hepatic) flexure forms.

(2) Averaging approximately 50 cm in length, **the transverse colon** (横结肠) is the longest segment of the colon and is located intraperitoneally. It extends with a downward convexity from the right hypochondriac region across the abdomen, traversing the epigastric and umbilical regions, and terminates in the left hypochondriac region. At this point, it sharply doubles back beneath the lower extremity of the spleen, creating the left colic (splenic) flexure. A peritoneal mesentery known as the transverse mesocolon is attached to the posterior wall of the omental bursa, thereby dividing the abdominal cavity into supracolic and infracolic compartments.

The descending colon (降结肠) is 25−30 cm long, and passes downward through the left hypochondriac and lumbar regions along the lateral border of the left kidney. It is retroperitoneal. Toldt's fascia fixes the descending colon to the posterior abdominal wall.

The sigmoid colon (乙状结肠) is characterized by its S-shaped configuration and is situated in the left iliac fossa, adjacent to the rectum and the anus. Serving as the continuation of the descending colon, it extends from the greater pelvis to the commencement of the rectum. Its primary function is to facilitate the elimination of solid and gaseous waste from the gastrointestinal tract. As an intraperitoneal structure, the sigmoid colon is tethered to the pelvic wall by the sigmoid mesocolon.

3. The Rectum

The rectum (直肠) constitutes the terminal segment of the alimentary canal within the pelvic cavity. Approximately 15 cm in length, it originates at the recto-sigmoid junction, situated at the level of the S3 vertebra, and terminates at the pelvic diaphragm. The rectum exhibits a distinct S-shaped configuration characterized by several bends or flexures, including the sacral and perineal flexures. The latter flexure is associated with three transverse rectal folds. The rectum concludes with a widened portion known as the ampulla. In males, the peritoneum extends from the rectum toward the bladder, forming the rectovesical pouch, while in females, it extends toward the vaginal fornix, creating the recto-uterine pouch or pouch of Douglas. These spaces represent potential sites for infections, abscess formation, and various pathological conditions.

4. The Anal Canal

The anal canal (肛管) (Fig. 2-14) represents the terminal segment of the gastrointestinal tract, measuring approximately 3—4 cm in adults. Situated between the rectum and the anus below the level of the pelvic diaphragm, it is entirely extraperitoneal. The anal canal is divided into three distinct parts: the columnar, the intermediate, and the cutaneous regions. Within its lumen, folds of mucous membrane known as the anal columns (肛柱) are present by arterial cavernous bodies, or anal cushions, located in the submucosa. These columns are interconnected at their distal ends by transverse folds called the anal valves (肛瓣). Positioned behind the anal valves are crypts known as the crypts of Morgagni, which receive the excretory ducts of the anal glands. Collectively, the anal valves contribute to the formation of the dentate (or the pectinate) line (齿状线), a serrated demarcation where the intestinal mucosa transitions to the squamous epithelium of the anal canal. This line divides the anal canal into the upper (2/3) and the lower (1/3) segments, each supplied by distinct neurovascular structures.

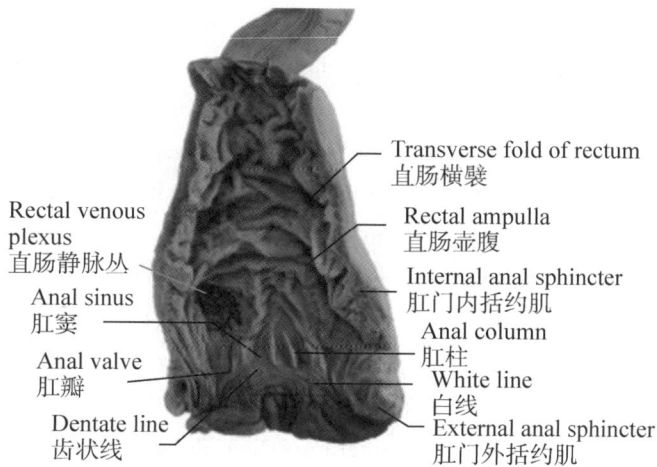

Fig.2-14 The rectum and anal canal

2.2.8 The Digestive Glands

The digestive glands (消化腺) encompass several important structures responsible for the secretion of digestive enzymes and fluids to aid in the breakdown of food. These glands include the salivary glands (唾液腺), the parotid gland (腮腺), the submandibular gland (下颌下腺), the ublingual gland (舌下腺), the liver (肝脏) and the pancreas (胰腺).

1. The Salivary Glands

The salivary glands are paired structures in the oral cavity that secrete saliva and other enzymes mixed with the masticated food to form the bolus. They help to lubricate the oral cavity and aid in the chemical digestion of food. The saliva also coats the food bolus, which makes it easier to swallow. There are three major salivary glands in the oral cavity: the parotid gland (腮腺), the submandibular gland (下颌下腺) and the sublingual gland (舌下腺).

(1) The parotid glands

A pair of parotid glands (腮腺) are situated in the preauricular area on each side of the facc. They are the largest of the three major salivary glands, weighing around 15−30 grams each. Each gland has an irregular shape resembling an inverted pyramid and is divided into superficial and deep lobes by the facial nerve (CN VII). The gland exhibits anteromedial, posteromedial, and superficial surfaces.

The main duct of each gland, approximately 7 cm long, exits from the superior part of the gland. It travels horizontally over the surface of the masseter muscle before coursing medially toward the muscle's anterior border. Eventually, the duct pierces the buccal mucosa to enter the oral cavity via a papilla adjacent to the upper second molar tooth.

(2) The submandibular glands

They are small, paired exocrine glands, each located within the submandibular (digastric) triangle of the neck. On average, the submandibular glands measure about 3—4 cm along its long axis and weigh roughly 10—15 g each. The submandibular duct or Wharton's duct is a relatively short conduit that drains the contents of the submandibular gland into the buccal cavity, about 5 cm long, eventually emerges from the sublingual papilla, adjacent to the lingual frenulum on either side of the floor of the mouth.

(3) The sublingual gland

It is the smallest one of the three major pairs of head salivary glands, lies bilaterally in the floor of the mouth and within the sublingual folds. It is covered superiorly by the tongue. Numerous ducts can be seen secreting saliva along the margin of the sublingual folds.

2. The Liver

The liver (肝脏), which is the largest accessory gland of the digestive system in the body, performs both external and internal secretions through its hepatic cells. Positioned in the right upper quadrant of the abdomen, beneath the right hemidiaphragm, the liver is anatomically divided into two lobes but functionally consists of eight segments. Apart from producing bile for fat digestion, the liver receives all nutrients absorbed from the small intestine via the hepatic portal venous system.

The bile, the liver's external secretion, is collected after passing through bile capillaries and is transported through bile ducts. The liver's external appearance divides it into four lobes: right, left, caudate, and quadrate. The right lobe is the largest, while the left lobe is smaller and flattened. These lobes are separated by a fossae for the gallbladder and the inferior vena cava. The caudate lobe is positioned between the fissure for the ligamentum venosum and the inferior vena cava, while the quadrate lobe lies between the gallbladder and the fissure for the ligamentum teres hepatis. The liver exhibits two surfaces—the diaphragmatic surface (膈面) and the visceral surface (脏面)—as well as two borders, the anterior and posterior borders.

(1) The diaphragmatic (superior) surface

The diaphragmatic (superior) surface. It consists of the superior, anterior, and right surfaces. It lies against the inferior surface of the diaphragm and is covered by visceral peritoneum, except in the bare area. The diaphragm serves as a partition separating the liver from the lower part of the lungs and pleurae, as well as from the heart, pericardium, and the right costal arches from the seventh to the eleventh inclusive.

The falciform ligament (镰状韧带) is a peritoneal reflection that connects the liver to the upper anterior abdominal wall. It divides the liver into right and left lobes on the superior surface and contains the round ligament of the liver on its free edge. The coronary ligament (冠状韧带) is formed by folds of peritoneum that reflect from the inferior surface of the diaphragm, connecting this structure to the liver. It consists of two layers: the anterior layer and the posterior layer.

The left and the right triangular ligaments (三角韧带) are lateral extensions of the coronary ligaments and also connect the diaphragm to the left and right lobes of the liver, respectively.

(2) The visceral (inferior) surface

The visceral (inferior) surface (Fig.2-15) of the liver features an "H" shaped groove. The ligamentum teres hepatis (the round ligament) of the liver, a fibrous remnant of the umbilical vein, is located anterior left and extends from the internal aspect of the umbilicus up to the liver. The ligamentum venosum (the ductus venosus of the fetal circulation) is positioned posterior right. Additionally, there are two fossae for the gallbladder (anterior right) and vena cava (the secondary porta hepatis, posterior left).

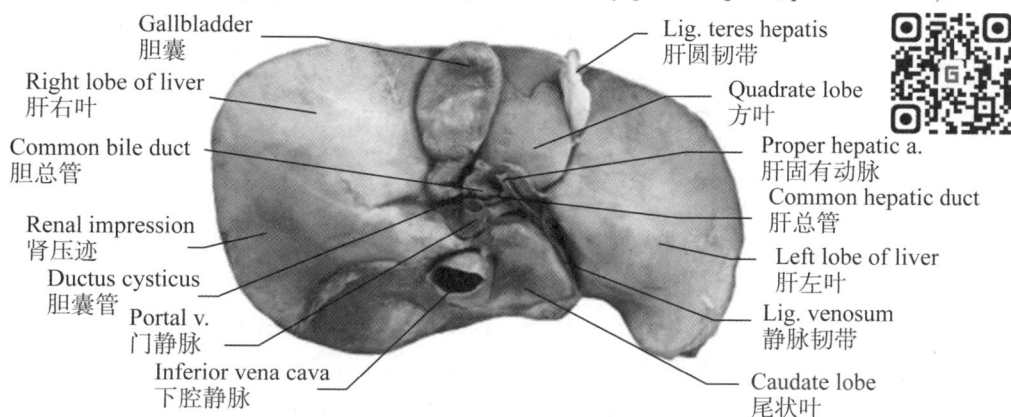

Fig.2-15　Visceral (inferior) surface of the liver
(v.: vein; Lig: ligamentum; a.: artery)

The transverse fissure is known as the porta hepatis (肝门), where the proper hepatic artery, hepatic ducts, hepatic portal vein, nerves, and lymphatic vessels are all located on the visceral surface. The "H" shaped groove divides the liver into four lobes: the right lobe (肝右叶), the left lobe (肝左叶), the caudate lobe (尾状叶), and the quadrate lobe (方叶).

(3) Position and relations

The liver is situated in the right hypochondriac and epigastric regions, positioned beneath the diaphragm and above the stomach, right kidney, and intestines. Its upper boundary aligns with the diaphragm, typically reaching up to the level of the fifth rib on the right side. Normally, the lower edge of the liver does not extend beyond the costal margin, although it may occasionally be palpable under the xiphoid process, typically not exceeding 3 cm. In children, it may be palpable beneath the costal margin.

The inferior surface of the liver is in proximity to the beginning of the transverse colon, while its posterior aspect is usually adjacent to the upper part of the descending portion of the duodenum, although at times it may be closer to the superior portion of the duodenum or the pyloric end of the stomach. Anteriorly, it rests against the abdominal wall, immediately below the ninth costal cartilage, with the transverse colon situated behind it.

(4) Functions

The liver performs a multitude of functions, making it a vital organ in the body. One of its primary functions is the secretion of bile, which aids in the digestion and absorption of fats from the diet. Additionally, the liver plays a crucial role in maintaining homeostasis through various metabolic activities.

Such activity involves the removal and breakdown of toxic substances from the bloodstream, ensuring that harmful compounds are eliminated from the body efficiently. The liver also regulates blood glucose levels by storing excess glucose as glycogen or releasing it into the bloodstream when it needs to maintain a steady supply of energy for the body. Furthermore, the liver is involved in lipid metabolism, including the synthesis, breakdown, and transport of lipids throughout the body. It helps to regulate lipid levels in the bloodstream, contributing to overall metabolic health.

Moreover, the liver serves as a storage site for essential micronutrients, such as vitamins and minerals, ensuring that they are readily available when needed for various metabolic processes. Overall, the liver's multifaceted functions are essential for maintaining metabolic balance, detoxification, and overall health and well-being.

(5) The extrahepatic apparatus

The extrahepatic apparatus (肝 外 胆 道), also known as the biliary system, encompasses several anatomical structures involved in the storage and transportation of bile. These structures include: the right and the left hepatic ducts, the common hepatic duct, the gallbladder and cystic duct, the common bile duct, the hepatopancreatic ampulla (sphincter of hepatopancreatic ampulla), the major duodenal papilla. These components of the extrahepatic apparatus play a crucial role in the storage, secretion, and delivery of bile for the digestion and absorption of dietary fats in the small intestine.

The gallbladder (胆囊) is a pear-shaped sac situated on the inferior aspect of the gallbladder fossa in the right lobe of the liver. It communicates with the common hepatic ducts via the cystic duct. This organ, measuring 7.5 — 12.0 cm in length, typically holds 25 — 30 mL of bile under normal conditions.

Anatomically, the gallbladder is divided into three parts: the fundus, the body, and the neck (or infundibulum). The fundus is clinically located at the level of the 9th costal cartilage, at the intersection of the lateral border of the right rectus abdominis and the costal margin. The body of the gallbladder tapers medially into the neck or infundibulum. The neck of the gallbladder narrows into the cystic duct, which contains slanted grooves that progress into the spiral valve of the cystic duct. The cystic duct mucosa forms the valves of Heister due to its spirally folded structure. Subsequently, the cystic duct takes a posterior course along with the common hepatic duct before their union.

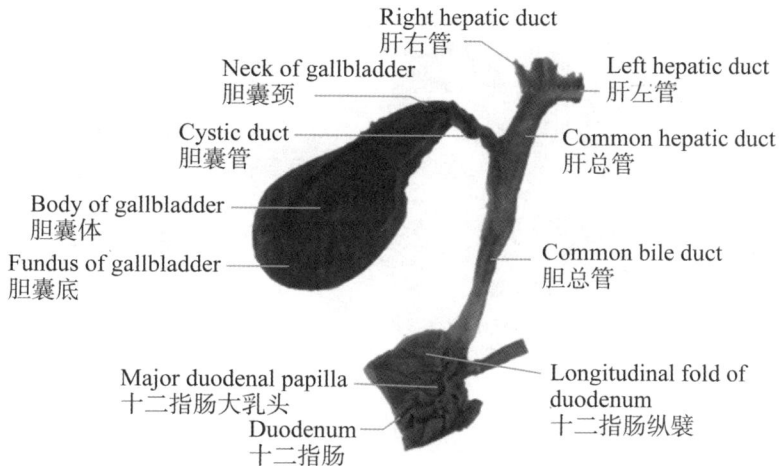

Fig.2-16　The extrahepatic apparatus

The union of the cystic and common hepatic ducts forms the common bile duct, which measures approximately 6－8 cm in length. The intraduodenal portion of the common bile duct pierces the medial wall of the second part (pars descendens) of the duodenum along with the pancreatic duct, forming the hepatopancreatic duct. This duct emerges on the luminal surface of the second part of the duodenum as the hepatopancreatic ampulla of Vater, which is regulated by the hepatopancreatic sphincter of Oddi (Fig.2-16).

2. The Pancreas

The pancreas (胰腺) is a dual-function organ situated in the retroperitoneal space, serving both as an exocrine gland of the digestive system, secreting pancreatic juice into the duodenum via the pancreatic duct, and as an endocrine gland, producing hormones. Anatomically, it consists of five parts and an internal system of ducts. The pancreas exhibits an irregularly lobulated shape and is yellowish in color. Its right extremity, known as the head of the pancreas, is broad and connects to the body via the neck, a slight constriction. Projecting inferiorly from the head is the uncinate process, which extends posteriorly toward the superior mesenteric artery. The body gradually tapers to form the tail, the narrowest part of the pancreas.

The main pancreatic duct, also known as the Wirsung duct, traverses the entire pancreatic parenchyma from the tail to the head. In the head region, it merges with the bile duct to form into the hepatopancreatic duct, which opens into the descending part of the duodenum at the major duodenal papilla. Additionally, the pancreas contains an accessory duct, which communicates with the main pancreatic duct at the level of the pancreatic neck and opens into the descending part of the duodenum at the minor duodenal papilla (Fig.2-17).

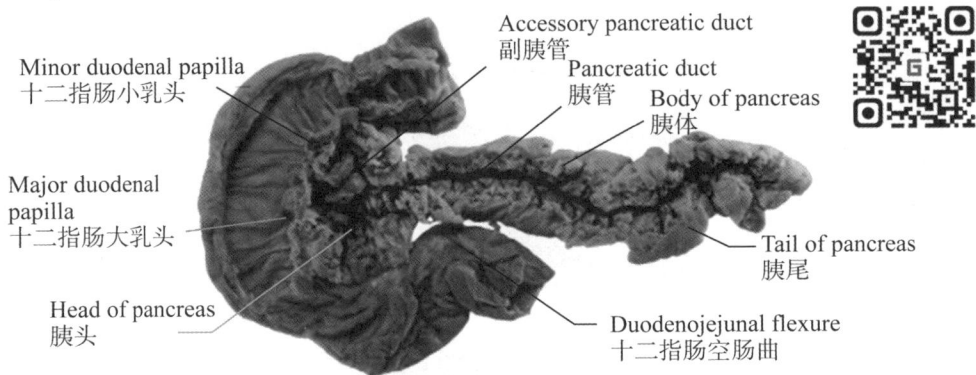

Fig.2-17   The pancreas

Positionally, the pancreas is located transversely across the posterior wall of the abdomen, spanning the epigastric and left hypochondriac regions at the level of L1—L2 vertebrae. It lies adjacent to several major blood vessels, including the abdominal aorta, inferior vena cava, and hepatic portal vein. Anteriorly, it is closely associated with the posterior wall of the stomach, with the head of the pancreas surrounded by the duodenum. The tail of the pancreas is in contact with the hilum of the spleen.

(福建医科大学   罗道枢)

Exercise

1. A 6-year-old child was hospitalized with severe vomiting and abdominal pain. He had a history of annular pancreas. This was a congenital malformation of the pancreas in which the head of the pancreas surrounded the duodenum and formed a ring. Which of the following structures was most often obstructed by this condition?

(A) The pylorus of the stomach.

(B) The first part of the duodenum.

(C) The second part of the duodenum.

(D) The third part of the duodenum.

(E) The jejunum.

2. A 60-year-old man was admitted to hospital after diagnosed with tumor. CT examination revealed that this tumor was located at the posterior abdominal wall and invaded the superior mesenteric plexus. Which of the following structures was most likely affected?

(A) The ascending colon.

(B) The rectum.

(C) The stomach.

(D) The descending colon.

(E) The kidney.

Answer

1. The correct answer is C.

Annular pancreas is a kind of pancreatic morphology "where" or "in which" the pancreas surrounds the descending part of duodenum (the second part of the duodenum), which is easy to compress the duodenum and cause obstruction.

2. The correct answer is A.

The superior mesenteric artery supplies the ascending colon (Choice A) and some of the pancreas. The inferior mesenteric and inter mesenteric arteries supply the descending colon (Choice D) and the rectum (Choice B), respectively.

The Respiratory System

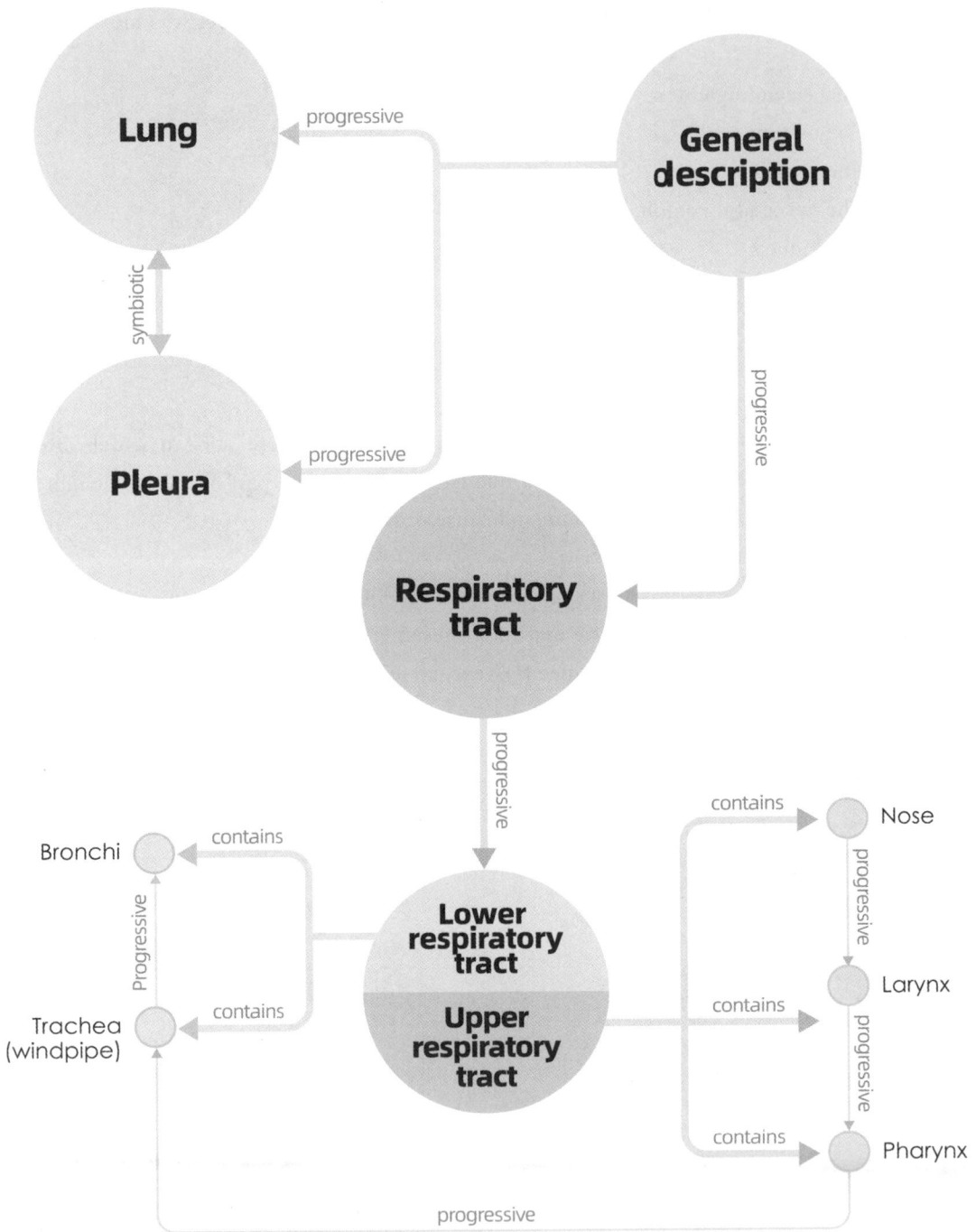

The Respiratory System

Chapter 3　Respiratory System

3.1　General Introduction

The respiratory system (呼吸系统) (Fig. 3-1) facilitates the exchange of gases, supplying oxygen to living cells and eliminating carbon dioxide produced during cellular metabolism. It consists of the respiratory tract (呼吸道) and the lungs (肺).

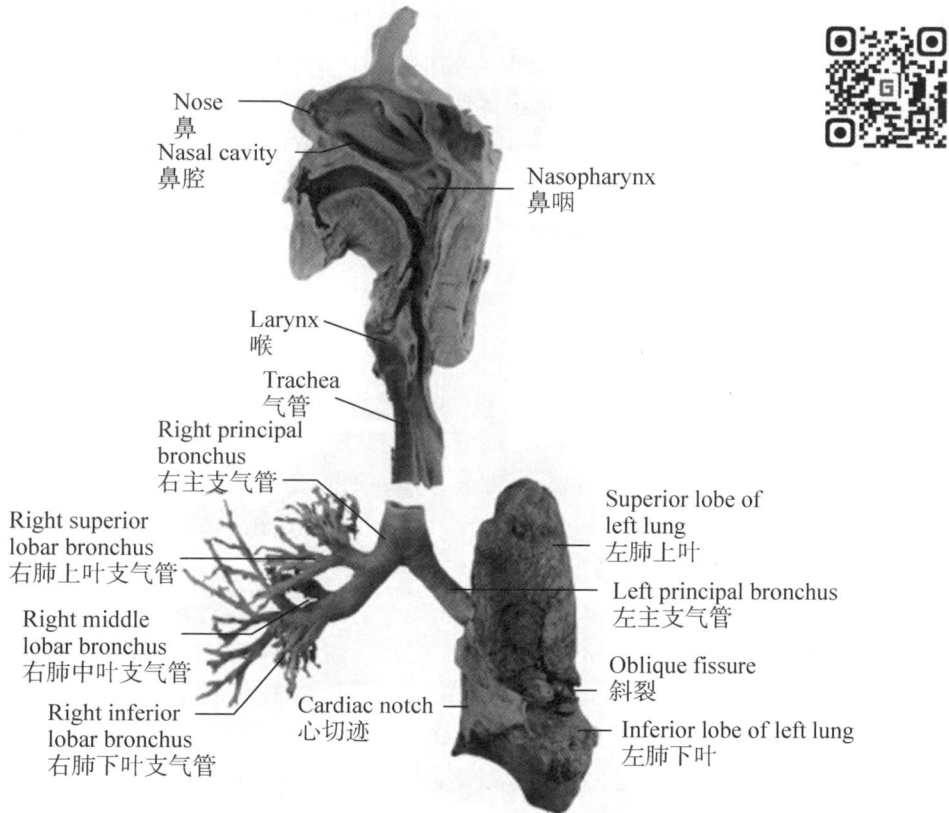

Fig.3-1　The respiratory system

1.The Respiratory Tract (呼吸道)

The respiratory tract includes the nose, the pharynx, the larynx, the trachea, and the bronchi. The upper respiratory tract consists of the nose, the pharynx, and the larynx, while the lower respiratory tract includes the trachea and the bronchi.

2.Lungs (肺)

Lungs are paired organs located in the thoracic cavity responsible for respiration. Their primary function is to provide oxygen to the body and expel excess carbon dioxide generated by cellular metabolism.

3.2　Nose

3.2.1　External Nose (外鼻)

The external anatomy of the nose forms a pyramidal structure, with its root continuing from the anterior surface of the head, and the area between the root and the apex is known as the dorsum of the nose. Below the apex are the two nares (nostrils), which serve as the entrance to the nasal cavity. These nares are separated by the nasal septum and bordered laterally by the ala nasi (nostril wings).

The external nose comprises both bony and cartilaginous components. The bony portion shapes the nose root and is formed by the nasal, maxillary, and frontal bones. The cartilaginous part, located inferiorly, consists of several alar cartilages, two lateral cartilages, and one septal cartilage.

3.2.2　Nasal Cavity (鼻腔)

The nasal cavity is divided into the left and right halves by a vertical, midline, osseocartilaginous septum. The nasal septum (鼻中隔) is composed of two parts: a bony septum and a cartilaginous septum. The posterosuperior part of the septum and its posterior border are made up by the vomer, which extends from the body of the sphenoid to the nasal crest of the palatine bones and maxilla.

The nasal cavity is further divided into three regions. The vestibule is located just inside the anterior external opening of the nose (the first floor) and contains hair follicles. The largest region is the respiratory region, which is lined with respiratory epithelium (the second floor). The olfactory region is a small area located inside the skull at the superior apex of the cavity, lined with olfactory cells and receptors. The two nasal cavities communicate with four bony recesses called the paranasal sinuses, named according to the bones they are within: the sphenoidal, maxillary, and frontal sinuses, and the ethmoidal sinus.

The openings of the paranasal sinuses and the nasolacrimal duct (鼻旁窦和鼻泪管的 开口) (Fig. 3-2) are divided into the nasal vestibule and the proper nasal cavity by the limen nasi. These boundaries include: the roof, which is formed by the cribriform plate of the ethmoid bone;the floor, which is the hard palate; the medial wall, which is the nasal septum; the lateral wall, which comprises the nasal conchae (superior, middle, and inferior), the nasal meatus (superior, middle, and inferior), and the sphenoethmoidal recess. The paranasal sinuses and their site of drainage into the nose are concluded in Table 3-1.

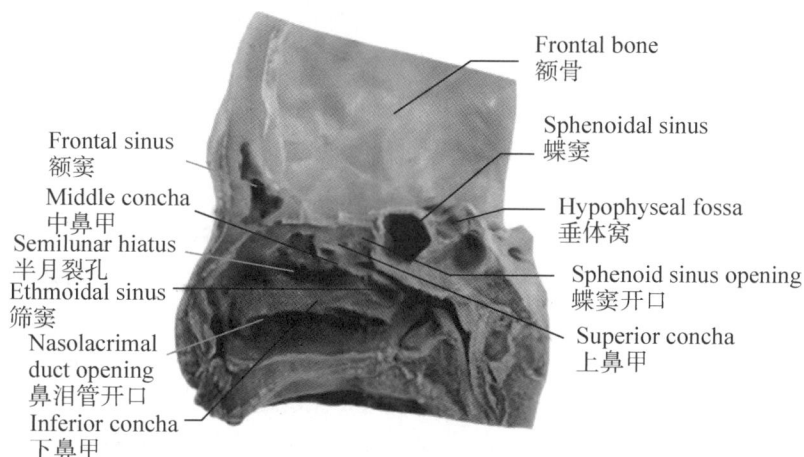

Frontal bone
额骨

Sphenoidal sinus
蝶窦

Frontal sinus
额窦

Middle concha
中鼻甲

Semilunar hiatus
半月裂孔

Ethmoidal sinus
筛窦

Nasolacrimal
duct opening
鼻泪管开口

Inferior concha
下鼻甲

Hypophyseal fossa
垂体窝

Sphenoid sinus opening
蝶窦开口

Superior concha
上鼻甲

Fig.3-2   The paranasal sinuses

Table 3-1   The paranasal sinuses and their sites of drainage into the nose

Name of sinus		Site of drainage
Frontal sinus		Middle meatus via ethmoidal infundibulum or medial to the hiatus semilunaris
Maxillary sinus		Into the inferior part of the ethmoidal infundibulum, and then into the middle meatus through semilunar hiatus
Sphenoid sinus		Sphenoethmoidal recess
Ethmoidal sinuses	Anterior group	Middle meatus
	Middle group	Middle meatus
	Posterior group	Superior nasal meatus

3.2.3   Mucous Membrane of Nose

On one hand, the olfactory region (嗅区) is situated in the upper nasal cavity, above the superior nasal conchae, and contains olfactory cells responsible for the sense of smell.

On the other hand, the function of the respiratory region is to warm, moisten, and clean the inspired air.

Additionally, there is a notable anatomical feature known as Little's area or Kiesselbach's plexus, which is located in the nasal mucous membrane of both the olfactory and respiratory regions.

3.2.4 Nasal Septal Blood Supply

The nasal septal blood supply is provided by several vessels, including the anterior ethmoid artery, the posterior ethmoid artery, the sphenopalatine artery, the greater palatine artery, and the superior labial artery.

The anterior and posterior ethmoidal branches of the ophthalmic artery primarily supply the ethmoidal and frontal sinuses and the roof of the nose. Additionally, a middle ethmoid artery may be present in about 20%−30% of sinus cavities.

The sphenopalatine branch of the maxillary artery serves as the principal vessel supplying the nasal mucosa. It provides blood to the mucosa of the turbinates, meatuses, and posteroinferior parts of the nasal septum.

The greater palatine branch of the maxillary artery supplies the region of the inferior meatus, while the infraorbital artery and the superior, anterior, and posterior alveolar branches of the maxillary artery contribute to the blood supply of the maxillary sinus. Furthermore, the pharyngeal branch of the maxillary artery is responsible for supplying the sphenoidal sinus, and the external nasal artery, originating from the superior labial artery, is responsible for supplying the skin covering the external nose.

3.3 Larynx

The larynx (喉) is a complex hollow structure situated in the anterior midline region of the neck, positioned between the trachea and the nasal cavity. It lies anterior to the esophagus and typically spans from the level of the third to the sixth cervical vertebrae. Comprised of a cartilaginous framework connected by membranes, ligaments, and associated muscles, the larynx is suspended from surrounding structures. It notably protrudes ventrally between the major vessels of the neck and is covered anteriorly by skin, fasciae, and the infrahyoid strap muscles, which lower both the hyoid bone and the larynx.

3.3.1 Laryngeal Cartilages (喉软骨)

The larynx (Fig.3-3) consists of three major unpaired cartilages (cricoid, thyroid, and epiglottis) and a pair of smaller cartilages (arytenoid cartilages).

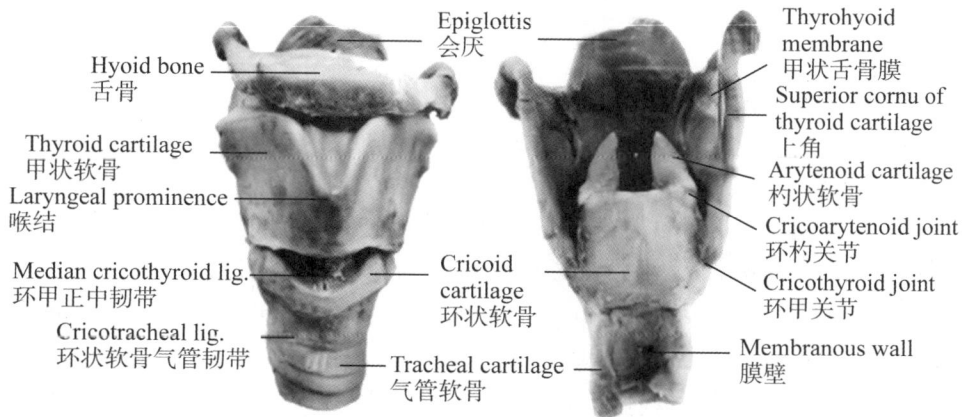

Fig.3-3   The larynx (lig.: ligamentum)

1. Thyroid Cartilage

The thyroid cartilage (甲状软骨) is shield-shaped and is the largest cartilage of the larynx. It consists of two laminae, the anterior borders of which are fused with each other at an acute angle in the middle line of the neck, forming a subcutaneous projection named the laryngeal prominence (喉结节). This prominence is most distinct at its upper part and is larger in males than that in females. Immediately above it, the laminae are separated by a V-shaped notch, known as the superior thyroid notch. The laminae are irregularly quadrilateral in shape, and their posterior angles are prolonged into processes termed the superior and inferior cornu.

2. Cricoid Cartilage

The cricoid cartilage (环状软骨) is smaller but thicker and stronger than the thyroid. It consists of two parts: a posterior quadrate lamina and a narrow anterior arch, which is 1/4 or 1/5 of the depth of the lamina. It is the only complete ring of cartilage that encircles the airway.

3. Epiglottic Cartilage

The epiglottic cartilage (会厌软骨) is a thin lamella of elastic fibrocartilage with a yellowish color. It is shaped like a leaf and projects obliquely upward behind the root of the tongue, in front of the entrance to the larynx. This leaf-shaped cartilage, covered by a mucous membrane, forms the epiglottis.

4. Arytenoid Cartilage

The arytenoid cartilage (杓状软骨) is paired, pyramid-shaped, and articulates with the lateral parts of the superior border of the lamina of the cricoid cartilage. It is attached to the vocalis and thyroarytenoid muscles. The vocal process, located anteriorly, is the site of posterior attachment of the vocal fold and muscular process.

3.3.2　Articulation of Larynx (喉的连接)

Cricothyroid joint (环甲关节) is a paired synovial articulation that connects the cricoid and thyroid cartilages. It forms between the inferior horn of the thyroid cartilage and the laterally located thyroid articular surface on the cricoid cartilage. The rotation moves the cricoid and thyroid cartilage relative to one another, bringing together or close the lamina of the thyroid cartilage and the arch of the cricoid cartilage. The joints connect the cricoid cartilage with the first ring of the trachea. It resembles the fibrous membrane which connects the cartilaginous rings of the trachea.

Cricoarytenoid joints (环杓关节) is a paired synovial articulation between the cricoid and arytenoid cartilages of the larynx. There are two articular facets that form this joint: superior arytenoid and inferior cricoid facets. It rotates around the vertical axis.

Conus elasticus (弹性圆锥) is an elastic fibrous membrane with an anterior and two lateral portions, arising from the posterior aspect of thyroid cartilage anterior horn, and then terminating at the vocal process of the arytenoid cartilage and the superior border of the cricoid cartilage outwards and posteriorly. The superior border of conus elasticus liberates and thickens, and tenses between the thyroid cartilage and the vocal process of arytenoid cartilage, which is called the vocal ligament. It is composed mainly of yellow elastic tissue.

Quadrangular membrane (方形膜) extends between the lateral borders of the epiglottis and the anterolateral margins of the arytenoid cartilage. Its free lower edge is thickened and forms the vestibular ligament. This ligament is enclosed by a fold of mucous membrane to form the vestibular fold (false vocal cord), which extends from the thyroid cartilage to the arytenoid cartilage. It is located among the epiglottic, thyroid, and arytenoid cartilages.

Thyrohyoid membrane (甲状舌骨膜) is a broad, fibroelastic layer extending from the hyoid bone to the thyroid cartilage.

3.3.3　Muscles of Larynx (喉肌)

The muscles of the larynx are categorized as extrinsic, passing between the larynx and surrounding parts, and intrinsic, confined entirely to the larynx.

Extrinsic Muscles, posterior cricoarytenoid muscle (环杓后肌), opens the glottis. Transverse arytenoid muscle (杓横肌) closes the glottis. Oblique arytenoid muscle(杓斜肌) closes the glottis. Lateral cricoarytenoid muscle (环杓侧肌) closes the glottis.

Intrinsic Muscles, cricothyroid muscle (环甲肌), lengthens and tenses the vocal fold. Posterior cricoarytenoid muscle (环杓后肌) opens the glottis. Thyroarytenoid muscle relaxes and shortens the vocal fold.

Conus elasticus (弹性圆锥) is located among the arytenoid, the thyroid, and the cricoid cartilages. Its upper free border forms the vocal ligament. The median cricothyroid ligament may be the site of cricothyrotomy during acute respiratory obstruction.

Cricotracheal ligament (环状软骨气管韧带), triangular in form, arises from the front and lateral part of the cricoid cartilage. Its fibers diverge and are arranged in two groups.

3.3.4　Laryngeal Cavity (喉腔)

The mucosa-lined cavity of the larynx extends from its superior opening, known as the laryngeal inlet, to the inferior border of the cricoid cartilage, which is continuous with the lumen of the trachea. The aperture of the larynx is bounded by the upper border of the epiglottic cartilage, the aryepiglottic folds, and the interarytenoid notch. It contains two pairs of shelf-like folds and three parts (Fig.3-4).

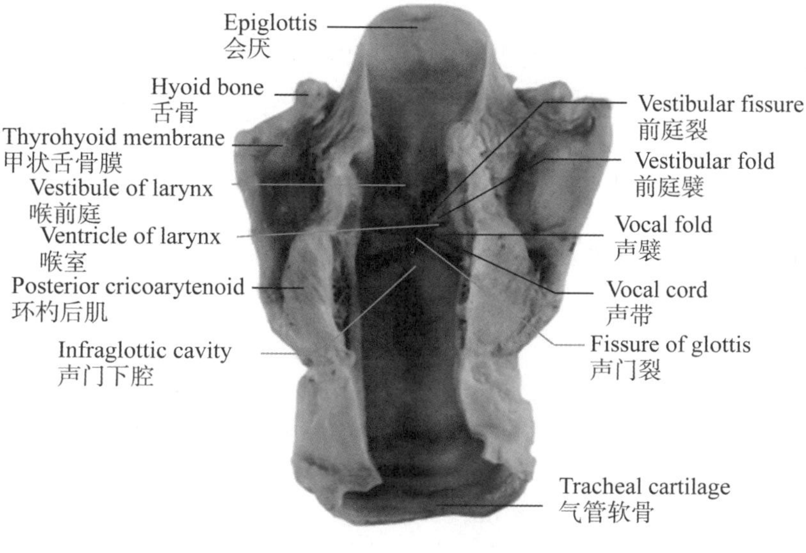

Fig.3-4　Laryngeal cavity (posterior view)

Two pairs of shelf-like folds consist of vestibular folds (前庭襞) and vocal folds(声襞). Each mucous membrane-covered vocal fold contains a vocal ligament that extends from the inner surface of the thyroid cartilage to the vocal process of the corresponding arytenoid cartilage. The vocal folds are the "true" structures that produce sound as air passes over them, whereas the vestibular folds (false vocal cords, which extends from the thyroid cartilage to the arytenoid cartilage) have no role in sound production but protect the vocal cords.

Two fissures include rima vestibuli (vestibular fissure) and fissure of glottis. The lateral walls of the middle part of the laryngeal cavity bulge outward to form lateral recesses (laryngeal ventricle) between the vestibular fold and the vocal fold. The vocal apparatus of the larynx is called the fissure of glottis (between two vocal folds, the narrowest part of larynx) and the vestibular fissure (between two vestibular folds).

Three parts are as follows: i) Vestibule of larynx (喉前庭): This area lies between the aperture of the larynx and the rima vestibuli (the vestibular fold). It serves as the entrance to the larynx and is involved in the initial passage of air into the respiratory system. ii) Intermediary cavity of larynx (喉中间腔): This portion is situated between the vocal folds and the vestibular fold. It plays a role in modulating airflow and sound production during speech and phonation. iii) Infraglottic cavity (声门下腔): It refers to the cavity between the vocal folds and the lower border of the cricoid cartilage. It facilitates the passage of air into the lower respiratory tract, including the trachea and lungs.

3.3.5　Sound Production

Air passing through the glottis vibrates the vocal folds and produces sound waves.

Sound variation: Sound is varied by tension on vocal folds and voluntary muscles (position arytenoid cartilage relative to thyroid cartilage).

Speech is produced by phonation which is sound production at the larynx and articulation is the modification of sound by other structures.

3.4　Trachea and Bronchi

3.4.1　Trachea

The trachea (windpipe, 气管) (Fig. 3-5) is a fibrocartilaginous tube of the lower respiratory tract, measuring approximately 10—11 cm in length. It extends from the lower part of the larynx, at a level with the sixth cervical vertebra in females or the seventh cervical vertebra in males, to the upper border of the fifth or the sixth thoracic vertebra. At this point, it divides into the right and left main bronchi, each leading to the right lung and the left lung respectively.

The trachea is composed of about 16—20 incomplete horseshoe-shaped tracheal cartilages, which are interconnected by intervening annular ligaments consisting of fibroelastic tissue. These cartilages provide structural support and maintain the patency of the tracheal lumen. Additionally, the cartilages are surrounded by smooth muscle tissue, which allows for flexibility during respiration. The carina of the trachea is a prominent ridge of cartilage located at the bifurcation point into the principal bronchi. It serves as a landmark and plays a role in directing airflow into the right and left main bronchi.

Epiglottic cartilage
会厌软骨

Hyoid bone
舌骨

Arytenoid cartilage
杓状软骨

Corniculate cartilage
小角软骨

Cricoarytenoid joint
环杓关节

Cricoid cartilage
环状软骨

Cricothyroid joint
环甲关节

Tracheal cartilage
气管软骨

Membranous wall
膜壁

Carina of trachea
气管隆嵴

Bifurcation of trachea
气管杈

Right principal bronchus
右主支气管

Right superior
lobar bronchus
右肺上叶支气管

Left principal bronchus
左主支气管

Right middle
lobar bronchus
右肺中叶支气管

Left superior
lobar bronchus
左肺上叶支气管

Right inferior
lobar bronchus
右肺下叶支气管

Left inferior
lobar bronchus
左肺下叶支气管

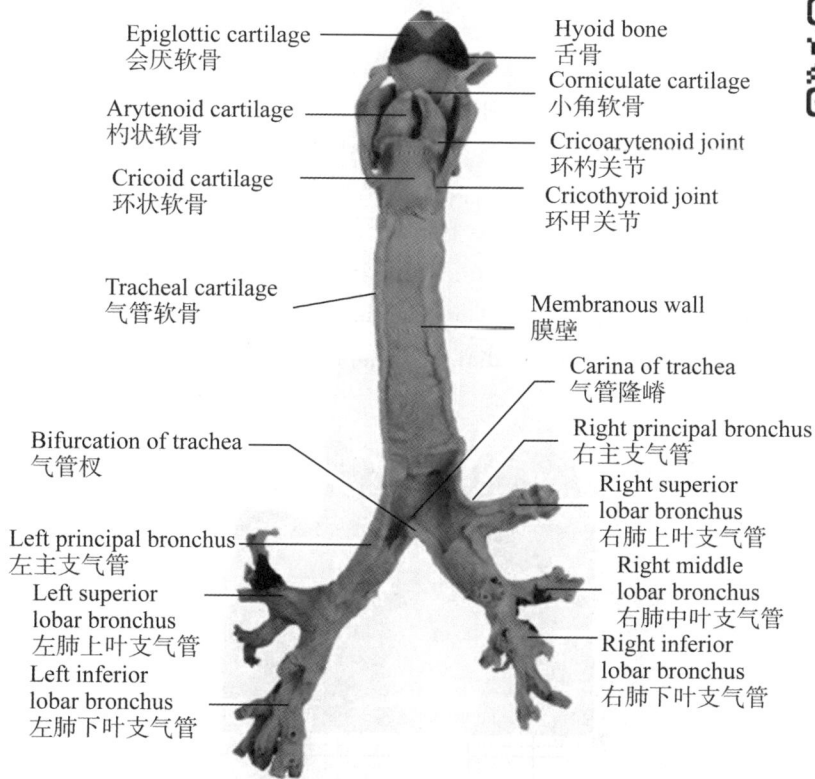

Fig.3-5   The respiratory tract

3.4.2   Bronchi

The bronchi (支气管) are the plural form of bronchus and serve as the passage-ways leading into the lungs. The first bronchi branch from the trachea, known as the right and left main bronchi. The right principal bronchus is shorter, wider, and more vertical than the left. It measures about 2.5 cm in length and leaves the extended line of the middle of the trachea at an angle of approximately 22° to 25°. Conversely, the left principal bronchus is narrower, longer, and more horizontal than the right. It is approximately 5 cm long and departs from the extended line of the middle of the trachea at an angle of about 35° to 36°.

Upon entering the lungs, the bronchi are further divided into secondary bronchi, also known as lobar bronchi, which then branch into tertiary (segmental) bronchi. Segmental bronchi continue to branch until they reach the terminal bronchioles, which in turn lead into respiratory bronchioles. These respiratory bronchioles are divided into 2 to 11 alveolar ducts, each of which is associated with 5 or 6 alveolar sacs.

3.5　Lungs

　　The lungs (肺) (Fig. 3-6) are vital organs of respiration, spongy and expandable, situated bilaterally within the thoracic cavity. They are separated from each other by the heart and other structures within the mediastinum. The surface of the lungs is smooth, shiny, and is subdivided into numerous polyhedral areas, representing the lobules of the organ. Each lung is in a cone-like shape, with the right lung being shorter and broader, while the left lung is longer and narrower. Each lung is characterized by its apex and base, as well as three surfaces—costal, medial, and diaphragmatic—divided by three borders—anterior, posterior, and inferior.

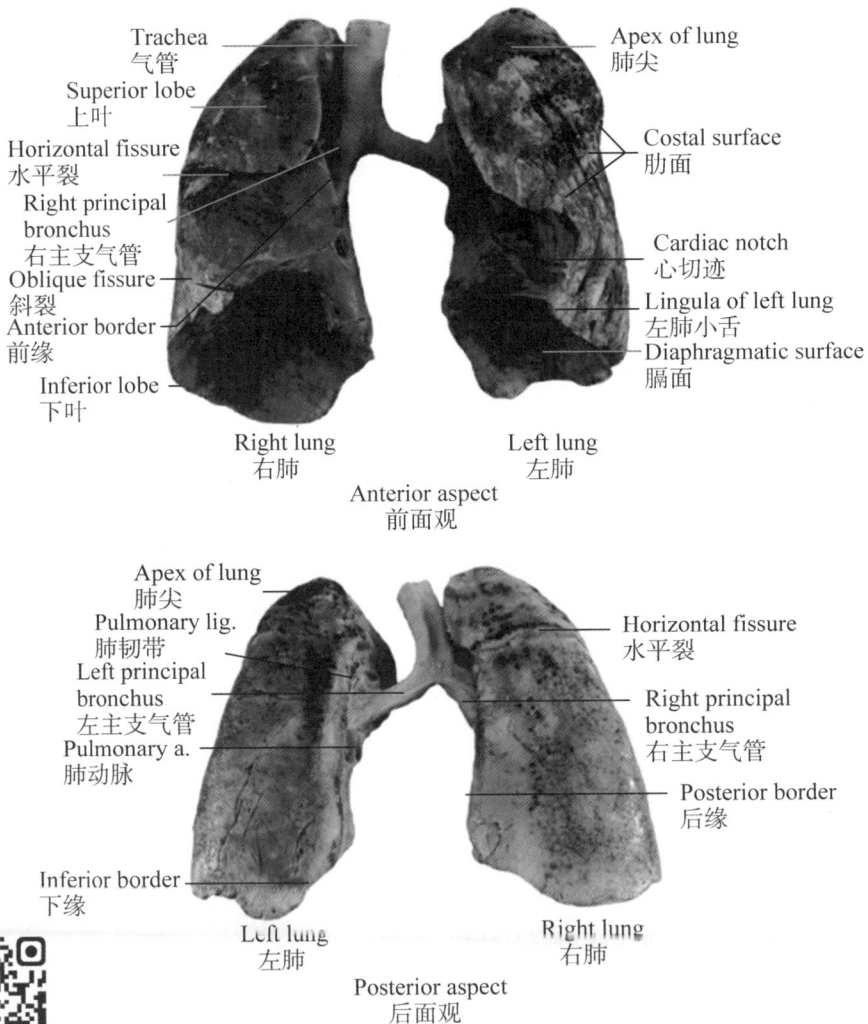

Fig.3-6　The lungs

3.5.1   Apex of Lung

The apex of the lung (肺尖) is the highest point of the lung, rounded in shape, and extends to the point of contact between the superior thoracic aperture and the cervical pleura. It reaches approximately 3—4 cm above the first costal cartilage and lies within the medial third one of the clavicle.

3.5.2   Diaphragmatic Surface

The diaphragmatic surface or base of the lung is broad and concave. It rests upon the convex surface of the diaphragm, which serves to separate the right lung from the right lobe of the liver, and the left lung from the left lobe of the liver, the gastric fundus, and the spleen.

3.5.3   Costal Surface (External or Thoracic Surface)

The costal surface (肋面) (external or thoracic surface) is smooth, convex, and of considerable extent, mirroring the shape of the chest cavity. It is deeper posteriorly and is in contact with the costal pleura. In specimens that have been hardened *in situ*, slight grooves corresponding with the overlying ribs may be observed.

3.5.4   Mediastinal Surface (Inner Surface)

The mediastinal surface (纵隔面) is in contact with the mediastinal pleura. It presents a deep concavity because of the adaption to the cardiac impression, which accommodates the pericardium; this is larger and deeper on the left than that on the right of the lungs, on account of the heart projecting farther to the left than to the right side of the median plane. The mediastinal surface is the presence of the hilum of lung (肺门) (T5—T7), the roots of the lungs through which the neurovascular and airway structures enter and leave the lung parenchyma. The structures found at the hilum of both lungs are the same, but their relationship to each other is slightly different. The following structures are found at each hilum.

The lung is connected to the heart and the trachea by its root. It is formed by the main bronchus (主支气管), the pulmonary artery (肺动脉), the pulmonary veins (肺静脉), the bronchial arteries and veins (支气管动脉和静脉), the pulmonary plexuses of nerves (肺神经丛), the lymphatic vessels (淋巴管), the bronchopulmonary hilar lymph node (支气管肺门淋巴结), and the areolar tissue, all of which are enclosed by a double-layered sleeve of the pleura. The root of the right lung lies posterior to the superior vena cava and part of the right atrium, and inferior to the azygos vein, while that of the left lung passes beneath the aortic arch and in front of the descending aorta; the phrenic nerve, the pericardiophrenic artery and vein, and the anterior pulmonary plexus, lie in front, and the vagus and posterior pulmonary plexus behind; below is the pulmonary ligament.

The root of each lung (Fig.3-7) are arranged in a similar manner on both sides: the upper of the two pulmonary veins in front; the pulmonary artery in the middle; and the bronchus, together with the bronchial vessels at the back. From the above downward, on the two sides, their arrangement differs. Thus, on the right side there are principal bronchi, pulmonary arteries, pulmonary veins, but on the left side there are pulmonary arteries, bronchi, pulmonary veins.

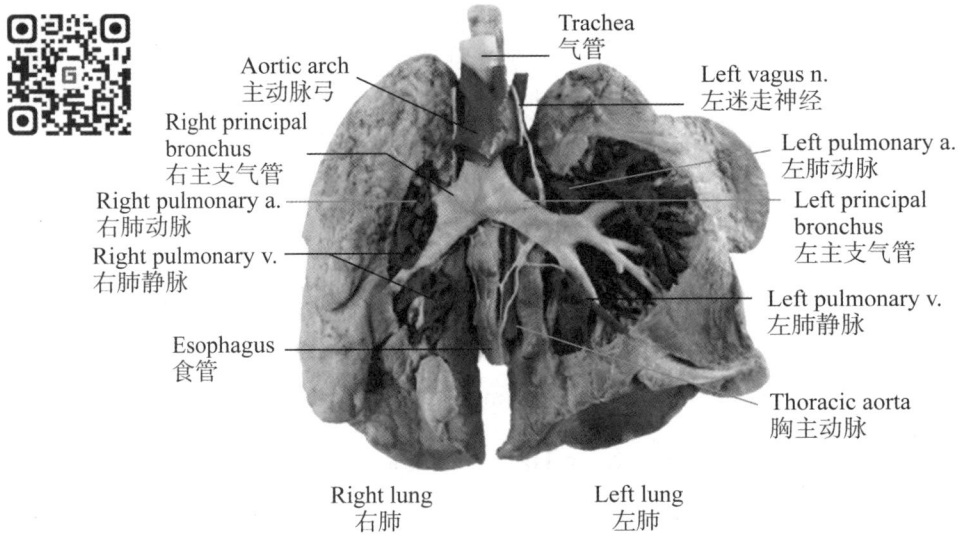

Fig.3-7　The root of the lungs

3.5.5　Borders

The posterior border is broad and rounded, and is received into the deep concavity on either side of the vertebral column. It is much longer than the anterior border, and projects, into the phrenicocostal sinus below. It is not recognizable, manifesting as a rounded region where the costal and vertebral surfaces of the lung meet. The inferior border is thin and sharp where it separates the base from the costal surface and extends into the phrenicocostal sinus; medially it is blunt and rounded where the diaphragmatic and mediastinal surfaces meet. The anterior border is thin and sharp, and overlaps the front of the pericardium. The anterior border of the right lung is almost vertical, and projects into the costomediastinal sinus; that of the left presents, below, an angular notch, the cardiac notch, in which the pericardium is exposed. Opposite to this notch, the anterior margin of the left lung is situated lateral to the line of the reflection of the corresponding part of the pleura.

3.5.6　Lobes and Fissures

The right lung is divided into three lobes: the superior, middle, and inferior lobes by two interlobular fissures. The two fissures are horizontal and oblique. The oblique fissure separates the inferior from the superior lobe and the middle lobe; the horizontal fissure presents as a curvilinear band passing from the lateral aspect of the costal surface to the hilum.

The left lung is divided into two lobes, an upper one and a lower one, by an interlobular fissure, which extends from the costal to the mediastinal surface of the lung both above and below the hilus. The fissure is oblique. The two lobes are superior and inferior. The superior lobe locates anterosuperior to the oblique fissure, consisting of the apex, anterior border, and much of the costal and most of the mediastinal surfaces of the lungs.

3.5.7　Bronchial Tree (支气管树)

Each principal bronchus is divided into lobar bronchi (two on the left, three on the right), each of which supplies a lobe of the lung. Each lobar bronchus is then divided into segmental bronchi, which supply specific segments of the lung (肺段) (Fig. 3-8). The lobes of lung are subdivided into smaller units called the bronchopulmonary segments. Bronchopulmonary segments (支气管肺段) are wedge-shaped, with the base lying peripherally and the apex lying towards the root of the lungs. Each lung has ten segments, which contains a segmental bronchus and branches of the pulmonary arteries and veins.

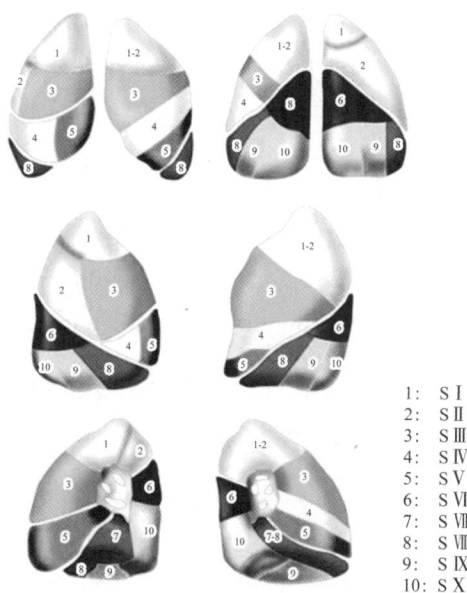

1:	S I
2:	S II
3:	S III
4:	S IV
5:	S V
6:	S VI
7:	S VII
8:	S VIII
9:	S IX
10:	S X

Fig.3-8　Pulmonary segmental bronchi

3.6　Pleura

Each lung is invested by an exceedingly delicate, double-layered serous membrane, the pleura (胸膜). The pleura is reflected from the mediastinum to the surface of the lung, where it is called visceral pleura (脏层胸膜) coveting the lungs and extending into the fissures of the lung between its lobes. The rest of the membrane lines the inner surface of the chest wall, covers the diaphragm, and is reflected over the structures occupying the middle of the thorax; this portion is termed the parietal pleura (壁胸膜). Two pleural layers continue with each other at the root of the lung forming a closed potential space — pleural cavity (胸膜腔). The pleura cavity contains a small amount of pleural fluid, which allows close sliding contact between the two layers of the pleura. There is subatmospheric pressure in the pleural cavity.

3.6.1　Parietal Pleura

The parietal pleura is divided into four portions: the costal pleura, the diaphragmatic pleura, the mediastinal pleura and the cupula of pleura.

The costal pleura (肋胸膜) lines the inner surface of the wall of the chest, including the sternum, the lateral margins of the vertebral bodies and the intervening intervertebral discs, the ribs, and the transversus thoracis, and the intercostal muscles.

The diaphragmatic pleura (膈胸膜) lines the diaphragm, covering most of the superior surface of the respiratory diaphragm.

The mediastinal pleura (纵隔胸膜) lines mediastinum, continuously covering the part above the hilum of the lung, from the sternum to the vertebral column. It is applied to the other thoracic viscera.

The cupula of pleura (胸膜顶) extends from the internal border of the first rib, up into the neck, over the apex of the lung, 2—3 cm above the medial third of the clavicle.

The pulmonary ligament (肺韧带) is redundant pleura at the root of the lung appearing as a double-layered fold, which extends downward and allows movement of structures forming the root of the lung.

3.6.2　Pleural Recesses (胸膜隐窝)

Pleural recesses (胸膜隐窝) are potential space within the pleural cavity where the inferior border of the lung does not completely extend to the inferior margin of the pleural reflection during quiet respiration. Costodiaphragmatic recess (肋膈隐窝), often referred to as the costophrenic angle, is a slit-like interval between the costal and diaphragmatic pleurae on each side, representing the lowest point of the pleural cavity. Typically, the lowest point of the recess is located about 5 cm inferior to the lower limit of the lung during quiet inspiration.

A similar recess exists behind the sternum, between the costal and mediastinal pleurae, known as the costomediastinal recess (肋纵隔隐窝).

The surface projection of the lower border of the lung and the pleurae (Table 3-2, Fig.3-9).

Table 3-2   The lower border of the lung and the pleurae

Lower border	Midclavicular lines	Midaxillary lines	Sides of the vertebral column
Lungs	6th rib	8th rib	10th rib
Pleurae	8th rib	10th rib	12th rib

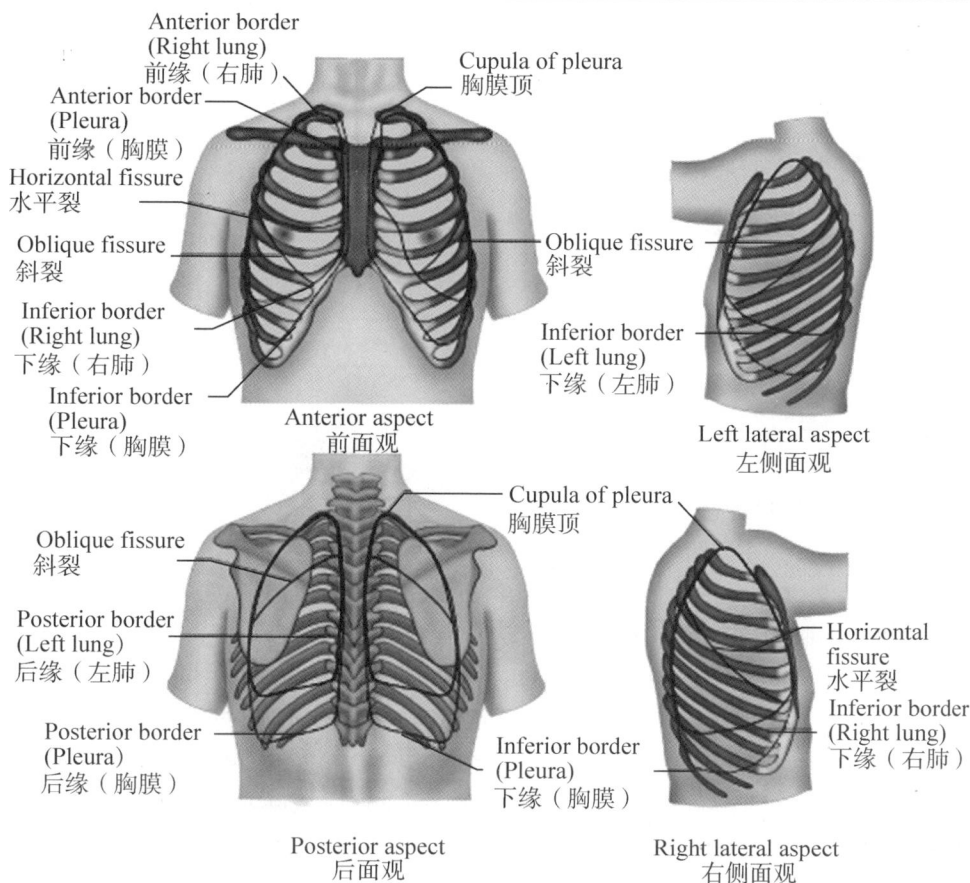

Fig.3-9   The surface projection of pleura and lungs

（浙江大学医学院   方马荣）

Exercise

1. A 90-year-old man was admitted to the department of orthopedics due to femoral fracture. Since he cannot sit up, his daughter had to feed him while he was lying on his back. However, the patient aspirated the liquid and subsequently developed pneumonia. Which of the following structures is the most likely site of the pneumonia?

(A) The anterior segment of the right upper lobe.

(B) The apical segment of the right lower lobe.

(C) The inferior lingular segment of the left upper lobe.

(D) The lateral segment of the right middle lobe.

(E) The superior lingular segment of the left upper lobe.

2. A 19-year-old boy complained a fever and runny nose. He had been diagnosed with maxillary sinusitis. Mucopurulent exudates were most likely to drain through an ostium in the_____?

(A) bulla ethmoidalis.

(B) hiatus semilunaris.

(C) inferior nasal meatus.

(D) sphenoethmoidal recess.

(E) superior nasal meatus.

Answer

1. The correct answer is B.

In supine patients, the fluid firstly flows into the trachea, then into the right main bronchus since the right main bronchus is thicker and shorter compared with the left main bronchus. The first posterior branch is the apical segment of the lower lobe (Choice B), and the most probable site of fluid flowing. The lateral segments of the lower lobes are also supplied by posteriorly branching segmental bronchi. In contrast, the anterior or inferior segment of the upper lobes are somewhat protected by an initial anteriorly directly bifurcation before their segmental bronchi arise. All other segments of the bronchial tree are not easily flooded by liquid.

2. The correct answer is B.

In maxillary sinusitis, exudate drains into the middle meatus through an ostium in the hiatus semilunaris (Choice B), which contains openings to the frontal and maxillary sinuses and anterior ethmoidal cells.

The bulla ethmoidalis (Choice A) is a part of the middle channel which contains an opening to the air cell of the middle sieve. The inferior nasal meatus (Choice C) receives liquid from the nasolacrimal duct. The sphenoethmoidal recess (Choice D) is located above the superior concha and contains an opening for the sphenoid sinus. The superior nasal meatus (Choice E) is located above the superior concha and contains an opening for the posterior ethmoidal cells.

The Urinary System

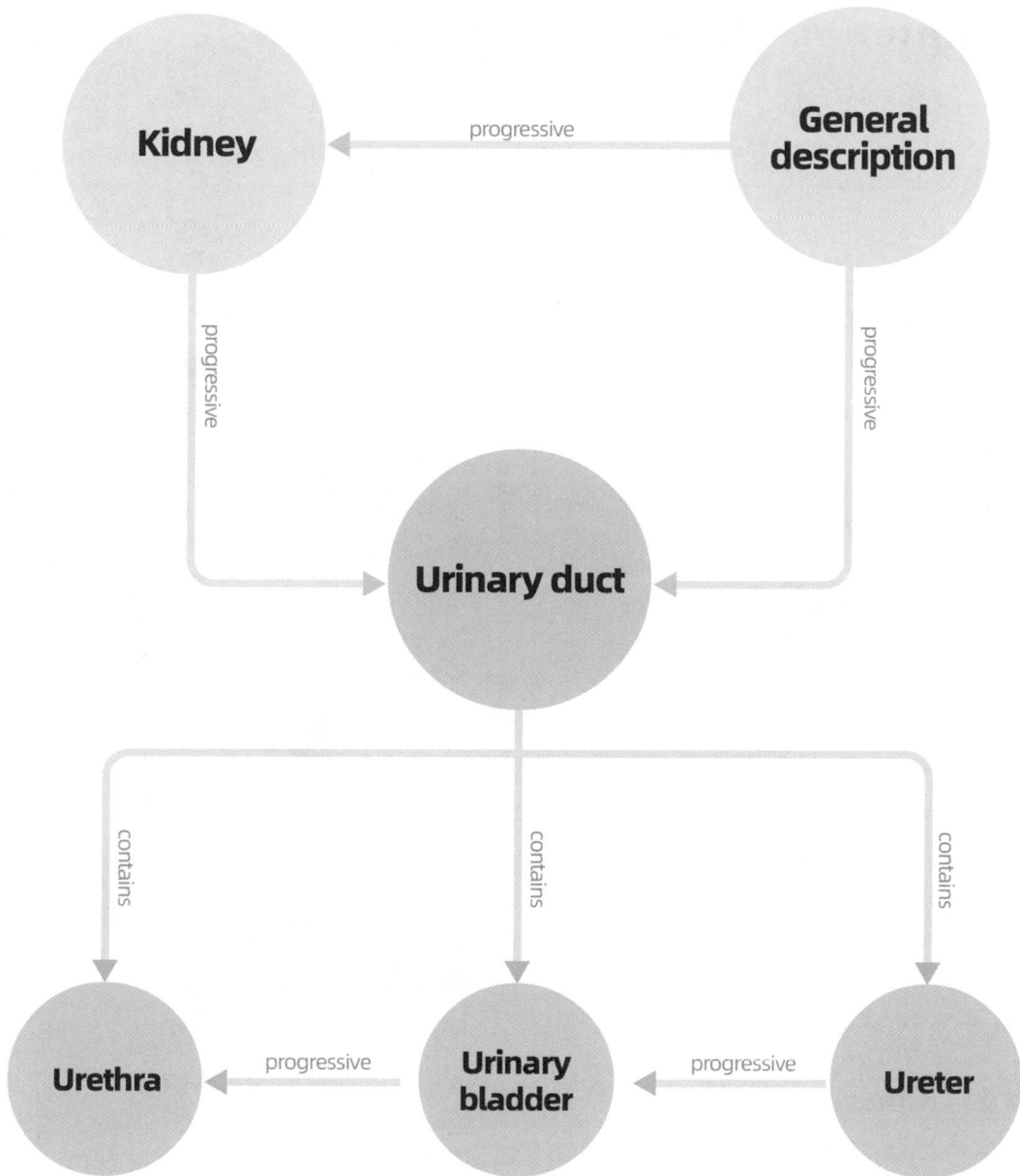

Kidney

General description

progressive

progressive

progressive

Urinary duct

contains

contains

contains

Urethra

progressive

Urinary bladder

progressive

Ureter

The Urinary System

Chapter 4   Urinary System

4.1   General Introduction

The urinary system(Fig.4-1), also known as the excretory system, is responsible for eliminating waste products from the body, including urea, uric acid, drugs, excess fluids, and electrolytes. It comprises several organs, including two kidneys, which produce urine, two ureters that transport urine to the urinary bladder for temporary storage, and the urethra, through which urine is expelled from the body. The urinary system is divided into the upper tract consisting of the kidneys and ureters, and the lower tract comprising the bladder and the urethra.

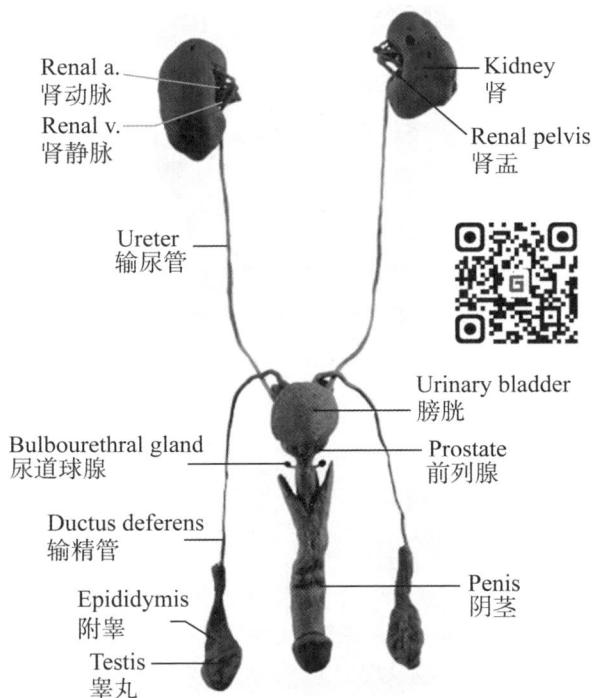

Fig.4-1   The urinary system

4.2   Kidneys

The kidneys (肾脏) (Fig.4-2) play a vital role in maintaining the body's internal environment by excreting waste products in the form of urine, which includes substances like urea, uric acid, excess water, and certain inorganic salts. This process helps regulate the balance of various components within the body. Additionally, the kidneys serve an endocrine function by producing and releasing erythropoietin (EPO), a hormone that regulates the production of red blood cells in the bone marrow.

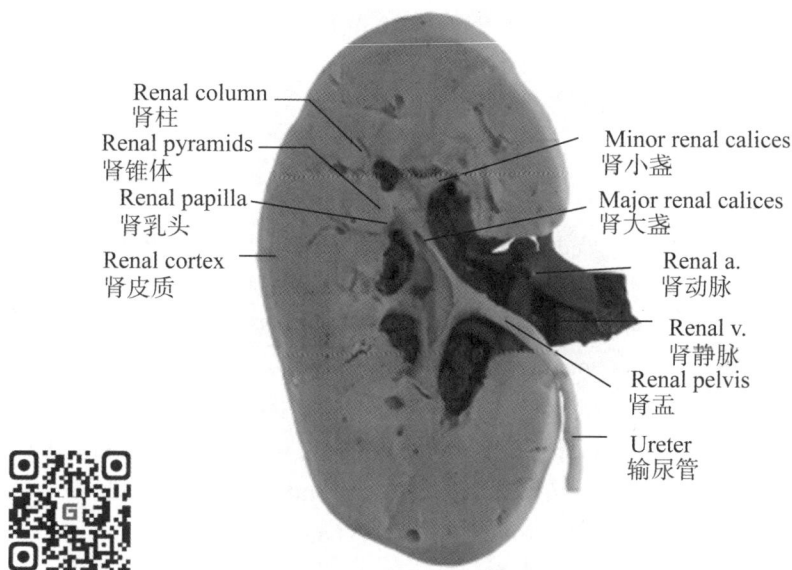

Renal column
肾柱
Renal pyramids
肾锥体
Renal papilla
肾乳头
Renal cortex
肾皮质

Minor renal calices
肾小盏
Major renal calices
肾大盏
Renal a.
肾动脉
Renal v.
肾静脉
Renal pelvis
肾盂
Ureter
输尿管

Fig.4-2　The kidney

4.2.1　General Features

The kidneys are bean-shaped, paired retroperitoneal organs located anterolateral to both sides of the vertebral column, close to the posterior body wall. Typically, they measure approximately 12 cm in length and 6 cm in width. The upper extremities of the kidneys align with the upper border of the twelfth thoracic vertebra on the left side and the first lumbar vertebra on the right side, while their lower extremities correspond to the level of the third lumbar vertebra on the left and the fourth lumbar vertebra on the right. The position of the liver relative to the kidneys results in the right kidney slightly inferior to the left one.

Each kidney features two extremities, two surfaces, and two borders, along with a renal hilum (肾门) and a renal pedicle (肾蒂). The renal pedicle consists of the renal vein, the renal artery, and the renal pelvis, arranged anterior to posterior, and the renal artery, renal vein, and renal pelvis, arranged superior to inferior.

The anterior surface of each kidney is convex, projects forward and lateralward. Its relations to adjacent viscera completely differ on the two sides.

The posterior surface of each kidney is directed backward and medialward. It is imbedded in areolar and fatty tissue and entirely devoid of peritoneal covering. It lies below the diaphragm, the medial and lateral lumbocostal arches, the Psoas major, the Quadratus lumborum, and the tendon of the transversus abdominis, the subcostal, and one or two of the upper lumbar arteries, and the last thoracic, iliohypogastric, and ilioinguinal nerves.

The lateral border, also known as the external border, of the kidney is convex and faces towards the postero-lateral wall of the abdomen. On the left side, it comes into contact with the spleen at its upper part.

The medial border, also known as the internal border, of the kidney is concave in the center and convex toward both extremities. It is directed forward and slightly downward. In its central part, there is a deep longitudinal fissure bounded by prominent overhanging anterior and posterior lips. This fissure is known as the hilum, which serves as a passage for the renal artery and vein, nerves, lymphatic vessels, renal pelvis, and adipose tissue enclosed in a connective tissue layer known as the renal pedicle. These structures enter and leave the kidney at the hilum. Above the hilum, the medial border is in relation with the suprarenal gland, and below the hilum, it is in relation with the ureter.

Renal sinus (肾窦) is a fat-filled cavity in the middle of the kidney, serving to cushion important structures. It is formed by the expansion of the hilum into a central cavity, lined by a prolongation of the fibrous tunic that continues around the lips of the hilum. Within the renal sinus are major and minor calyces, the renal artery and vein, renal pelvis, nerves, lymphatic vessels, and adipose tissue.

4.2.2　Structure (构造)

The kidney is comprised of two main regions: an internal medullary region and an external cortical region.

The renal cortex (肾皮质), characterized by its reddish-brown color and soft, granular texture, is situated directly beneath the fibrous tunic of the kidney. It arches over the bases of the renal pyramids and extends into the space between adjacent pyramids, reaching toward the renal sinus. These extensions of the cortex, known as renal columns, divide the renal medulla into triangular segments called renal pyramids. Together, the renal cortex and pyramids constitute the renal parenchyma, which is the functional tissue of the kidney. Within the cortex are found the glomeruli of all renal nephrons, as well as the proximal and distal convoluted tubules. Additionally, collecting ducts extend from the cortex into the medulla, ultimately leading towards the renal papillae located at the tapered ends of the renal pyramids in the medulla.

The renal medulla (肾髓质) consists of a series of pale, striated conical masses known as renal pyramids. The bases of these pyramids are directed towards the circumference of the kidney, while their apices converge towards the renal sinus. Within the renal sinus, they form prominent papillae that project into the minor calyces. These minor calyces, numbering from seven to thirteen, are funnel-shaped tubes that expand from the upper urinary tract, each embracing one or more of the renal papillae. They unite to form two or three short tubes known as the major calyces, which in turn drain into the infundibula. Eventually, they coalesce to form into a funnel-shaped sac called the renal pelvis. Passing through the hilum, the renal pelvis is wider above and narrower below, where it joins the ureter.

4.2.3　Renal Segment (肾段)

The kidney is divided into five renal segments, and each is supplied by a branch of the renal artery. The segments are apical segment, superior segment, middle segment, inferior segment, and posterior segment.

4.2.4　Coverings (被膜)

The kidneys are enveloped by three layers. These are the fibrous capsule, adipose capsule, and renal fascia, arranged from the innermost to the outermost layer (Fig.4-3).

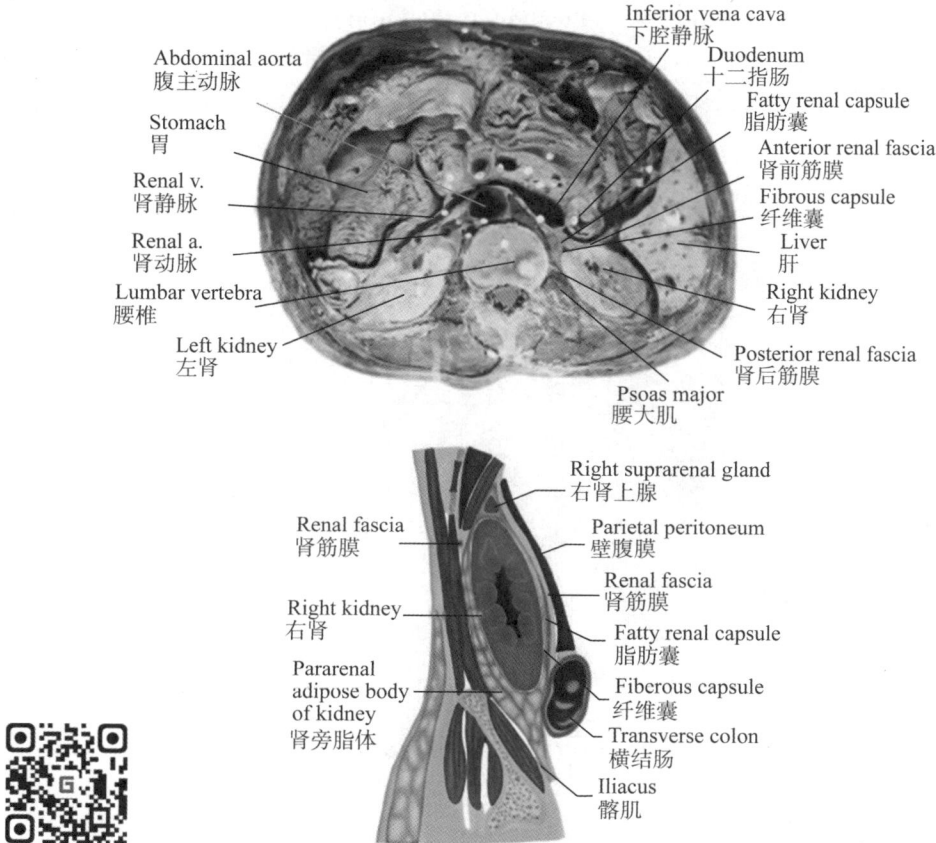

Fig.4-3　The capsule of the kidney

(1) Fibrous capsule (纤维囊). This is the innermost layer, a strong fibrous memb-rane. It can be easily separated from a healthy kidney surface but adheres firmly to an inflamed organ.

(2) Fatty renal capsule (脂肪囊). Positioned in the middle, the adipose capsule is a thick layer of adipose (fat) tissue that surrounds the fibrous capsule. It functions as a cushion, protecting the kidney from mechanical shocks and jolts.

(3) Renal fascia (肾筋膜). The outermost layer is the renal fascia, which is a dense layer of elastic connective tissue. It surrounds both the kidney and the suprarenal gland, holding these organs securely in place within the abdominal cavity.

4.2.5 Position

The kidneys measure approximately 12 cm in length and 6 cm in width. They are situated behind the peritoneum, with one kidney on each side of the vertebral column (Table 4-1). The upper pole of each kidney is positioned closer to the median plane of the body than the lower pole (Fig.4-4).

Table 4-1　Position of the kidneys

Kidney	The upper pole	The lower pole
Left	T12	L3 or L4
Right	L1	L4

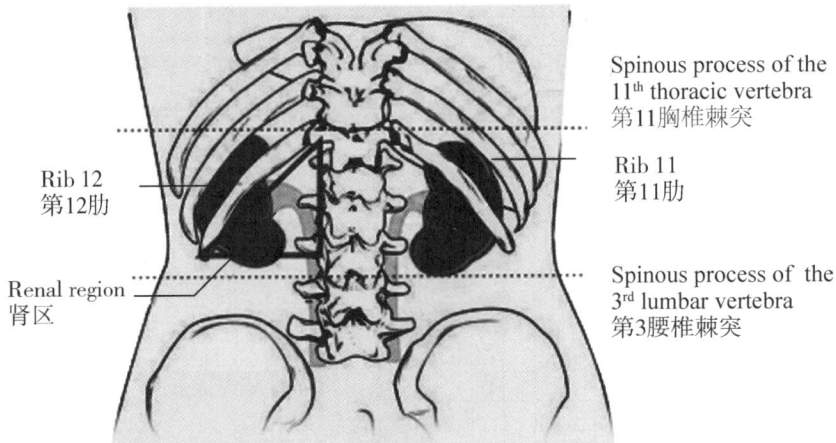

Spinous process of the 11th thoracic vertebra
第11胸椎棘突

Rib 12
第12肋

Rib 11
第11肋

Renal region
肾区

Spinous process of the 3rd lumbar vertebra
第3腰椎棘突

Fig.4-4　The body surface projection of the kidneys

4.2.6 Relation

Each kidney, along with its adrenal gland, is enveloped by two layers of fat known as the perirenal and pararenal fat, and enclosed within the renal fascia. Approximately 3/4 of the surface of the right kidney is nestled in the renal impression on the inferior surface of the liver, demarcated by a layer of parietal peritoneum. Adjacent to the medial border, there is typically a narrow but somewhat variable area that makes contact with the descending part of the duodenum. The lower portion of the anterior surface comes into lateral contact with the right colic flexure and, medially, typically interacts with the small intestine. The regions associated with the liver and the small intestine are covered by peritoneum, while the areas related to the suprarenal gland, the duodenum, and the colic flexure lack peritoneal covering.

On the posterior aspect, each kidney rests against the diaphragm, the medial and lateral lumbocostal arches, the psoas major and quadratus lumborum muscles, and the tendon of the transversus abdominis. Additionally, it is adjacent to the subcostal and one or two of the upper lumbar arteries, as well as the last thoracic, iliohypogastric, and ilioinguinal nerves.

4.3   Ureter

The ureter (输尿管) (Fig.4-5) measures from 25 cm to 30 cm in length, and is a thick-walled narrow cylindrical tube which is directly continuous near the lower end of the kidney with the renal pelvis. It runs downward and slightly medialward in front of the psoas major, enters the pelvic cavity, and finally opens into the fundus of the bladder. The ureter can be divided into three parts: the abdominal part, the pelvic part, and the mural part.

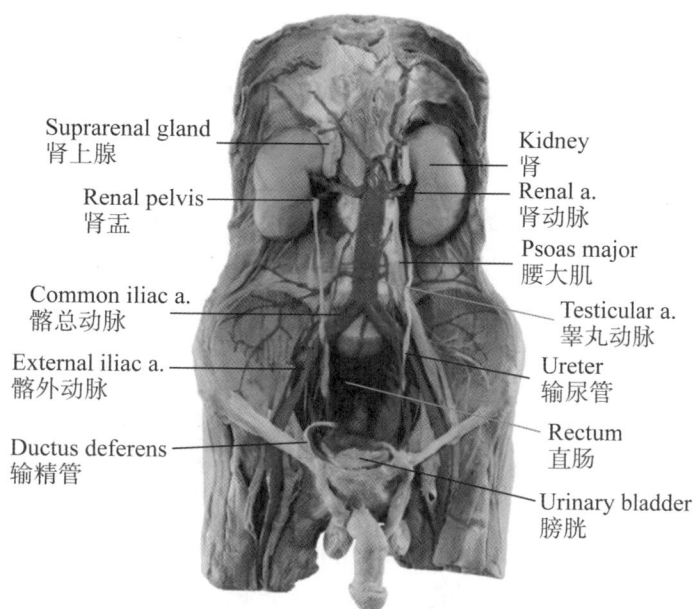

Fig.4-5   The ureter

There are three strictures in the ureter, which are the most common sites for renal stone impaction: at its junction with the renal pelvis, at the terminal line near the medial border of the psoas major muscle, and where it traverses within the wall of the urinary.

4.3.1   Abdominal Part of the Ureter

The abdominal part of ureter (输尿管腹部) lies behind the peritoneum on the medial part of the psoas major and is crossed obliquely by the internal spermatic vessels. It extends from the renal pelvis to the terminal line, then descends backward to the peritoneum on the medial part of psoas major. It enters the pelvic cavity by crossing either the termination of the common or the commencement of the external, iliac vessels.

4.3.2   Pelvic Part of the Ureter

The pelvic part of ureter (输尿管盆部) runs at first downward on the lateral wall of the pelvic cavity, along the anterior border of the greater sciatic notch and under the cover of the peritoneum. It lies in front of the hypogastric artery medial to the obturator nerve and the umbilical, obturator, inferior vesical, and middle hemorrhoidal arteries. In the female, the ureters are accompanied by the uterine artery. The artery crosses over the ureter about 2 cm distant from the side of the uterine cervix.

4.3.3   Intramural Part of the Ureter

The intramural part of the ureter (输尿管壁内部) passes obliquely through the bladder wall of 2 cm long. Three constrictions are point conjoined with the renal pelvis, the point crossed with iliac artery and the intramural part.

4.4   Urinary Bladder

The urinary bladder (Fig.4-6) is a musculomembranous sac which acts as a reservoir for the urine. It is located in the anterior portion of the lesser pelvic cavity. In adults, the bladder typically holds an average volume of 300 mL to 500 mL of urine. In its empty state, the urinary bladder has a pyramidal shape, consisting of the apex of the bladder (膀胱尖), the fundus of the bladder (膀胱底), the body of bladder (膀胱体) and the neck of the bladder (膀胱颈). The apex of the bladder is directed anteriorly and lies at the level of the upper border of the pubic symphysis. The fundus of the bladder is triangular and directed backward towards the rectum. The body of the bladder is situated between the apex and the fundus. The neck of the bladder is the lower part of the bladder. In men, the neck rests on the prostate gland, while in women, it is related to the pelvic fascia around the urethra.

Vesical fold
膀胱襞

Apex of bladder
膀胱尖

Ureter
输尿管

Body of bladder
膀胱体

Ductus deferens
输精管

Interureteric fold
输尿管间襞

Ureteric orifice
输尿管口

Vesicular gland
精囊腺

Trigone of bladder
膀胱三角

Prostate
前列腺

Internal urethral orifice
尿道内口

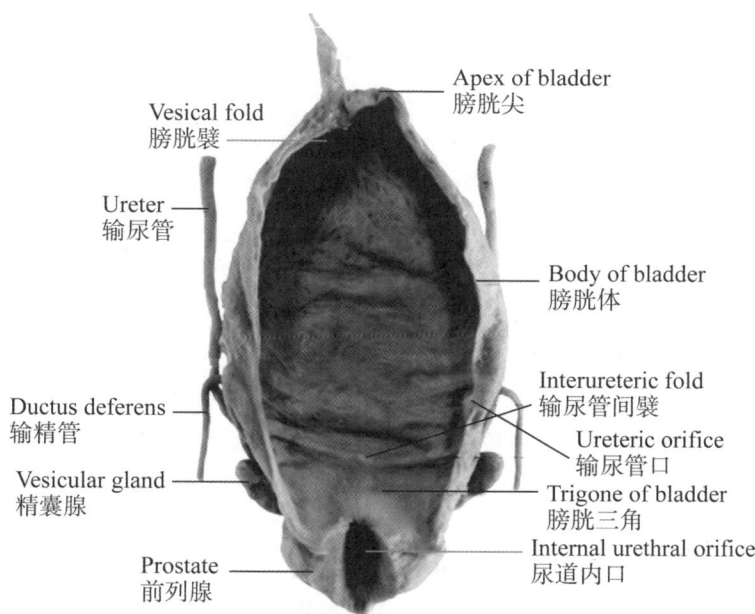

Fig.4-6   The urinary bladder

In its empty state, the mucosa of the urinary bladder exhibits numerous folds. However, a smooth triangular area persists at its base, known as the trigone of the bladder. This smooth triangular region is formed by the two ureteral orifices and the internal urethral orifice. The trigone is highly sensitive to expansion, and infections (trigonitis) tend to persist in this area.

The ureteric orifices are slit-like openings located at the posterolateral corners of the trigone. When the bladder fills and the pressure increases, the distal ureter is compressed, acting as a flap valve to prevent the reflux of urine.

The internal urethral orifice is situated at the apex of the trigone, which is the lowest part of the bladder. The interureteric fold serves as the superior boundary of the trigone, connecting the two ureteric orifices. This fold is a crucial landmark for identifying the ureteric orifices when examining the bladder with a cystoscope while the patient is alive.

4.5   Urethra

The urethra (Fig.4-7) is a single thin-walled tube responsible for carrying urine from the bladder to the outside of the body. It is associated with two urethral sphincters: an internal smooth muscle (involuntary) urethral sphincter and an external skeletal muscle (voluntary) urethral sphincter. The structure of the urethra varies between sexes.

1. Female Urethra

The female urethra is significantly shorter (approximately 4 cm), broader (approximately 6 mm), and lacks curvature. Positioned behind the symphysis pubis, it is embedded in the anterior wall of the vagina. Crossing the perineal membrane, it terminates at the external urethral orifice located in the vestibule of the vagina.

2. Male Urethra

The male urethra is longer (approximately 18—20 cm), narrower, and curved. It consists of two curvatures, three portions, and three constrictions. Clinically, the prostatic portion and the membranous portion are collectively referred to as the posterior urethra, while the spongy or cavernous portion is known as the anterior urethra. The prostatic urethra is the part passing through the prostate gland.

The prostatic part (前列腺部), the widest and most dilatable part of the canal, is about 3—4 cm long, It runs almost vertically through the prostate from its base to its apex. There is a midline ridge at its posterior wall throughout most of its length called the urethral crest, which projects into the lumen and makes its transverse section crescentic.

The membranous part (膜部) is the shortest and the narrowest part of the canal. It is located between the apex of the prostate and the bulb of the urethra, perforating the urogenital diaphragm about 2.5 cm below and behind the pubic symphysis.

The spongy part (海绵体部) is the longest part of the urethra and is contained in the corpus cavernosum penis. It is about 15 cm long in the flaccid penis and extends from the termination of the membranous portion to the external urethral orifice on the glans penis.

There are three constrictions including the internal urethral orifice (尿道内口), the membranous part (膜部), the external urethral orifice (尿道外口) and the three dilations including the prostatic part (前列腺部), the bulbous urethra (尿道球部) of urethra, the navicular fossa of urethra (尿道舟状窝). It also has two curvatures including the subpubic curvature and the prepubic curvature.

(新疆医科大学　董建江)

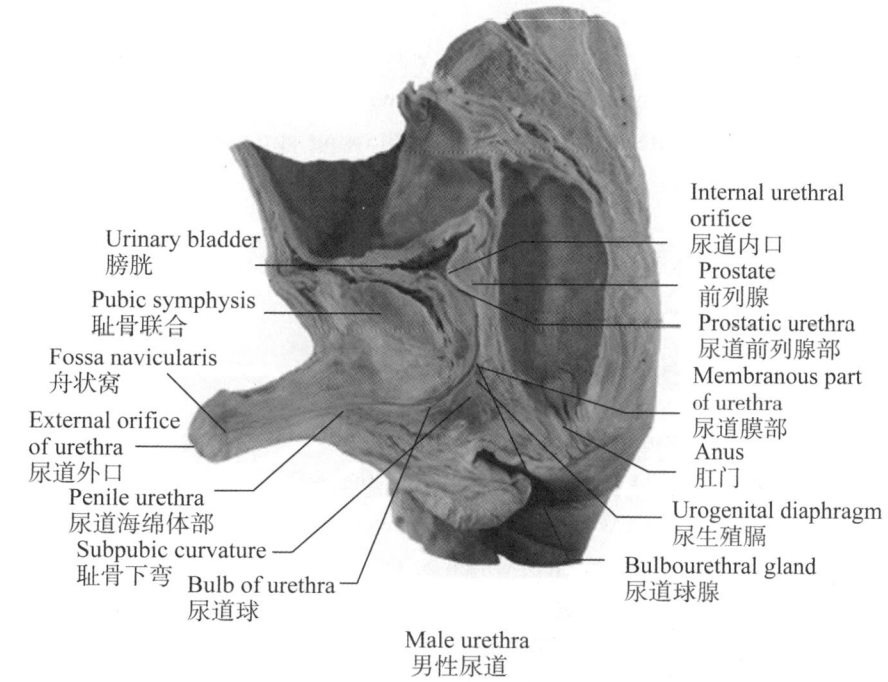

Internal urethral orifice
尿道内口
Prostate
前列腺
Prostatic urethra
尿道前列腺部
Membranous part of urethra
尿道膜部
Anus
肛门
Urogenital diaphragm
尿生殖膈
Bulbourethral gland
尿道球腺

Urinary bladder
膀胱
Pubic symphysis
耻骨联合
Fossa navicularis
舟状窝
External orifice of urethra
尿道外口
Penile urethra
尿道海绵体部
Subpubic curvature
耻骨下弯
Bulb of urethra
尿道球

Male urethra
男性尿道

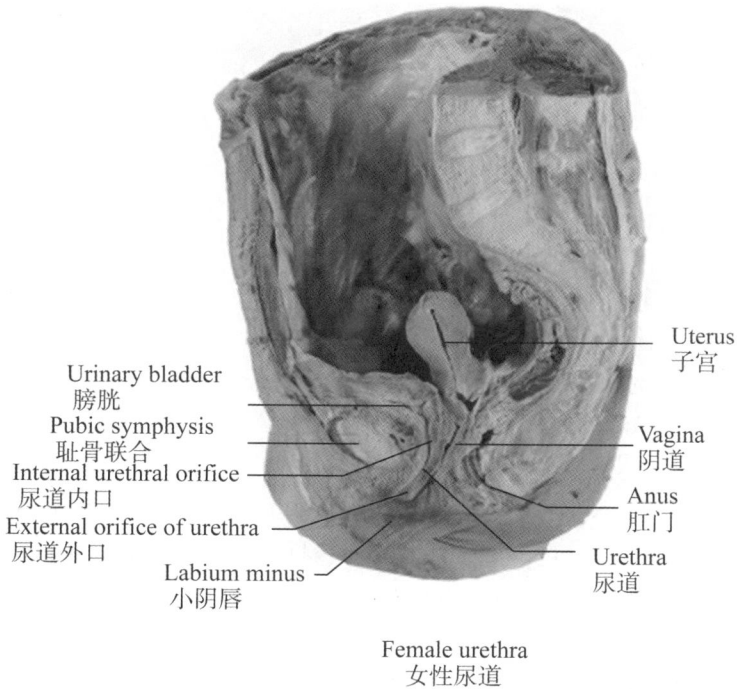

Uterus
子宫
Vagina
阴道
Anus
肛门
Urethra
尿道

Urinary bladder
膀胱
Pubic symphysis
耻骨联合
Internal urethral orifice
尿道内口
External orifice of urethra
尿道外口
Labium minus
小阴唇

Female urethra
女性尿道

Fig.4-7   The urethra

Exercise

1. A 40-year-old woman was diagnosed with hysteromyoma. The gynecologist suggested to remove the uterus. Which of the following structure was most likely to be inadvertently ligated during surgery?

(A) The uterine tube.

(B) The internal iliac vein.

(C) The ovarian artery.

(D) The ureter.

(E) The uterine vein.

2. A 22-year-old woman was diagnosed with bladder tumor. The examination of voiding cystourethrogram (VCUG) revealed that the reflux was present. Therefore, an intravenous pyelogram (IVP) was performed. However, it showed that the renal anatomy was normal. During IVP performance, which of the following structures would have been seen emptying into the renal pelvis?

(A) Major calyx.

(B) Minor calyx.

(C) Renal pyramid.

(D) Ureter.

(E) Renal papillae.

Answer

1. The correct answer is D.

The ureter (Choice D) crosses the uterine artery posteriorly and passes laterally to the body of the uterus near its junction with the cervix. During a hysterectomy, therefore, the ureter may be inadvertently ligated.

2. The correct answer is A.

The minor calyces (Choice B), of which there are usually 7 to 14, first unite into 2 major calyces before emptying into the renal pelvis. The renal pyramids (Choice C) is located in renal medulla which collects tubules of the kidney, the bottom of renal pyramids is formed renal papillae (Choice E) which enter the minor calyces (Choice B), several minor calyces unite into major calyces (Choice A), 2－3 major calyces empty into the renal pelvis.

The Reproductive System

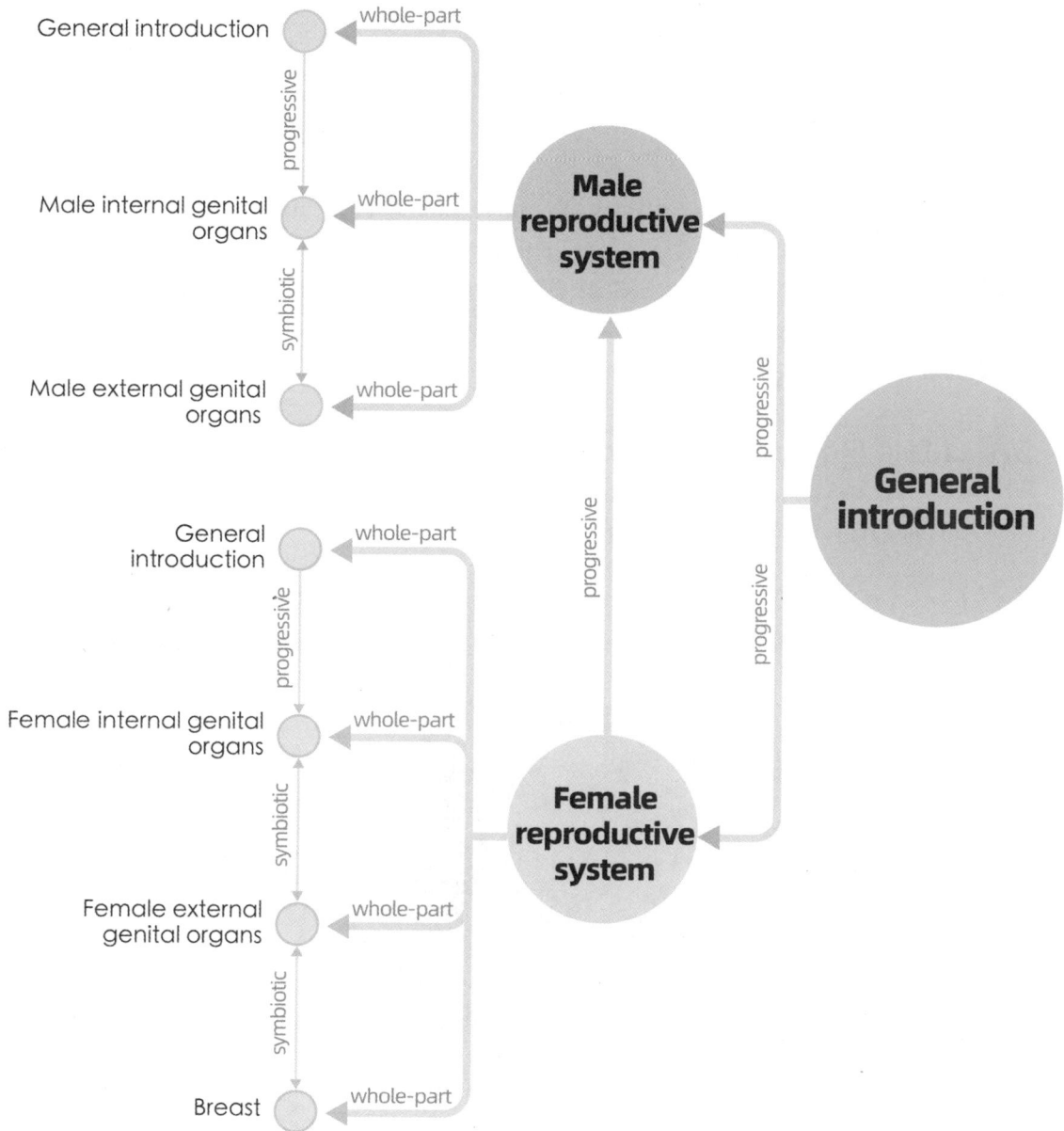

General introduction —— whole-part —— ○

progressive

Male internal genital organs —— whole-part —— ○

symbiotic

Male external genital organs —— whole-part —— ○

Male reproductive system

progressive

General introduction —— whole-part —— ○

progressive

Female internal genital organs —— whole-part —— ○

symbiotic

Female external genital organs —— whole-part —— ○

symbiotic

Breast —— whole-part —— ○

Female reproductive system

progressive

progressive

General introduction

The Reproductive System

Chapter 5   Reproductive System

The reproductive system plays roles in reproduction and sexuality. It consists of the internal and external genitalia (生殖器). The internal genitalia include the gonads(生殖腺), the ductal system (管道系统), and the accessory sex glands (附属腺). The breast (or mamma) (乳房) in females is a part of the integumentary system but is closely related to the reproductive system, thus it will be introduced in this chapter.

5.1   Male Reproductive System

The male reproductive system is shown in Fig.5-1.

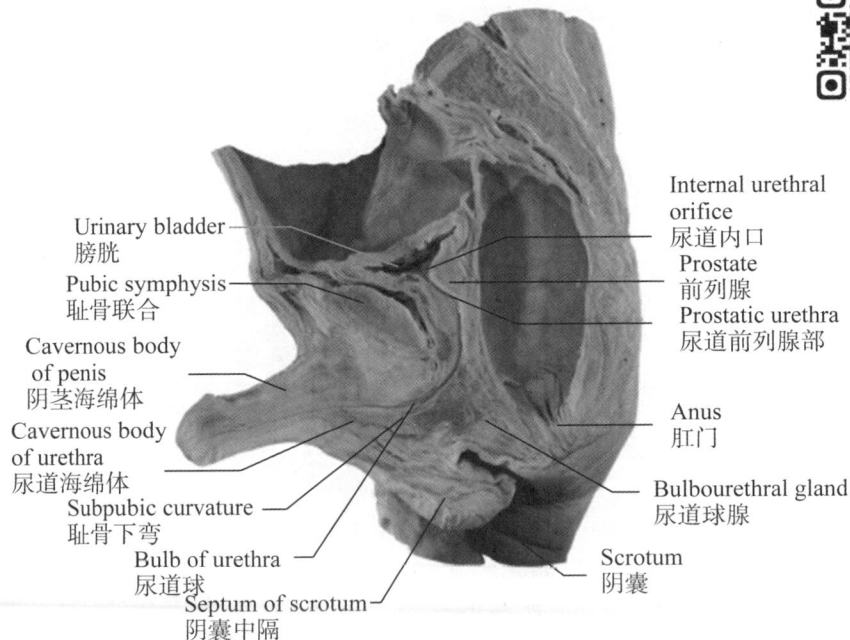

Fig.5-1   The male reproductive system

5.1.1　General Introduction

In the male internal genitalia, the gonads are the testis (睾丸), the ductal system includes the epididymis (附睾), the ductus deferens (输精管), the ejaculatory ducts (射精管), and the urethra (尿道), while the accessory sex glands include the seminal vesicles (精囊腺或精囊), the prostate (前列腺), and the bulbourethral glands (尿道球腺). The male external genitalia consist of the scrotum (阴囊) and the penis (阴茎).

The gonads are responsible for producing sperms and secreting androgens. The ductal system plays major roles in sperms and seminal fluid storage, as well as the sperms maturation, and propelling from the body on ejaculation. Sperms that are not ejaculated are ultimately reabsorbed. The accessory sex glands mainly secrete fluid to join semen, which supplies nutrients to sperms and facilitates sperms movement.

5.1.2　The Internal Genitalia

1.The Testes (睾丸)

The testes (Fig. 5-2) are paired oval-shaped glandular organs, suspended in the scrotum by the spermatic cords. The testis is about 5.0 cm in length, 2.5 cm in width, and 10－15 g in weight. It has two extremities and two borders: The upper extremity is covered by the head of the epididymis, the posterior border (called the mesorchial border) is connected with the epididymis, and penetrated by blood vessels, nerves and lymphatic vessels, while both the lower extremity and the anterior border are free.

The glandular structure of the testis consists of 100－200 lobules. Each lobule is contained in one of the intervals between the fibrous septa (called the septulum testis,睾丸小隔), which extends from the mediastinum testis. And the mediastinum testis is the thickening part of a dense white fibrous capsule (called the tunica albuginea,白膜) at the posterior border of the testis. This tunica albuginea locates internally to the tunica vaginalis, which is a serous membrane derived from the peritoneum. There are 2－4 tightly and highly coiled tubules (called the contorted seminiferous tubules, 精曲小管) within each lobule and interstitial tissues in the spaces between adjacent seminiferous tubules. The seminiferous tubules are lined with a layer of germ cells, producing sperm cells. And the interstitial tissue contains clusters of Leydig cells (睾丸间质细胞), secreting testosterone and other androgens. These androgens play important roles in the growth, development, and function of the male reproductive system, as well as the development and maintenance of the secondary male characteristics. The seminiferous tubules converge into the straight seminiferous tubules (精直小管), further form the rete testis (睾丸网) in the mediastinum testis. Then there are about 12－15 efferent ductules of the testis (睾丸输出小管) extending from the rete testis and joining the epididymis.

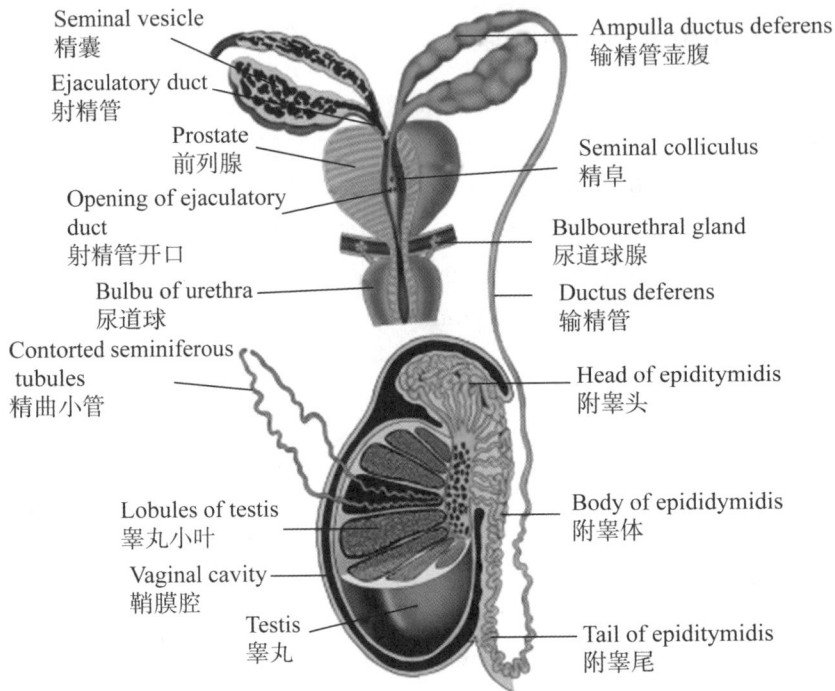

Fig.5-2　The structure of testes and epididymis

2. The Epididymis (附睾)

The epididymis is a comma-shaped organ enclosed in the scrotum, clasping the posterior border of the testis. The epididymis consists of the tightly coiled ductus-epididymis about 600 cm in length. It begins at the top of the testis, where the efferent ductules of testis join and which is called the head. It descends narrow in the midportion (called the body) and ends at the tail, which is at the distal end of the body and continuous with the ductus deferens (or vas deferens).

3. The Ductus Deferens (输精管)

The ductus deferens (or vas deferens), the excretory duct of the testis, ascends along the posterior border of the testis in loose coils and enters the abdomen through the inguinal canal. Then it curves medially across the external iliac vessels towards the pelvic and crosses over the ureter. At the base of bladder in front of the rectum, the ductus deferens dilates as the ampulla and becomes thinner at the ends, finally meets with the duct of the seminal vesicle to form the ejaculatory duct (射精管). It is about 50 cm in length and 3 mm in diameter. According to the structures which it goes through, the ductus deferens is divided into four parts: the testicular part (睾丸部), the funicular (spermatic) part (精索部), the inguinal part (腹股沟管部), and the pelvic part (盆部).

4. The Spermatic Cords (精索)

The spermatic cords are soft round ropes between the upper extremity of the testis and the deep ring of the inguinal canal, suspending the testis in the scrotum. They are composed of the ductus deferens, the testicular arteries, the pampiniform plexus, the lymphatic vessels, and the nerves. These structures are wrapped up by the areolar tissues and the cremaster muscles.

5. The Ejaculatory Duct (射精管)

The paired ejaculatory ducts lie on either side of the middle line, which is about 2 cm in length. Each is formed by the union of the duct of the seminal gland with the ampulla of the ductus deferens at the base of the prostate. They pass inferiorly and anteriorly through the prostate, finally open into the prostatic urethra.

6. The Urethra (尿道)

The urethra is located between the internal urethral orifice in the floor of the urinary bladder and the external urethral orifice at the glans penis. It is about 16—22 cm in length and 5—7 mm in diameter. The urethra serves as the shared terminal duct of the reproductive and urinary system. It is divided into three parts according to the structures which it passes through, including the prostatic part (前列腺部), the membranous part (膜部) and the cavernous part (海绵体部, also called the spongy or penile urethra). The openings of the ejaculatory ducts are at the prostatic utricle (前列腺小囊) on the summit of the seminal colliculus (精阜), which is the middle of the urethral crest (尿道嵴) on the posterior wall of the prostatic urethra. There are three constrictions (the internal orifice, the membranous portion, and the external orifice) and three dilations (the prostatic portion, the bulbar portion, and the navicular fossa) in the male urethra. In addition, it has two curvatures: the subpubic curvature and the prepubic curvature. The subpubic curvature is fixed whereas the prepubic curvature may straighten or disappear upon erection of the penis.

7. The Prostate (前列腺)

The prostate is a wedge-shaped organ surrounding the prostatic urethra, with the base attached to the urinary bladder and the apex inferiorly pointing to the superior fascia of the urogenital diaphragm. It is behind the symphysis pubis, and in front of the rectum, through which it may be palpated when hypertrophy. The prostate is about the size of a chestnut and 8—20 g. Structurally, it is a partly glandular and partly muscular organ which has five lobes, the anterior, posterior, middle and two lateral lobes. The anterior prostate is composed mostly of fibromuscular tissue, while the two lateral lobes are glandular tissues. Prostatic secretion contributes up to 15% of the volume of the seminal fluid.

8. The Seminal Vesicle (精囊腺或精囊)

The paired seminal vesicles are oval sacculated and lobulated membranous pouches about 5 cm in length, placed between the base of the bladder and the rectum. They serve as reservoirs for the semen and produce approximately 50% — 60% of the volume of the seminal fluid.

9. The Bulbourethral Gland (尿道球腺)

The paired bulbourethral glands (also called the Cowper's glands) are about the size of a pea, and lie behind and lateral to the membranous urethra within the urogenital diaphragm. Their ducts open into the spongy urethra (Fig.5-3).

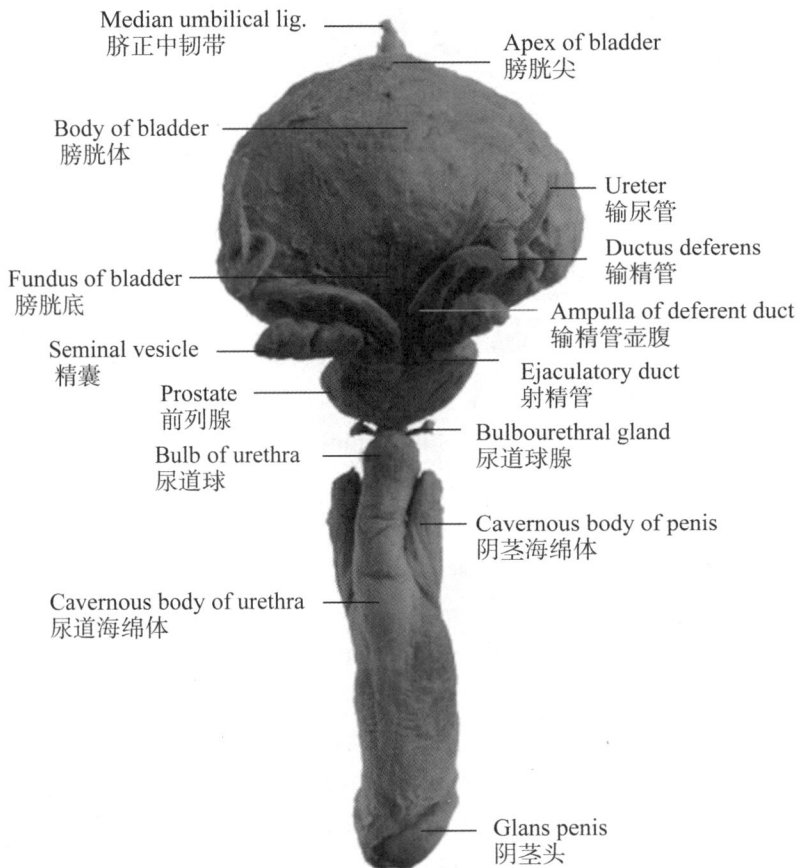

Fig.5-3   Accessory gland (posterior view)

5.1.3   External Genitalia

1. The Scrotum

The scrotum (阴囊) (Fig. 5-4) is a cutaneous pouch which contains the testes, the epididymis and parts of the spermatic cords. It is separated into two lateral portions by a ridge or raphe on its surface and divided into two lateral sacs by the scrotal septum internally. This scrotal septum extends between the raphe and the root of the penis. Each sac contains a single testis. The scrotum wall consists of the loose skin and superficial fascia (called the dartos coat,肉膜). The dartos coat is continuous with the subcutaneous tissue of the abdominal wall (the Scarpa's fascia) as well as the subcutaneous tissue of the groin and the perineum (the Camper's fascia). There is a thin layer of non-striped muscular fibers (called dartos muscle) in the superficial fascia, which pulls the testes upwards during contraction and regulates the temperature of the testes about $2-3$ ℃ below core body temperature. This temperature is required for normal sperm production.

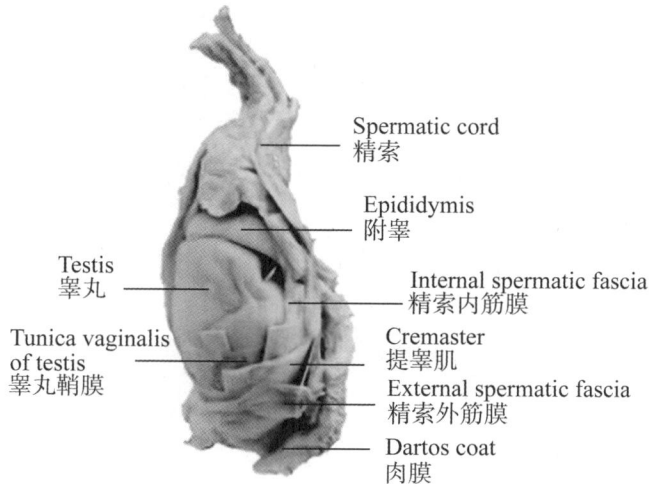

Fig.5-4   Structure and content of the scrotum

Under the dartos coat, there are four layers of tissues wrapping the testes and the spermatic cords. The outside-in layers are: the external spermatic fascia (精索外筋膜), the cremaster muscle (提睾肌), the internal spermatic fascia (精索内筋膜), and the parietal layer of tunica vaginalis testis (睾丸鞘膜壁层). The external spermatic fascia is continuous with the external oblique fascial of the abdominal wall. The cremaster muscle originates from the internal oblique muscle and transversus abdominus muscle. The internal spermatic fascia is continuous with the transversalis fascia. And the tunica vaginalis is continuous with the peritoneum, consisting of a viscera layer and a parietal layer. There is a space between these two layers, which is called vaginal cavity, containing a small amount of serous fluid.

2.Penis (阴茎)

The penis (Fig.5-5) is the male reproductive organ for the ejaculation of semen and the excretion of urine. It is cylindrical in shape, containing the urethra as well as consisting of two cavernous body of penis (阴茎海绵体) (or corpus cavernous penis) dorsolaterally and one cavernous body of urethra (尿道海绵体) (or corpus spongio-sum penis) midventrally. It can be divided into three parts: a head, a body and a root. The root of penis (阴茎根) is composed of the bulb of penis (阴茎球), the expanded portion of the base of the cavernous body of urethra, and the two crus of penis (阴茎脚), the separated and tapered portions of the cavernous body of penis. The root of the penis is fixed because of the attachment of the crus of penis to the ischial and inferior pubic rami, as well as the attachment of the bulb of the penis to the inferior surface of the urogenital diaphragm. The

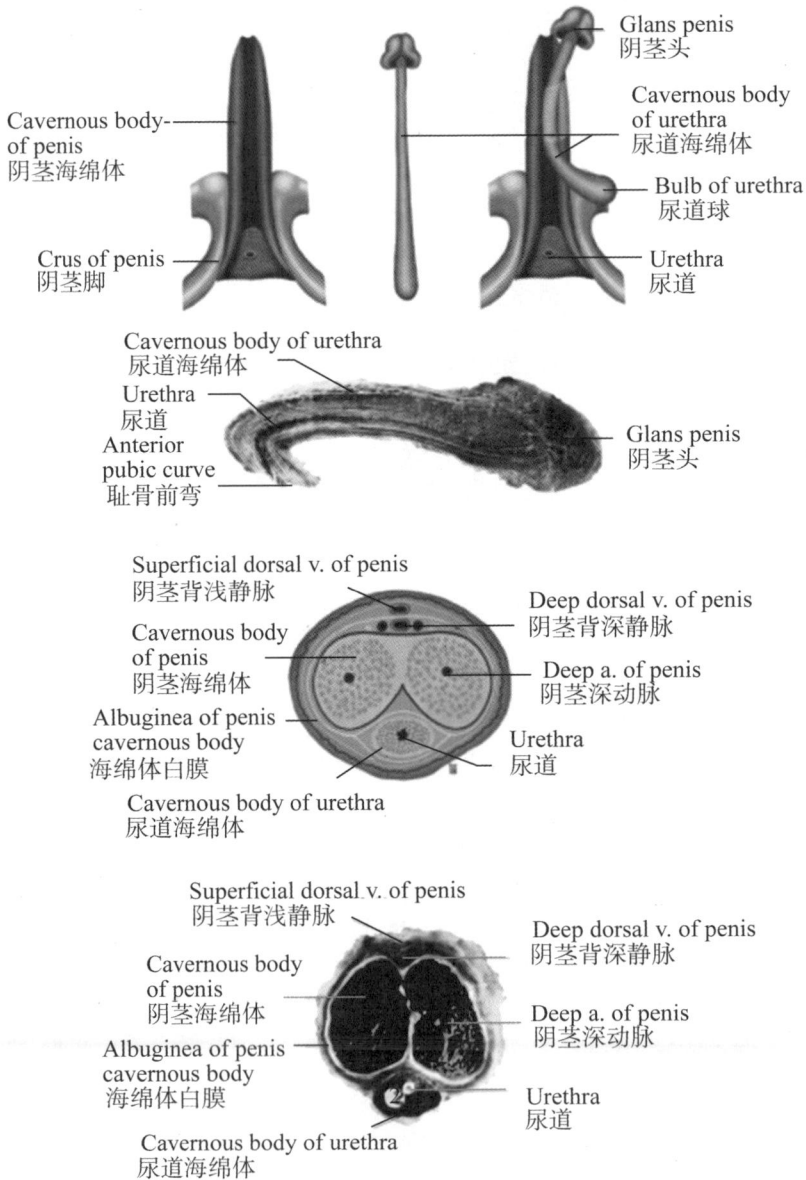

Fig.5-5　The corpus cavernosum of the penis

bulb of the penis is enclosed by the bulbospongiosus muscle.

The body of the penis suspended by the fundiform ligament from the inferior part of the linea alba and the suspensory ligament of the penis from the pubic symphysis, containing the greater part of the urethra, the cavernous body of the urethra and the cavernous body of the penis. Each cavernous body is surrounded by the fibrous tissue called tunica albuginea (白膜). All three cavernous bodies are erectile tissues, which are composed of numerous irregular blood sinuses lined by endothelium, as well as surrounded by smooth muscles, fascia and skin. The blood sinuses fill with blood during penile erection.

The head of the penis (glans, 阴茎头) is the enlarged end of the cavernous body of the urethra. The distal urethra enlarges within the glans penis and forms a terminal slit-like opening, the external urethral orifice. There is the loosely fitting prepuce (or foreskin) covering the glans in an uncircumcised penis.

5.2 Female Reproductive System

5.2.1 General Introduction

In the female internal genitalia, the gonads are the ovaries (卵巢); the ductal system includes the uterine tubes (输卵管), the uterus (子宫), and the vagina (阴道); while the accessory sex glands include the greater vestibular glands (前庭大腺). The female external genitalia is termed as the female pudendum (or vulva)(女阴), consisting of the mons pubis (阴阜), the greater lips of pudendum or the labium majus (大阴唇), the lesser lip of pudendum (or the labium minus) (小阴唇), the vaginal vestibule (阴道前庭), the clitoris (阴蒂), and the bulb of vestibule (前庭球) (Fig.5-6).

The gonads are responsible for producing mature ova and secreting steroid hormones. The ductal system plays various roles for the reproduction. The uterine tubes retrieve ovulated eggs, provide a site for fertilization of eggs and sperms, as well as transport the secondary oocytes and the fertilized zygote to the uterine. The uterus supports the implantation of fertilized zygote and the growth of fetus. The vagina holds the penis during intercourse, serves as a temporary receptacle for semen and a passageway for childbirth and menstrual flow. The accessory sex glands secrete mucus for vaginal and vulvar lubrication.

Peritoneum
腹膜

Uterus
子宫

Vesicouterine pouch
膀胱子宫陷凹

Urinary bladder
膀胱

Pubic symphysis
耻骨联合

Internal urethral orifice
尿道内口

External orifice of urethra
尿道外口

Labium minus
小阴唇

Uterine tube
输卵管

Fundus of uterus
子宫底

Cavity of uterus
子宫腔

Neck of uterus
子宫颈

Rectouterine pouch
直肠子宫陷凹

Vagina
阴道

Anus
肛门

Urethra
尿道

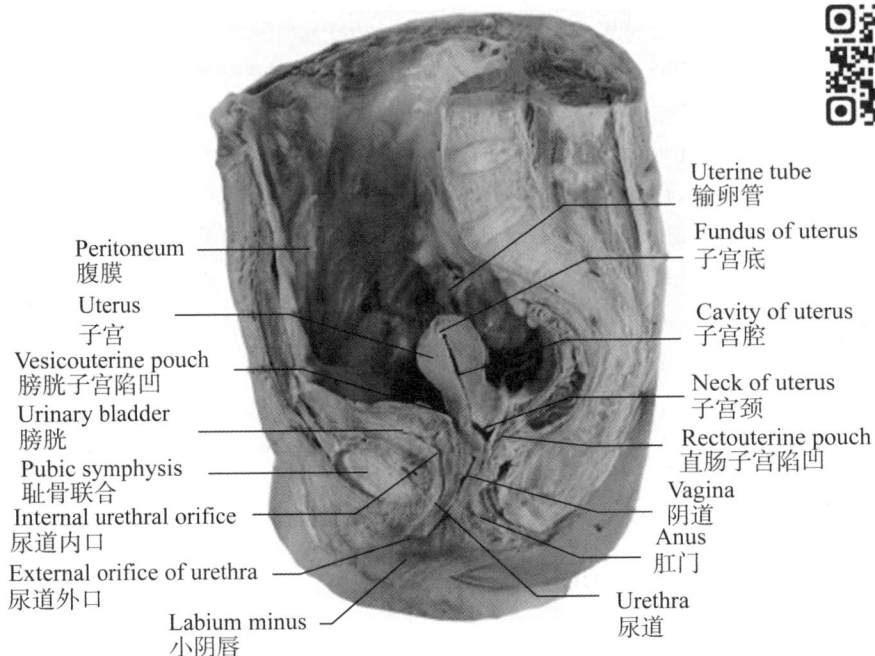

Fig.5-6   The female reproductive system

5.2.2　Internal Genitalia

1. Ovaries (卵巢)

The ovaries (Fig. 5-7) are homologous with the testes in the male. They are paired greyish-red nodular bodies, situating on either side of the uterus in the ovarian fossa(卵巢窝). The ovarian fossa is the shallow depression on the lateral wall of the pelvis between the external iliac artery and the internal iliac artery, which is about 4 cm×3 cm×2 cm in size. The ovaries have lateral and medial surfaces; superior and inferior extremities; as well as anterior and posterior borders. The medial surface of each ovary is close to the loops of the small intestine, while the lateral surface of each ovary is close to the lateral wall of the pelvis. Its superior extremity (called the tubal extremity, 输卵管端) is in contact with the fimbriae of the uterine tube, and its inferior extremity (called the uterine extremity) is connected with the uterus by the proper ligament of the ovary or the ovarian ligament (卵巢固有韧带). Its anterior border called the mesovarian border of ovary (卵巢系膜缘) is attached to the posterior surface of the broad ligament by the mesovarium, while the posterior border of each ovary is free. In the middle portion of the anterior border, there is the hilus of ovary(卵巢门) which the ovarian blood vessels and nerves pass through, as well as the point of the ovary attaches to the mesovarium. The mesovarium (卵

巢系膜) is a double-layered fold of the peritoneum, which is a part of the broad ligament. Besides the mesovarium and the proper ligament of the ovary, the suspensory ligament of ovary(卵巢悬韧带) attaches the ovary to the pelvic wall. All these ligaments hold ovaries in position.

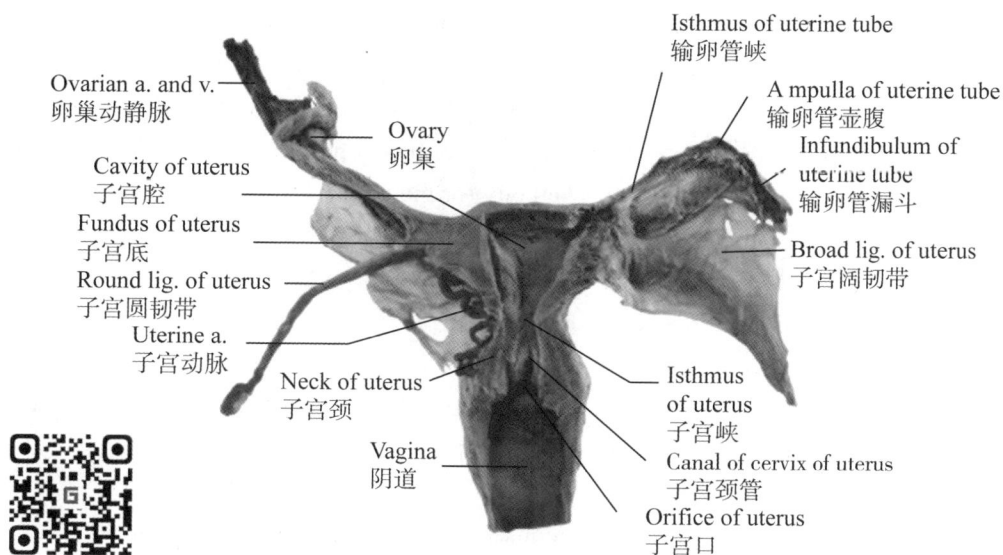

Fig.5-7　Internal female genital organs

2. Uterine Tubes (输卵管)

The paired uterine tubes (or the fallopian tubes, the oviducts) extend laterally from the fundus of the uterus to the upper extremity of the ovary. Each tube is about 10－14 cm in length and goes between the folds of the broad ligament of the uterus. The uterine tubes are divided into four sections, which are the uterine part (子宫部), the isthmus (峡部), the ampulla (壶腹部) and the infundibulum (输卵管漏斗) in the sequence of the distance increase from the uterus. The uterine part is the narrowest (1 mm in diameter) and transverses the uterine musculature. It opens into the uterine cavity at the uterine orifice (输卵管子宫口). The isthmus is the short, narrow and thick-wall portion where the ligation of the uterine tube is usually performed. The ampulla is the widest, thin-walled and longest portion with plenty of blood supply. It is the lateral 2/3 of the uterine tube where the fertilization often occurs. The infundibulum is funnel-shaped and open to the pelvic cavity. The opening of the infundibulum is called the abdominal orifice of fallopian tube (输卵管腹腔口), surrounded by a fringe of fingerlike projections called fimbria of uterine tube (输卵管伞). The longest fimbriae, which is attached to the ovary, is called the ovarian fimbria (卵巢伞).

3. Uterus (子宫)

The uterus is a hollow, thick-walled, inverted pear-shaped, muscular organ that situates in the middle of the pelvic cavity in the frontal plane. Normally, it locates between the bladder and rectum, does not extend above the linea terminalis, nor below the level of ischial spines. In an adult woman who has never been pregnant, it is about 7—9 cm in length, 4 cm in width, and 2—3 cm in thickness at the upper part. There are three subdivisions of the uterus: the fundus of uterus (子宫底), the body of uterus (子宫体) and the neck of uterus (子宫颈). The fundus is a dome-shaped portion between the fallopian tubes and superior to the uterine tubes. The body (or the corpus) is the largest and tapering portion of the uterus. The cervix is the inferior cylindrical portion of the uterus, half of which protrudes into the upper vagina. A constricted region of the cervix next to the body of uterus is called the isthmus of uterus (子宫峡), which is about 1 cm long in nonpregnancy and elongates up to 7—11 cm long in the late pregnancy. There are an interior cavity in the body (called the cavity of uterus,子宫腔) and a narrow spindle space inside the cervix (called the cervical canal,子宫颈管). The cervical canal opens into the vagina at the orifice of uterus (子宫口).

Histologically, the uterine wall is composed of three layers: the perimetrium (子宫外膜), the myometrium (子宫肌层) and the endometrium (子宫内膜). The perime-trium is the serosa outer layer and a part of parietal peritoneum. The myometrium is made up of three layers of smooth muscle tissues. And the endometrium is a mucous membrane which the function layer sloughs off during menstruation.

In most nonpregnant women, the uterus is in the anteverted and anteflexed positions when the bladder is empty. The uterus tilts forward at an angle of about 90 degrees between the long axis of the uterus and the vagina, and this position is termed as the anteversion (子宫前倾). While the long axis of the body of the uterus is bent forward at an angle of about 170° with the long axis of the cervix, this position is termed as the anteflexion (子宫前屈). To hold the uterus in normal place, there are several connective tissue ligaments, the pelvic diaphragm and the urogenital diaphragm. Among the ligaments, there are three paired fibromuscular cords: the round ligaments, the uterosacral ligaments and the cardinal ligaments. i) The round ligaments of the uterus (子宫圆韧带) extend from the lateral angle of the uterus inferior to the uterine tubes, traverse the pelvis, pass through the inguinal canals, finally attach to the soft tissues at the labia majora and the mons pubis. They normally maintain the anteverted position of the uterus. ii) The uterosacral ligaments of the uterus (子宫骶韧带) attach to the uterus posteriorly at the level of the cervix, travel from either side of the rectum, connect to the front of the sacrum. They coordinate with the round ligaments to maintain the anteverted and anteflexed positions of the uterus. iii) The cardinal ligaments of the uterus (子宫主韧带) are located at the base of the broad ligament of the uterus, as well as extend from the uterine cervix to the lateral walls of the pelvis. They provide strong support for the uterus from prolapse. Besides the three sets of ligaments, there are double folds of the parietal peritoneum attaching the uterus to either lateral pelvic walls, called the broad ligament of the uterus (子宫阔韧带). This ligament is a flat sheet covering the surface of the uterus, the uterine tubes, the round ligaments, the ovary, the proper ligament of the ovary, as well as the blood vessels, the lymphatic vessels and the nerves to the internal female genitalia. The lateral one third of the upper margin of the broad ligament is called the suspensory ligament of ovary (or the infundibulopelvic ligament), containing the ovarian blood and lymphatic vessels, as well as the ovarian nerve plexus. The broad ligament holds the uterus in the middle of the pelvic cavity from moving to either side of the pelvis. The broad ligament together with the uterus forms a septum across the female pelvis dividing the pelvic cavity into two portions: the vesicouterine pouch between the bladder and the uterus, and the rectouterine pouch (or the Douglas' pouch) between the uterus and the rectum.

4. Vagina (阴道)

The vagina is a closed tubular fibromuscular canal that travels upwards and backwards from the vestibule to the cervix, and is situated between the bladder and the rectum. Near the upper vagina, the cervix protrudes into the vagina on its front surface at approximately a 90° angle. Where the vaginal lumen surrounds the cervix of the uterus, it is a continuous recess divided into four parts: the anterior, posterior, left and right lateral fornices. The posterior fornix is deeper than the other fornices and is the anterior boundary of the rectouterine pouch. Furthermore, the rectouterine pouch is the deepest point of the female peritoneal cavity. The outer vaginal opening (the virginal orifice, 阴道口) to the vulva is normally partly covered by a thin layer and an irregular circle of mucosal tissue called the hymen(处女膜)before the first intercourse.

5. Greater Vestibular Gland (前庭大腺)

The great vestibular glands (or the Bartholin's glands,巴氏腺) are pea-sized mucus-secreting glands, located bilaterally at the posterior introitus, beneath the bulbospongiosus muscle, at the tail end of the vestibular bulb, and deep into the posterior labia majora. Their efferent ducts drain into a groove between the hymen and the labium minus.

5.2.3　External Genitalia

1. The Mons Pubis (阴阜)

The mons pubis is the rounded, hair-bearing prominence anterior to the pubic symphysis, formed by skin and a collection of fatty tissue beneath the integument.

2. The Greater Lips of Pudendum (大阴唇)

The greater lips of pudendum (or the labia majora) are two prominent longitudinal cutaneous folds, which extend inferiorly and posteriorly from the mons pubis to the perineum. They form the lateral boundaries of a fissure or cleft, into which the vagina and urethra open. Anteriorly, they meet below the mons pubis to form the anterior labial commissure (唇前连合). Posteriorly, they are close to each other and form the posterior labial commissure (唇后连合), which is the posterior boundary of the vulva.

3. The Lesser Lips of Pudendum (小阴唇)

The lesser lips of pudendum (or the labia minora) are two small cutaneous folds, situate between the labia majora, and extend from the clitoris obliquely downward, lateralward, and backward. Their anterior folds encircle the clitoris forming the clitoral hood and the frenulum of the clitoris. Their posterior ends are usually joined by a fold of skin, called the frenulum of pudendal labia or the fourchette (阴唇系带).

4. The Vaginal Vestibule (阴道前庭)

The vaginal vestibule is the region between the labia minora. Within the vaginal vestibule, there are the external urethral orifices anterior to the vaginal orifices, as well as the openings of the paraurethral glands and the greater vestibular glands on either side of the urethral and vaginal orifices respectively.

5. The Clitoris (阴蒂)

The clitoris is an erectile structure, homologous to the penis. It is situated beneath the anterior labial commissure, partially hidden between the anterior ends of the labia minora. It consists of the glans, the body and two crura. The crura are attached below the middle of the pubic arch, while the body is made up of two corpora cavernosa, which is composed of erectile tissue enclosed in thick fibroelastic tunica albuginea. The glans exists at the tip of the clitoral body as a fibrovascular cap and is highly innervated.

6. The Bulb of Vestibule (前庭球)

The bulb of vestibule is the homologue of the cavernous body of male urethra. It consists of two elongated masses of the trabecular and erectile tissue, placed one on either side of the vaginal orifice, beneath the labia majora, and united to each other in front by a narrow median band termed the pars intermedia (Fig.5-8).

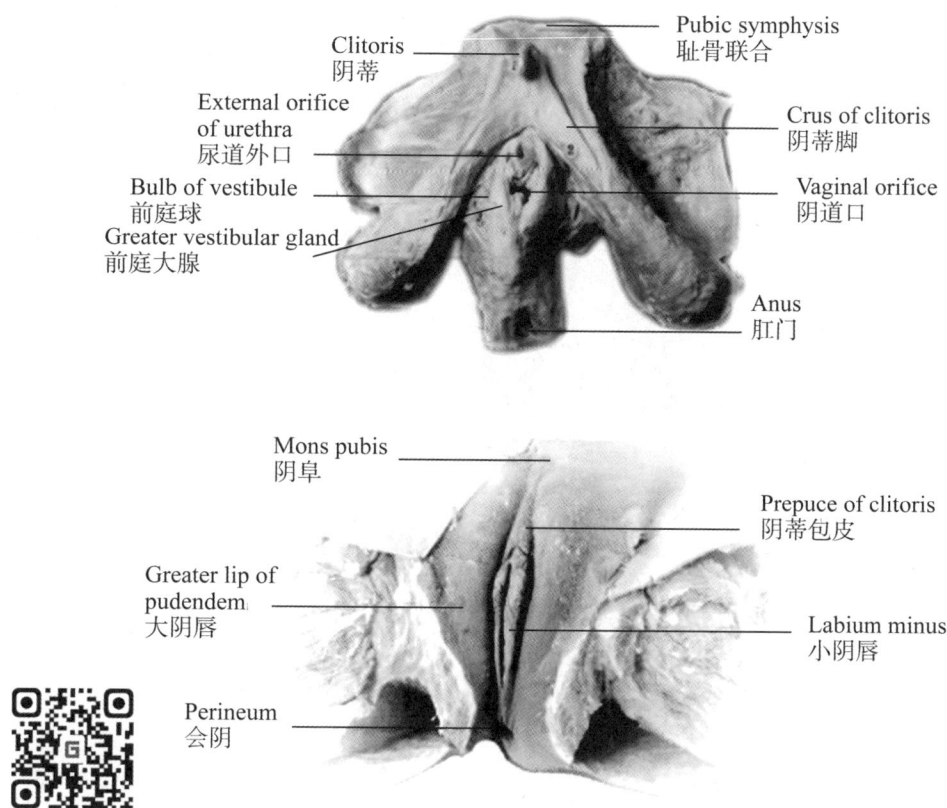

Clitoris
阴蒂

External orifice
of urethra
尿道外口

Bulb of vestibule
前庭球

Greater vestibular gland
前庭大腺

Pubic symphysis
耻骨联合

Crus of clitoris
阴蒂脚

Vaginal orifice
阴道口

Anus
肛门

Mons pubis
阴阜

Greater lip of
pudendem
大阴唇

Perineum
会阴

Prepuce of clitoris
阴蒂包皮

Labium minus
小阴唇

Fig.5-8　The female external genitalia

5.2.4　Breasts

The breasts (or mammae) (Fig. 5-9) are paired prominences located on the upper ventral region of the chest, normally well developed in females as a sexual characteristic and modified sudoriferous glands to produce milk during lactation. They extend from the level of the second to the third rib/costal cartilage to the level of the sixth to the seventh rib/costal cartilage in the front of the rib cage, and from the parasternal line to the midaxillary line.

On the surface of each breast, there is a pigmented projection with 15－20 "pores" on the top, called the nipple (乳头). The nipple is located at the intersection of the midclavicular line and the fifth rib or the fourth intercostal space. The circular pigmented area surrounding the nipple is called the areola of breast (乳晕). It is rough and contains protruding, modified sebaceous glands which secrete oily fluid to lubricate and protect the nipple.

Pectoralis major
胸大肌

Lobules of
mammary gland
乳腺小叶

Lactiferous ducts
输乳管

Suspensory lig.
of breast
乳房悬韧带

Nipple
乳头

Lactiferous sinuses
输乳管窦

Body of breast
乳房体

Pectoral fascia
胸肌筋膜

Costal bone
肋骨

Intercostal muscle
肋间肌

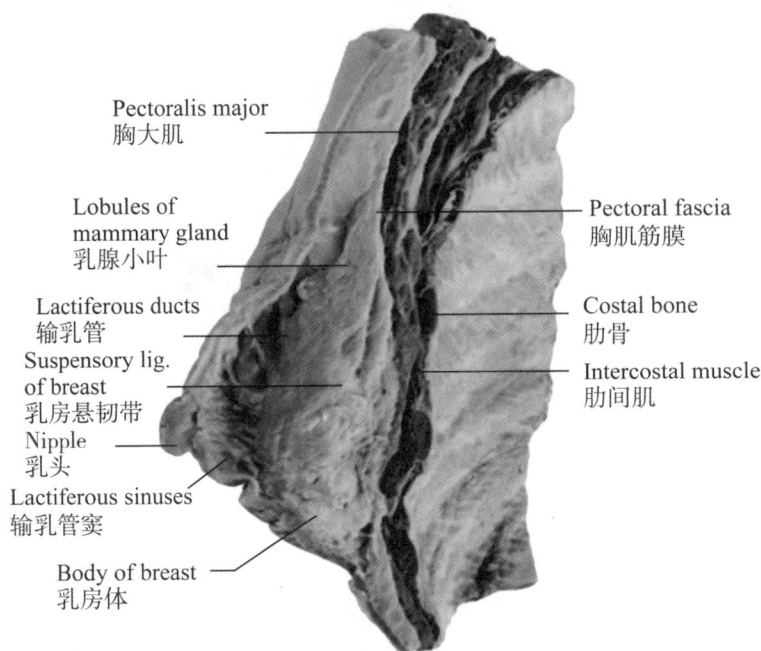

Fig.5-9　Adult female breasts

Histologically, the breasts are made up of skin, glandular tissue, fibrous tissue and adipose tissue. The glandular tissue affects the lactation functions of the breasts. It is embedded in subcutaneous adipose over the pectoral fascia and the pectoralis major, and it is connected by a network of ducts. Each mammary gland consists of 15－20 irregular lactiferous lobes, which are separated to several smaller compartments by fibrous tissues called lobules. These lobules are composed of grapelike clusters of milk-secreting glands (called alveoli) surrounded with myoepithelial cells. The alveoli produce and store milk in response to hormonal signals. When the myoepithelial cells contract, the milk will be propelled from the alveoli into a series of secondary tubules in lobules and then into the lactiferous ducts in lobes. These lactiferous ducts will expand to form sinuses near the nipple called lactiferous sinuses, which gradually taper, converge at the nipple, and finally open at the pores on the nipple. The fibrous tissue is important in maintaining the shape and the structure integrity of the breasts. It invests the entire surface of the breasts, wraps the ductal glandular components, sends down septa between the lobes, as well as forms strands of connective tissues that radiate from the superficial fascia to the skin envelope and the pectoral fascia respectively. These stands of connective tissues are called the suspensory ligaments of breast (乳房悬韧带) or the Cooper's ligaments (Cooper, 韧带), which assist in the diagnosis of breast diseases. When the breast carcinoma blocks the local lymphatic ducts leading to swelling of the breast, the skin takes on a dimpled appearance reminiscent of the peel of an orange because of the tethering of the skin to the pectoral fascia by the suspensory ligaments of Cooper. Besides, carcinomas can also shorten Cooper's ligaments leading to a dimpling. The adipose tissue is considerable abundance in the breasts, and determines the form and size of the breasts. It covers the surface of the mammary glands, and fills in the interval between the lobes. However, there is no fat immediately beneath the areola and the nipple.

（浙江大学医学院　柳华）

Exercise

1. A pregnant women found a small amount of dark red bleeding from the vagina accompanied by abdominal pain. The doctor diagnosed her with an ectopic pregnancy. Which of the following structure was the most likely site of ectopic pregnancy?

(A) Isthmus of uterine tube.

(B) Ampulla of uterine tube.

(C) Uterus.

(D) Infundibulum of uterine tube.

(E) Abdominal cavity.

2. A man wanted to perform a vasectomy. Which of the following structure was the most likely site for vasectomy?

(A) Testicular division of the ductus deferens.

(B) Spermatic cord division of the ductus deferens.

(C) Inguinal division of the ductus deferens.

(D) Pelvis division of the ductus deferens.

(E) Ejaculatory duct.

Answer

1. The correct answer is B.

The ectopic pregnancy is an abnormal pregnancy in which the egg lays outside the uterine cavity. This is mainly due to inflammation in or around the lumen of the uterine tube which causes poor patency of the lumen and prevents the movement of the fertilized egg. The fertilized egg is formed in ampulla of uterine tube. Therefore, the fertilized egg can easily develop in the ampulla of uterine tube (B) and lead to an ectopic pregnancy.

2. The correct answer is B.

The spermatic cord of the ductus deferens lies between the upper part of the testis and the subcutaneous ring of the inguinal canal. This segment is superficial and easily accessible, making it an ideal site for ligation of the ductus deferens.

The Cardiovascular System

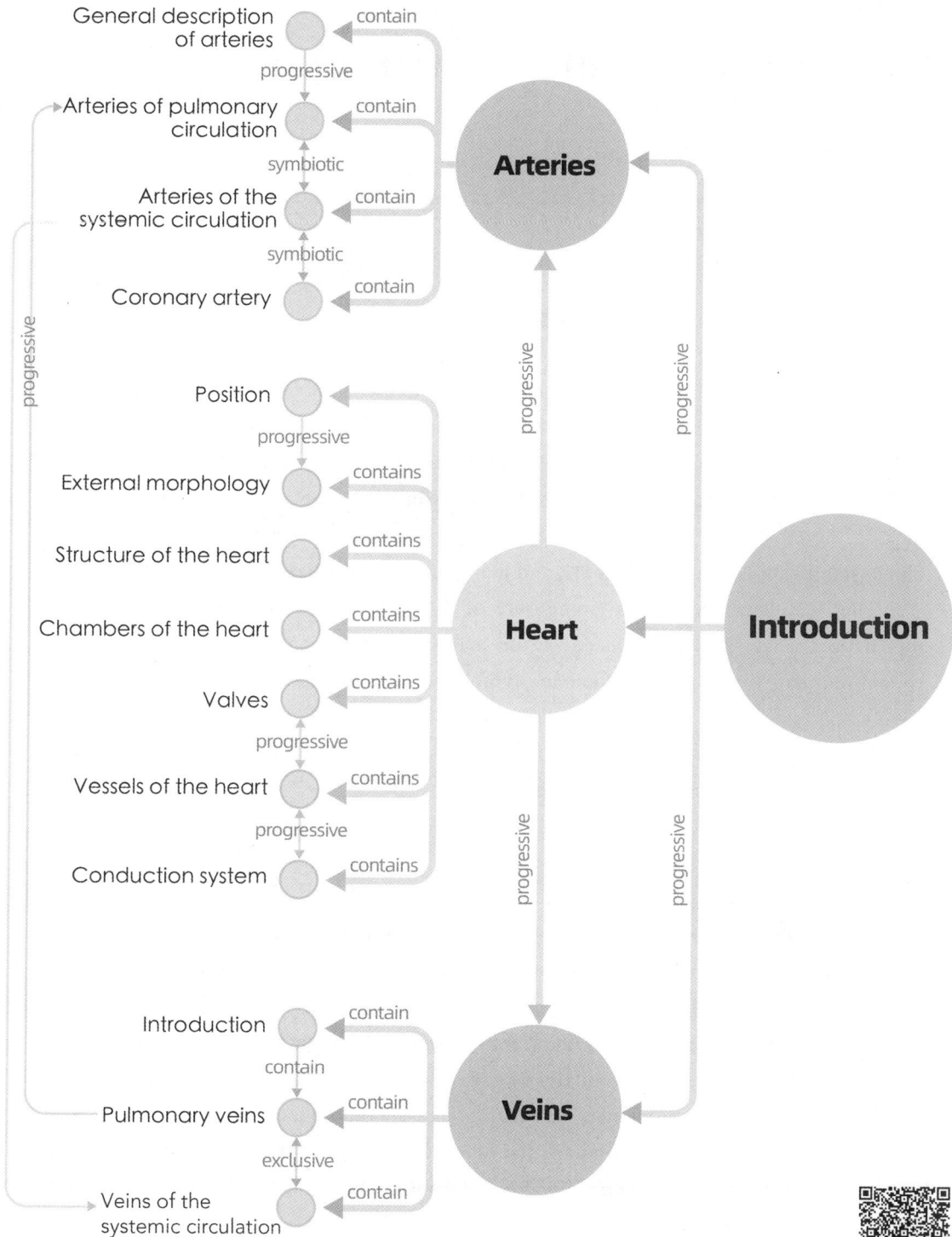

General description of arteries — contain — **Arteries**
progressive
Arteries of pulmonary circulation — contain
symbiotic
Arteries of the systemic circulation — contain
symbiotic
Coronary artery — contain

Position — progressive
External morphology — contains
Structure of the heart — contains
Chambers of the heart — contains — **Heart** ← **Introduction**
Valves — contains
progressive
Vessels of the heart — contains
progressive
Conduction system — contains

Introduction — contain — **Veins**
contain
Pulmonary veins — contain
exclusive
Veins of the systemic circulation — contain

progressive

The Cardiovascular System

Chapter 6 Cardiovascular System

Angiology

Angiology (脉管学) encompasses the cardiovascular system (心血管系统) and the lymphatic system (淋巴系统). The cardiovascular system consists of the heart and blood vessels, forming a tubular network that transports and distributes blood throughout the body (Fig. 6-1). It also circulates and transports nutrients, metabolites, oxygen, carbon dioxide, hormones, and blood cells, providing nourishment to all cells, redistributing blood, stabilizing temperature and pH, and maintaining homeostasis.

The lymphatic system is composed of lymphatic vessels, lymph organs, and lymphatic tissues, providing channels for leukocyte migration and the absorption of certain nutrients from the gut. Blood and lymph circulate through their respective vessels, but lymph circulation begins from lymphatic capillaries and ultimately rejoins the bloodstream. It's important to note that these two systems communicate with each other and are intimately associated developmentally.

6.1 General Introduction

The cardiovascular system (Fig. 6-2) is a network composed of the heart (心) as a centralised pump, blood vessels: arteries (动脉), veins (静脉) and capillaries (毛细血管) that distribute blood throughout the body, and the blood itself, for transportation of different substances. The heart is the central organ of the cardiovascular system, and consists of a hollow muscle. Essentially heart is a pair of muscular pumps, one feeding the low hydrostatic pressure pulmonary circulation, and the other feeding the high hydrostatic pressure systemic circulation. It pumps the blood to all parts of the body through a series of tubes. The arteries (动脉) carry blood away from the heart, and are composed of three coats: an internal or endothelial coat; a middle or muscular coat; and an external or connective-tissue coat. Arteries branch extensively to form a network of progressively

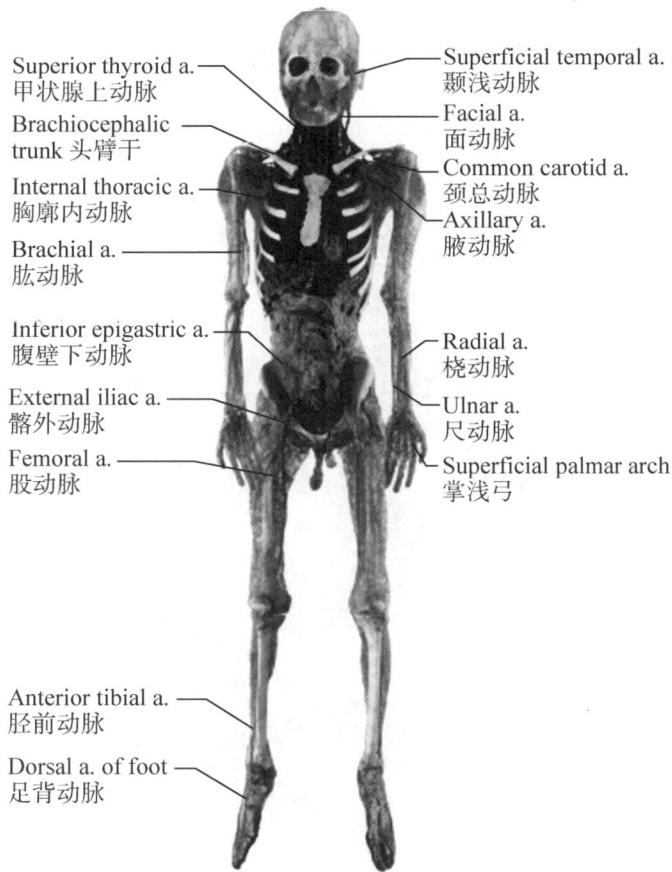

Fig.6-1   Systemic arterial distribution

smaller vessels. Capillaries (毛细血管) are the net-works of vessels that carry the blood from the arterial to the venous system. The wall of a capillary consists of a fine transparent endothelial layer and basement mem-brane, and is continuous with the endothelial cells which line the arteries and veins. All exchanges of fluid, nutrients, and wastes between the blood and tissue cells occur across the walls of capillaries. The veins (静脉) transport blood from the capillaries, and back to the heart. The microscopic veins deliver blood to progressively larger vessels that empty into the large veins.

Arteries and veins are primarily named according to their anatomical position. In functional terms, four main classes of vessel are described: conducting and distributing vessels (large arteries), resistance vessels (small arteries but mainly arterioles), exchange vessels (capillaries, sinusoids and small venules) and capacitance vessels (veins). Structurally, arteries can also divides into elastic and muscular types.

The cardiovascular system divides into two separate loops: the shorter pulmonary circuit that exchanges blood between the heart and the lungs for oxygenation, and the longer systemic circuit that distributes blood throughout all other systems and tissues of the body. Both of these circuits begin and end in the heart.

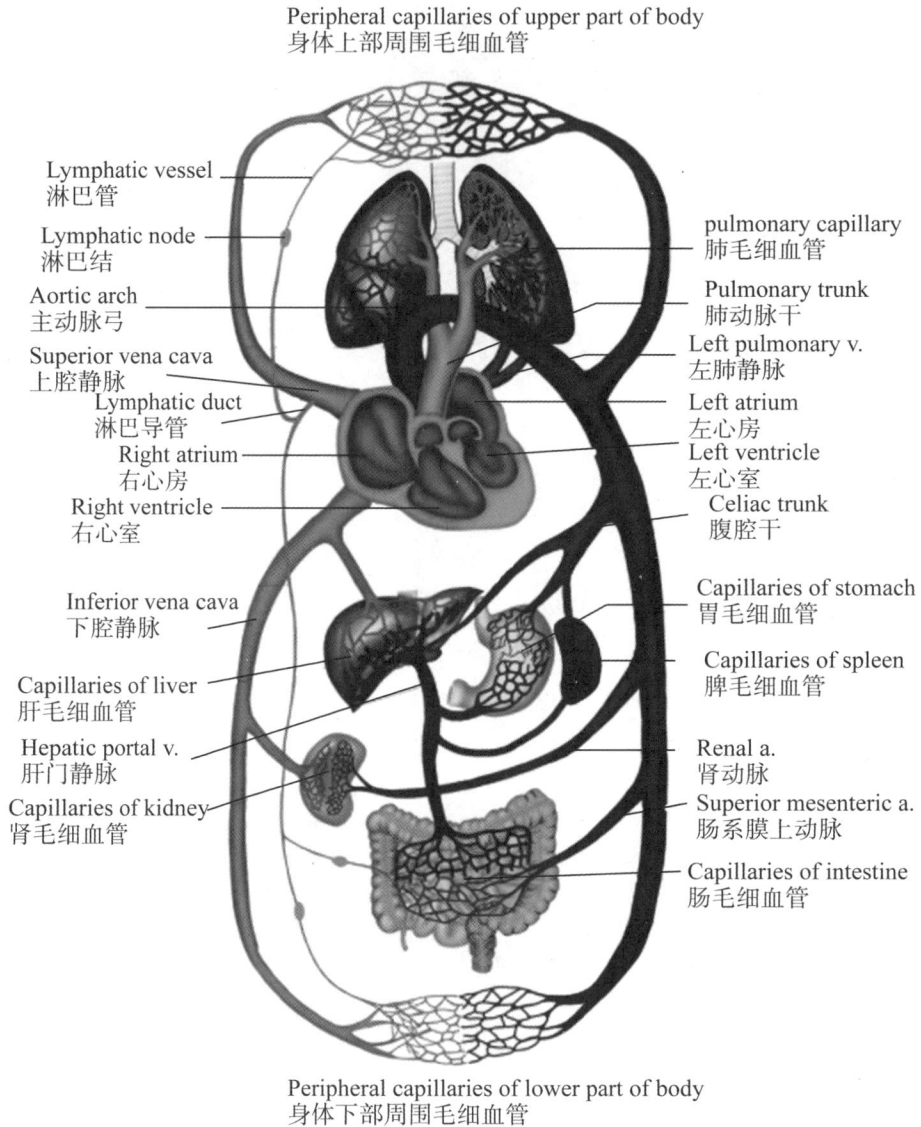

Fig.6-2　Blood circulation

6.1.1　Systemic (Greater) Circulation (体循环)

Left ventricle→aorta and its branches→capillaries of body→superior and inferior vena cava→right atrium.

The substance exchange between the blood and tissue cells through capillary wall takes place in the systemic circulation. The arteries carry the arterial blood (rich in oxygen and nutrients) to organs and tissues through capillaries, and after exchanging, systemic veins return the venous blood (rich in carbon dioxide and metabolic products) back to the right atrium.

From the heart to the periphery, the arteries increase in number, decrease in diameter and thickness. As a result, blood flow is faster near the heart than at the periphery. From the periphery to the heart, the venules return blood from the capillaries, converge on each other, forming a progressively smaller number of veins of increasingly large size and eventually, forming two largest veins, the superior and inferior vena cava, then back to the right atrium.

6.1.2 Pulmonary (Lesser) Circulation (肺循环)

Right ventricle → pulmonary trunk → right and left pulmonary Arteries → pulmonary capillaries (in lungs) → pulmonary veins → left atrium.

In the pulmonary circulation, the pulmonary arteries transport deoxygenated blood (venous blood) to the lungs for gas exchange, and then the pulmonary veins transport oxygenated blood (arterial blood) back to the left atrium.

Vascular anastomosis (血管吻合) (Fig.6-3): When blood vessels connect with each other to form a region of diffuse vascular supply, it is called an anastomosis. Anastomoses usually include the artery-artery, vein-vein, artery-vein, and collateral anastomoses, which provide critical alternative routes for blood to flow in case of blockages.

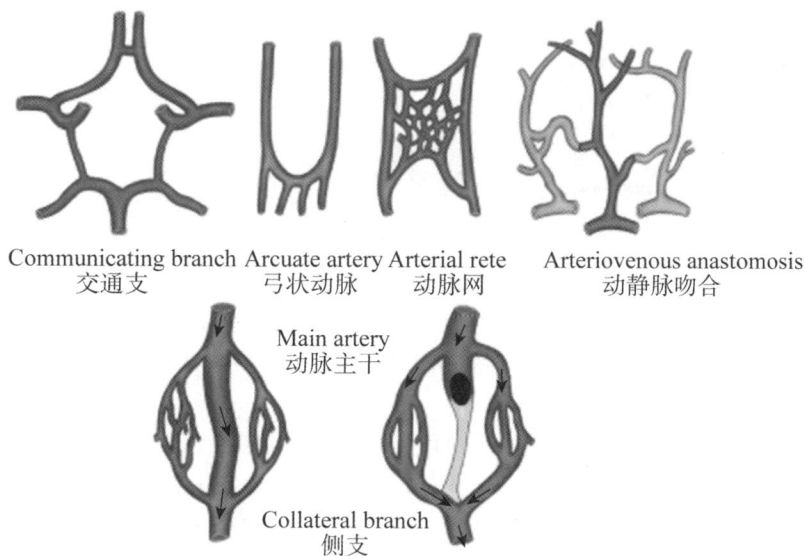

Communicating branch　Arcuate artery　Arterial rete
交通支　　　　　　弓状动脉　　动脉网

Arteriovenous anastomosis
动静脉吻合

Main artery
动脉主干

Collateral branch
侧支

Fig.6-3　Collateral circulation

6.2 Heart

The heart (心) serves as a transport system pump that keeps blood continuously circulating through the blood vessels of the body based of its structure as a hollow, four-chambered muscular organ. The pericardium (心 包) contains the heart and its great vessels. The heart is described as having one base, one apex, two surfaces and three borders.

6.2.1 Position

The heart is enclosed in the pericardium, and lies in the middle mediastinum between the lungs and mediastinal pleura. It is placed obliquely at around 45° to the sagittal plane behind the body of the sternum and adjoining costal cartilages. About 2/3 of the heart on the left and 1/3 on the right to the median plane. The weight of the heart varies from 280 to 340 g in males and from 250 to 280 g in females. An average size of adult heart is about 12 cm from base to apex, 6 cm from anterior to posterior, and 8 to 9 cm at the broadest transverse diameter and somewhat larger than a closed fist.

6.2.2 External Morphology

The heart is a hollow muscular organ, pyramidal in shape. It consists of four chambers including right and left atria, right and left ventricles. It contains one apex, one base, two surfaces, three borders, and four grooves (Figs. 6-4 & 6-5).

1. The Cardiac Apex (心尖)

The cardiac apex is formed by left ventricle and is directed anteroinferiorly to the left. It lies at the level of the left fifth intercostal space, $1-2$ cm medial to the left midclavicular line.

2. The Cardiac Base (心底)

The cardiac base is somewhat quadrilateral, and faces posteriorly and to the right. It is formed mainly by the left atrium, and only partly by the right atrium. Two pulmonary veins on each side open into the left atrium, and the superior and inferior vena cava open into the right atrium. It neighbors posteriorly to the pericardium, esophagus, thoracic aorta, vagus nerve, etc.

3. The Sternocostal Surface (胸肋面)

The sternocostal surface is formed mainly by the right atrium and right ventricle, and a lesser portion is formed by the left auricle and ventricle. It is directed anteriorly and superiorly to the inferior part of the body of sternum, and the 4th to the 6th left costal cartilages.

4. The Diaphragmatic Surface (膈面)

The diaphragmatic surface is formed by the ventricles (chiefly the left ventricle). It is largely horizontal, and gently directs downwards and backwards. It rests mainly upon the central tendon, and a small area of the left muscular part of the diaphragm.

5. The Right Border (右缘)

The right border is vertical and formed entirely by right atrium, and corresponds to a line running from the upper border of right third costal cartilage ±1.2 cm from the margin of sternum, downwards to the sixth sternocostal joint.

6. The Left Border (左缘)

The left border is round and mainly formed by the left ventricle and partly by the left auricle. It is represented by a line running from the apex upwards and medially to a point on lower border of the left second costal cartilage ±1.2 cm from sternal margin.

7. The Inferior Border (下缘)

The inferior border is horizontal and formed by the right ventricle and cardiac apex. It is represented by a line joint the lower end of right border to the apex.

8. Four Grooves

Coronary sulcus (冠状沟) (atrioventricular sulcus) is a groove on the external surface of the heart and marks the division between the atria and ventricles. It contains the main parts of the coronary vessels. It's almost circular, but superiorly, it is obliterated by the pulmonary trunk.

Anterior interventricular groove and posterior interventricular groove (前室间沟和后室间沟) mark the division between the left and right ventricles. The anterior interventricular groove is on the sternocostal surface, and the posterior interventricular groove is on the diaphragmatic surface of heart, and they are respectively consistent with the anterior and inferior borders of interventricular septum. These two grooves extend from the coronary sulcus to a notch right to the cardiac apex on the inferior border, which is called the cardiac apical incisure (心尖切迹).

Interatrial sulcus (房间沟) is a shallow groove between the right atrium and superior and inferior vena cava on the cardiac base and marks the division between the left and right atrium.

Atrioventricular crux (房室交点) is a junction area of the posterior interventricular groove, interatrial sulcus and coronary sulcus.

Aortic arch
主动脉弓

Arterial lig.
动脉韧带

Ascending aorta
升主动脉

Pulmonary trunk
肺动脉干

Superior vena cava
上腔静脉

Left auricle
左心耳

Right auricle
右心耳

Circumflex branch
旋支

Branch of arterial conus
动脉圆锥支

Anterior interventricular branch
前室间支

Right coronary a.
右冠状动脉

Great cardiac v.
心大静脉

Anterior right
ventricular branch
右室前支

Left interventricular branch
左室前支

Left ventricle
左心室

Right ventricle
右心室

Anterior interventricular groove
前室间沟

Right marginal branch
右缘支

Cardiac apex
心尖

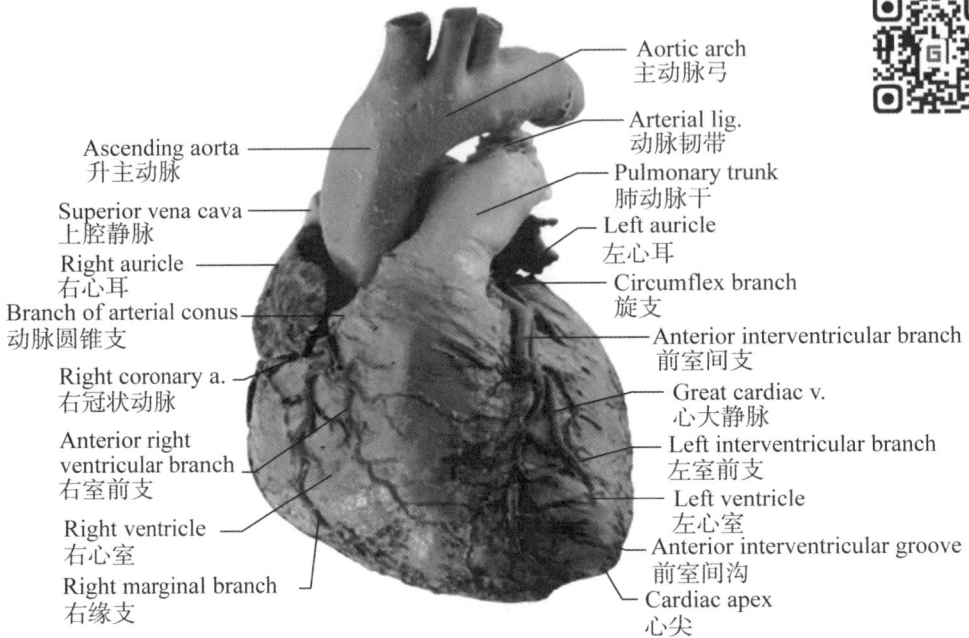

Fig.6-4　External features and blood vessels of the heart (anterior aspect)

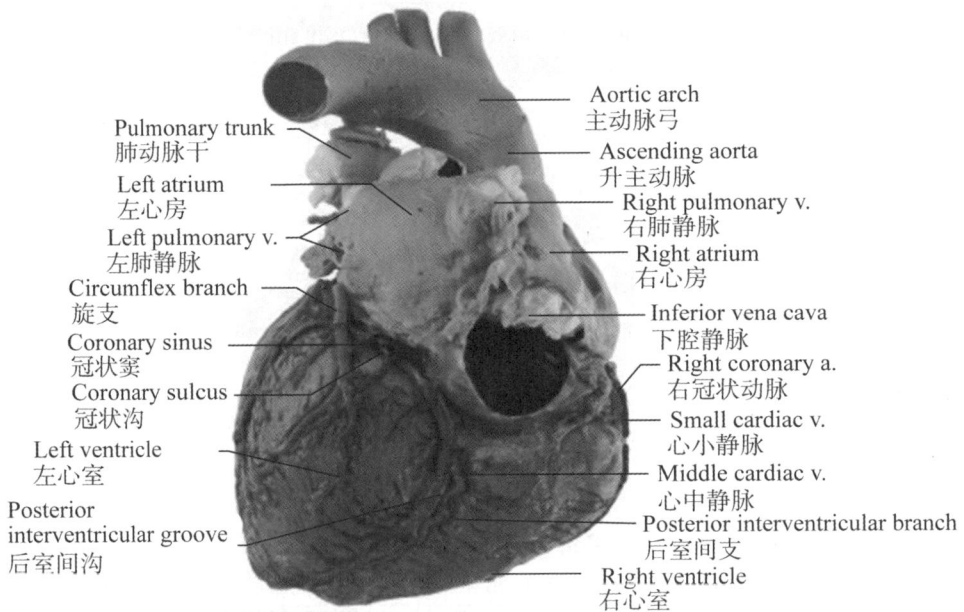

Pulmonary trunk
肺动脉干

Aortic arch
主动脉弓

Left atrium
左心房

Ascending aorta
升主动脉

Left pulmonary v.
左肺静脉

Right pulmonary v.
右肺静脉

Circumflex branch
旋支

Right atrium
右心房

Coronary sinus
冠状窦

Inferior vena cava
下腔静脉

Coronary sulcus
冠状沟

Right coronary a.
右冠状动脉

Small cardiac v.
心小静脉

Left ventricle
左心室

Middle cardiac v.
心中静脉

Posterior
interventricular groove
后室间沟

Posterior interventricular branch
后室间支

Right ventricle
右心室

Fig.6-5　External features and blood vessels of the heart (posterior aspect)

6.2.3　Chambers of Heart

1. The Right Atrium (RA) (右心房)

The right atrium is larger than the left one, but its walls are somewhat thinner. It consists of two parts including an anteriorly situated rough-walled atrium proper (固有心房) and a posteriorly situated smooth-walled sinus venarum cavarum (腔静脉窦). An anterior ear-shaped appendage of atrium proper is called the right auricle (右心耳).

(1) **Four orifices of the right atrium**

There are three inlets in the RA. Orifice of superior vena cava (上腔静脉口)opens into its roof returning blood to the heart from the head, neck and upper limbs and which has no valve. Orifice of inferior vena cava (下腔静脉口) opens into its inferoposterior part returning blood to the heart from the lower part of the body. A flap-like valve of inferior vena cava (Eustachian valve) (下腔静脉瓣) is at the anterior edge of the inferior vena cava. The valve of the inferior vena cava is large for fetus and serves to direct blood toward and through the foramen ovale of the interatrial septum and into the left atrium. The valve varies markedly degenarated in postnatal life as fossa ovalis (卵圆窝) . Orifice of coronary sinus (冠状窦口) opens into the right atrium between the inferior vena cava and the right atrioventricular orifice returning most of the blood from the cardiac muscle. A thin, semicircular valve of coronary sinus (冠状窦瓣) covers the lower part of the orifice. Many small orifices of small veins also drain the venous blood of the wall of heart and open directly into the right atrium. One outlet: right atrioventricular orifice (右房室口) lies anteroinferiorly in the right atrium and leads venous blood from the right atrium to the right ventricle.

(2) **Crista terminalis** (界嵴)

It is a vertical ridge that from superior vena cava to inferior vena cava. Sulcus terminalis (界沟) is a shallow groove running between the right sides of the opening of the superior and inferior vena cava on the outside of heart that corresponds to the crista terminalis, and it's the junction between the sinus venarum cavarum and the atrium proper.

(3) **Two parts of the right atrium**

They are separated externally by the sulcus terminalis and internally by the crista terminalis. The sinus venarum cavarum is the main part of the right atrium that lies posterior to the ridge and is derived embryologically from the sinus venosus. The smooth-walled sinus venarum cavarum receives the openings of the superior and inferior vena cava and the coronary sinus. The atrium proper is in front of the ridge, and is roughened or trabeculated by bundles of muscle fibers as the pectinate muscles. The pectinate muscles that arise from the crista terminalis and extend anterolaterally along the internal surface of the right atrial auricle. The right auricle is a small conical muscular pouch, projects to the left from the root of superior vena cava, pectinate muscles in wall. Orifice of coronary sinus lies posterior to the ridge. The posterior portion of the medial wall of right atrium is mainly formed by the interatrial septum (atrial septem) (房间隔) which separates the right atrium from the left atrium. Fossa ovalis is an oval depression on the lower part of the septal wall of right atrium and superior to the orifice of inferior vena cava, which is a remnant of the fetal foramen ovale, and it's also the most predilection site of atrial septal defects (ASD). The Koch Triangle (triangle of the trioventricular node) (科赫三角) is a triangular zone which presents between the attachment of the septal leaflet of the tricuspid valve, the anteromedial margin of the opening of the coronary sinus, and the Todaro tendon (a palpable round subendocardial tendon in front of the orifice of inferior vena cava) . Koch triangle is an important surgical landmark since it contains the atrioventricular node and its atrial connections.

2. The Right Ventricle (RV)

The right ventricle (右心室) (Fig.6-6) is triangular in shape and extends from the tricuspid valve in the right atrium. The convex anterosuperior surface makes up a large part of the anterior surface of the heart, and the inferior surface is flat and is related mainly to the central tendon of diaphragm. The wall of the right ventricle is relatively thin (about 0.3 to 0.5 cm), and the ratio of the thickness of the right to left ventricular walls usually is 1: 3. The inlet and outlet parts of the right ventricle are divided by the supraventricular crest (室上嵴), which is a prominent muscular ridge between the right atrioventricular orifice and the orifice of pulmonary trunk. The trabeculated inlet part located posterior to the body of sternum at the level of the fourth and fifth intercostal spaces. The tricuspid complex guards the venous blood running from the right atrium to the right ventricle through the right artrioventricular orifice. The smooth-walled outflow tract conus arteriosus (动脉圆锥或漏斗) is cone-shaped, leads upward to the orifice of pulmonary trunk.

The trabeculae carneae (肉柱) are rounded or irregular muscular columns which project from the whole of the inner surface of the ventricle, with the exception of the conus arteriosus. It is irregularly arranged bundles of myocardium. The septomar-ginal trabecula (隔缘肉柱) is also named as the moderator band (节制索), which extends from interventricular septum to the base of anterior papillary muscle, as part of the conduction system of the heart involves carrying the right bundle branch. The papillary muscles (乳头肌) are conical-shaped projections with bases attached to the ventricular wall and the tips with the chordae tendineae inserted on the free edge of the tricuspid valvular leaflets. Three groups of papillary muscles are located in anterior, posterior (inferior) and septal positions. The anterior papillary muscles are the largest, and arise from the right anterolateral ventricular wall between the anterior cusps of the tricuspid valve and the posterior ones. The posterior (inferior) papillary muscles, smaller than the anterior papillary muscles, arise from the myocardium inferior to the posterior cusps of the tricuspid valve. The smallest septal papillary muscles arise from the interventricular septum mainly to the septal cusps.

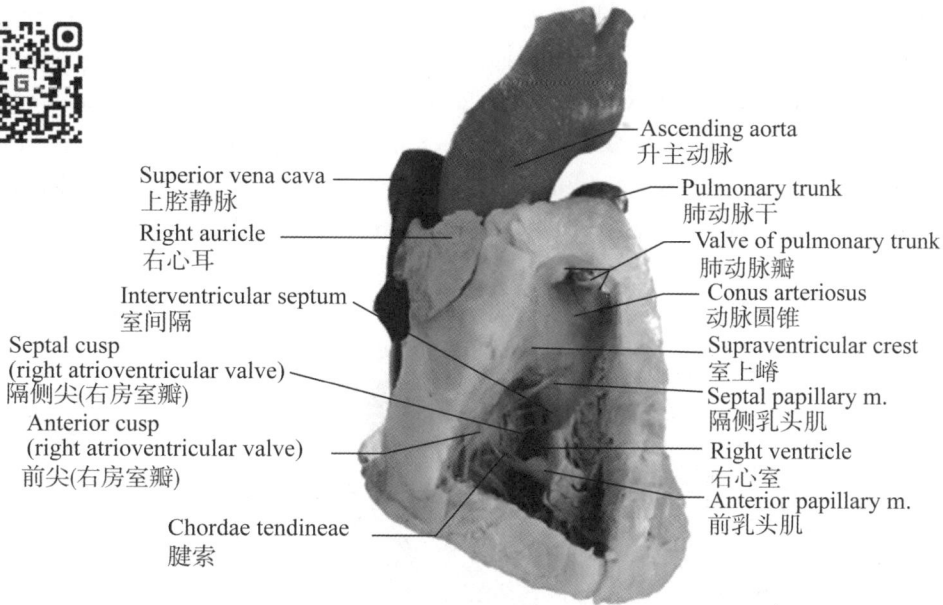

Fig.6-6   Internal view of the right ventricle (m.: muscle)

3. The Left Atrium

The left atrium (LA, 左心房, Fig.6-7) lies behind the right atrium and forms the greater part of the base of the heart. It's covered anteriorly by the pulmonary trunk and ascending aorta, and the pericardium separates it from the esophagus posteriorly. Left atrium is similar to the right atrium, it has a main cavity (vestibule) and an auricle. It's smaller in volume than the right atrium, but the walls are thicker (3mm on average). The left atrium lacks a crista terminalis, the muscle bundles are arranged in a whorl-like fashion. The left auricle (左心耳) is longer and narrower than the right auricle. It contains pectinate muscles which are smaller than the right one. The tip of the auricle has a variable position, often lying over the pulmonary trunk and anterior interventricular branch of the left coronary artery. It's a site for thrombus formation, especially in cases of atrial fibrillation.

Five orifices of left atrium

Four inlets are four orifices of pulmonary veins (left and right, superior and inferior), two from each lung, and open through the posterior wall. The orifices at their point of entry are smooth and oval. One outlet is the left atrioventricular orifice, blood leaves through the left atrioventricular orifice to the left ventricle.

4. The Left Ventricle

The cone-shaped left ventricle (LV, 左心室, Fig. 6-7) is located posteriorly and left to the right ventricle. The walls are three times thicker than those of the right ventricle. The anterior and inferior interventricular sulci indicate the lines of mural attachment of the ventricular septum and the limits of the ventricular territories. One inlet is the left atrioventricular orifice (左房室口) guarded by the mitral valve or left atrioventricular (二尖瓣). One outlet is the aortic orifice (主动脉口) guarded by the aortic valve (主动脉瓣).

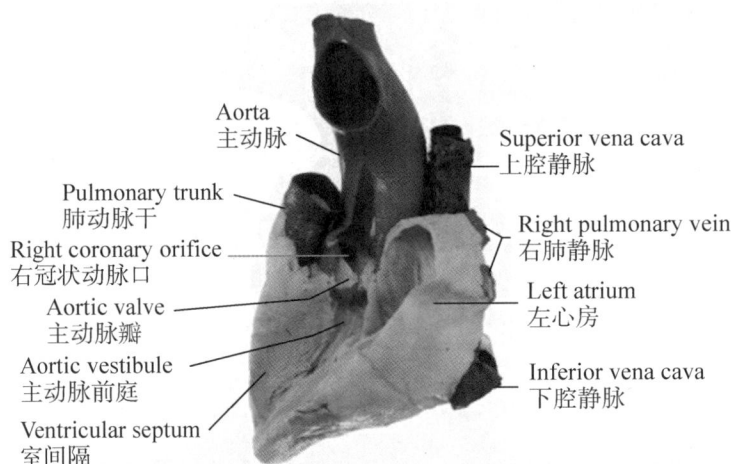

Fig.6-7   Internal view of the left ventricle

Two parts are divided by the anterior cusps of the mitral valve. The inflow tract is posterior and left to the anterior cusps of mitral valve. The walls are rough because there are well-developed trabeculae carneae and two groups of large papillary muscles, but no moderator band. The outflow tract is the anteromedial portion of the left ventricle and also called the aortic vestibule (主动脉前庭). It's a smooth area leading to the aortic orifice.

6.2.4   Valves

The heart valves are uniquely designed gates that promote the unidirectional flow of blood through the heart. They are attached to special muscular appendages that help to keep them stable.

1. The Tricuspid Valve

The tricuspid valve (the right atrioventricular valve, 三尖瓣) guards the right atrioventricular orifice and consists of three leaflets formed by a fold of endocardium with some enclosed connective tissue. Three triangular leaflets (cusp) are anterior, posterior (inferior) and septal leaflets. The bases of leaflets are attached to the fibrous ring (tricuspid anulus) surrounding the atrioventricular orifice, and the free margins and ventricular surfaces are attached to the chordae tendineae (腱索), fine and white fibrous collagenous structures, attach to papillary muscles. The tricuspid anulus, leaflets, chordae tendineae and papillary muscles constitute the right atrioventricular valvular complex.

2. The Mitral Valve

The mitral valve (the left atrioventricular valve, 二尖瓣) guards the left atrioventricular orifice, which has a structure similar to that of the tricuspid valve. Two triangular leaflets are anterior and posterior with commissural leaflets between them (posteromedial and anterolateral commissures). The anterior leaflet is the larger and intervenes between the atrioventricular and aortic orifices, and the posterolateral one is the posterior leaflet. The mitral anulus, leaflets, chordae tendineae and papillary muscles constitute the left atrioventricular valvular complex. The mitral, tricuspid and aortic orifices are intimately connected at the site of the central fibrous body.

Similar functions for the right and left atrioventricular valves: The valves are open during ventricular diastole to allow blood to enter ventricles from atria, and close during ventricular systole to prevent regurgitation of blood into atria.

3. The Pulmonary Valve

The pulmonary valve (肺动脉瓣, Fig.6-8) guards the orifice of pulmonary trunk(肺动脉口) at the top of the conus arteriosus. It has three semilunar leaflets, and each with a free border that has central nodules of semilunar valve. For a fetus, the leaflets are anterior, posterior and septal position before the heart has rotated to the left. In the adult, the leaflets become anterior, right and left, respectively. The curved lower margins and sides of each leaflet are attached to the arterial wall. The open mouths of the leaflets are directed upward into the pulmonary trunk.

4.T he Aortic Valve

The aortic valve (主动脉瓣, Fig.6-8) guards the aortic orifice and its structure is precisely similar to the pulmonary valve. It has three semilunar leaflets (right, left and post). One is situated on the anterior wall (right leaflet) and two are located on the posterior wall (left and posterior leaflets). Behind each cusp, the aortic wall bulges to form a corresponding aortic sinus (主动脉窦). The right aortic sinus gives rise to the right coronary artery, and the left posterior sinus gives rise to the left coronary artery. Linking the sinuses to the origins of the coronary arteries, three aortic sinuses are also named as right coronary, left coronary and non-adjacent (non-coronary) sinuses, respectively. The orifice of each coronary artery is beyond the level of the free border of aortic valvular leaflet.

Similar functions for pulmonary and aortic valves

During ventricular systole, the leaflets are pressed against the wall of the vessel by the outrushing blood, and allow the blood to force upward. During ventricular diastole, blood flows back toward the heart and enters the sinuses, and the valve leaflets fill, come into apposition in the center of the lumen, and close the corresponding orifice.

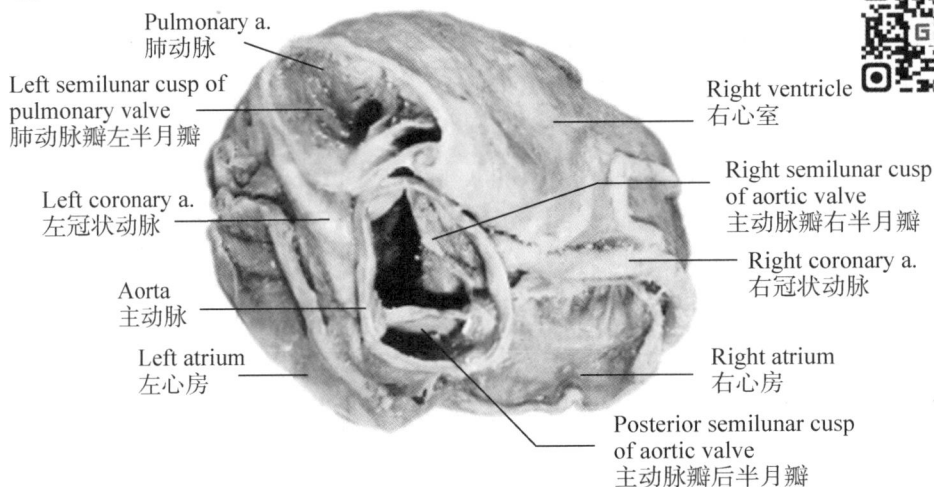

Pulmonary a.
肺动脉

Left semilunar cusp of
pulmonary valve
肺动脉瓣左半月瓣

Left coronary a.
左冠状动脉

Aorta
主动脉

Left atrium
左心房

Right ventricle
右心室

Right semilunar cusp
of aortic valve
主动脉瓣右半月瓣

Right coronary a.
右冠状动脉

Right atrium
右心房

Posterior semilunar cusp
of aortic valve
主动脉瓣后半月瓣

Fig.6-8 Aortic valve

6.2.5 Structure of Heart

The heart consists of muscular fibers, and of fibrous rings which serve for their attachment. It is covered by the visceral layer of the serous pericardium (浆膜心包) (epicardium) (心外膜) that also contains the juxtacardiac parts of its great vessels, and lined by the endocardium (心内膜). Between these two membranes is the muscular wall myocardium (心肌).

1. Walls of the Heart

Endocardium (心内膜) is the inner coat of the heart wall, and continuous with the valve flaps. It's formed by the endothelial tissue and a thick subendothelial layer of elastic and collagenous fibers and serves as protective inner lining of the chambers and valves. Myocardium (心肌层) is arranged spirally and attached to fibrous rings surrounding the four orifices of heart. The cardiac muscle tissue is separated by connective tissues and including blood capillaries, lymph capillaries, and nerve fibers. The thickness of the myocardium varies in accordance with the force needed to eject blood from the particular chamber. Epicardium (心外膜) is the visceral layer of serous membrane (visceral pericardium). The coronary vessels and their main branches are embedded in this layer.

2. Interatrial Septum

Interatrial Septum (房间隔) is located between the right and left atria, which faces forward and to the right. The fossa ovalis is clearly visible in the interatrial septum just above the orifice of the inferior vena cava. Interventricular septum (室间隔) is located between right and left ventricles. It has a thin upper membranous part (the most predilection site of ventricular septal defects, VSD) and a thick lower muscular part. Based on the attachment of the septal cusp of the tricuspid valve, the membranous part is considered to be divided into the upper atrioventricular part(between the left ventricle and the right atrium) and the lower interventricular part (between the left and right ventricles). The muscular part is the major part of the septum.

3. Fibrous Skeleton of the Heart

Fibrous skeleton of the heart (心纤维支架) consists of dense, fibrous connective tissue in the four fibrous rings and interconnecting areas between the atria and the ventricles. The four rings surround the two atrioventricular, pulmonary, and aortic orifices. The interconnecting areas include the right and left fibrous trigones. The right fibrous trigone (右纤维三角) is also named as the central fibrous body (中心纤维体), which is the thickened area of connective tissue among the rings of the bicuspid valve, the tricuspid valve and the aortic valve. It adheres inferiorly to the muscular part of the interventricular septum, and forwardly connects with the membranous part of the interventricular septum. The Todaro tendon (Todaro 腱) lies in the deep of endocardium of the right ventricle, and anteriorly connects with the central fibrous body. The left fibrous trigone (左纤维三角) is a thickened triangle area of the connective tissue between the aortic ring and the left atrioventricular ring. It's a landmark during the operation of the mitral valve.

6.2.6　Cardiac Conduction System

The cardiac conduction system (心传导系统, Fig.6-9) consists of specialized cardiac muscle cells that generate and distribute electrical impulses through the heart. The spread of excitation is very rapid, but different parts of the ventricles are excited at slightly different times. The five components of cardiac conduction system are sinoatrial node (窦房结), internodal atrial myocardium (internodal tracts) (结间束), atrioventricular node (房室结), atrioventricular bundle (房室束) with its left and right bundle branches, and subendocardial plexus of conduction cells (the purkinje fibers)(浦肯野纤维).

The sinoatrial node initiates the cardiac cycle by producing an electrical impulse (generated in the nodal cells) that spreads over both atria, causing them to contract simultaneously and force blood into the ventricles, function as the cardiac pacemaker. The basic depolarization rate of the sinoatrial node is 70 to 80 times per minute for adults. The impulse is transmitted over preferentially conducting to right and left atria, and then to internodal tracts, and passes to the atrioventricular node. The impulse is delayed by 40 ms at the atrioventricular node, and then the impulse continues through the atrioventricular bundle. The atrioventricular bundle divides into the right and the left bundle branches (左右束支), which are continuous with the conduction myofibers within the subendocardial plexus in ventricular walls —Purkinje fibers. Stimulation of these fibers causes the ventricles to contract simultaneously.

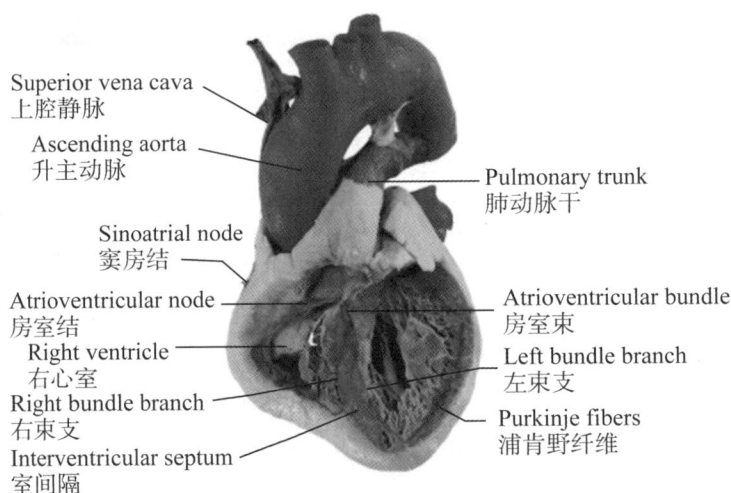

Superior vena cava 上腔静脉
Ascending aorta 升主动脉
Pulmonary trunk 肺动脉干
Sinoatrial node 窦房结
Atrioventricular node 房室结
Atrioventricular bundle 房室束
Right ventricle 右心室
Left bundle branch 左束支
Right bundle branch 右束支
Purkinje fibers 浦肯野纤维
Interventricular septum 室间隔

Fig.6-9　The conduction system of the heart

1. Sinoatrial Node

Sinoatrial node (SA node, 窦房结) is the cardiac pacemaker, and is a cigar-shaped structure, 8 to 25 mm long, located at the junction of right atrium and superior vena cava, upper part of the sulcus terminalis, under the epicardium, and penetrating the atrial myocardium.

2. Atrioventricular Node

Atrioventricular node (AV node, 房室结) is an oblique, half-oval atrial structure, located in the lower part of interatrial septum just above the orifice of coronary sinus, under the endocardium. The lower part related to the membranous part of the interventricular septum. Its anatomical landmarks are the boundaries of the triangle of Koch (the septal leaflet of the tricuspid valve, the opening of the coronary sinus and the tendon of Todaro).

3. Internodal Atrial Myocardium (Internodal Tracts)

Specialized pathways of the internodal atrial myocardium (internodal tracts) (结间束) have been considered to connect the sinuatrial and atrioventricular nodes, but there is no morphological evidence that tracts occur in the atrial walls.

4. Atrioventricular Bundle

Atrioventricular bundle (AV bundle, 房室束) is the direct continuation of the atrioventricular node. It passes forward through the right fibrous trigon to reach the inferior border of membranous part, and divides into right and left bundle branches at the upper border of the muscular part of interventricular septum. The right bundle branch (右束支) is a narrow, discrete and rounded group of fascicles, which passes down on the right side of interventricular septum to reach the septo-marginal trabecular and into the base of anterior papillary muscle. The left bundle branch (左束支) passes down on the left side of interventricular septum beneath the endocardium. It is usually divides into two branches, fine branches leave the sheets, forming subendocardial networks, firstly surround the papillary muscles and then curve back subendocardially to be distributed to all parts of the ventricle. The right and left bundle branches eventually become continuous with the Purkinje fibers.

5. Purkinje Fibers

Purkinje fibers (Purkinje, 浦肯野纤维) are continuous with myocardium. Stimulation of these fibers causes the ventricles to contract simultaneously

6.2.7   Vessels of the Heart

The myocardium is supplied with blood by the right and left coronary arteries (Fig.6-10). These two vessels arise from the ascending part of the aorta, at the location of the aortic (semilunar) valve. The level of the opening of each artery is variable. They also form a variable and often insignificant anastomosis via marginal and interventricular loops. The majority of the veins are drained by the coronary sinus into the right atrium. A portion of the veins directly drain into the right atrium.

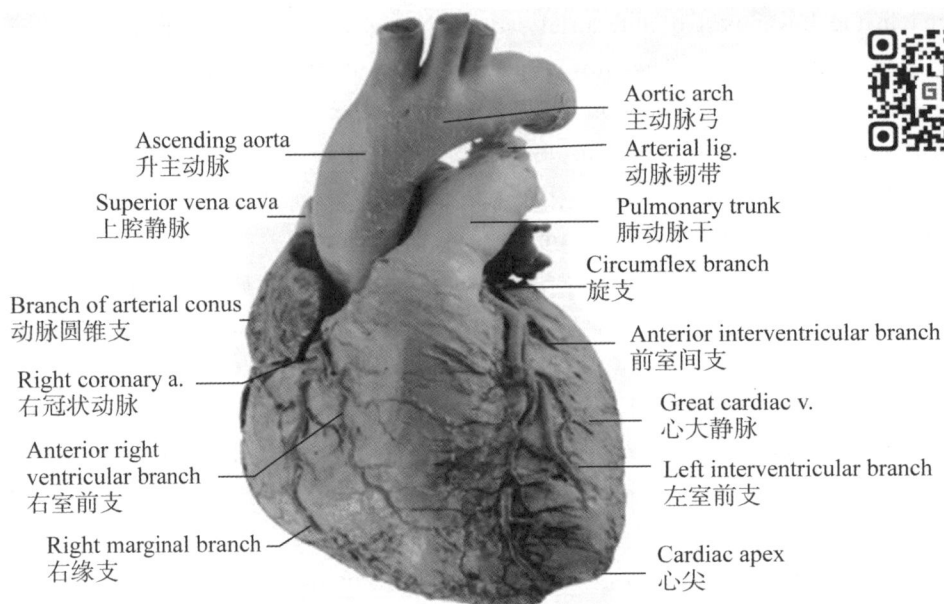

Fig.6-10　Blood supply of the heart

1. Coronary Arteries

The coronary arteries (冠状动脉) arise from the root of the ascending aorta. The left and right aortic sinus give rise to the corresponding left and right coronary arteries (respectively).

(1) Left coronary artery

The left coronary artery (左冠状动脉) arises from left aortic sinus and runs between pulmonary trunk and left auricle into coronary sulcus. Left coronary artery usually larger in calibre than the right, supplies almost all of the left ventricle and atrium, and 2/3 of the anterior interventricular septum, including the atrioventricular bundle and its branches.

Main branches. Anterior interventricular branch (前室间支) is commonly desc-ribed as the continuation of the left coronary artery. It travels downward in the anterior interventricular groove and reaches the cardiac apex, more frequently, it curves around the notch of the cardiac apex into the inferior interventricular sulcus, meeting the terminal parts of the inferior interventricular branches of the right coronary artery. The anterior interventricular artery gives off right and left anterior ventricular and interventricular septal branches. Circumflex branch (旋支) travels to left in coronary sulcus, and continues around the left cardiac border into the posterior and inferior aspect. Proximally, the left atrial auricle usually overlaps it. It gives off a larger left marginal artery and smaller anterior and inferior branches. The circumflex branch serves the left atrium and ventricle, lesser portion of anterior wall of right ventricle.

(2) **Right coronary artery**

The right coronary artery (右冠状动脉) arises from the right aortic sinus and runs between right auricle and pulmonary trunk into the coronary sulcus. It gives the right circumflex and posterior interventricular branches approximately at the atrioventricular crux. The right coronary artery supplies the right atrium and right ventricle, the sinoatrial and atrioventricular nodes, the interatrial septum, a portion of the left atrium, the posterior one third of the interventricular septum, and a portion of the posterior part of the left ventricle. The right coronary artery more often reaches the left border by anastomosing with the circumflex branch of the left coronary artery.

Main branches. Posterior interventricular branch (后室间支) travels downward in the posterior interventricular groove and anastomoses near the apex with the anterior interventricular branch of the left coronary artery. It may flank either to the right or left, or on both sides, by these parallel branches. It supplies the inferior walls of both ventricles on bilateral sides of the interventricular groove and posterior one third of interventricular septum. Right marginal branch (右缘支) is larger in calibre and travels along inferior border, and reaches the cardiac apex in most cases. Branch of sinuatrial node (窦房结支) passes posteriorly around the superior vena cava to supply the sinoatrial node. Its origin is variable and sometimes from the left coronary artery (40%).

2. Cardiac Veins

The heart is drained by three sets of veins as the coronary sinus and its tributaries, the anterior cardiac veins and the smallest cardiac veins.

The coronary sinus (冠状窦) lies the inferior atrioventricular sulcus between the left atrium and ventricle on the posterior surface of the heart. It carries most of venous blood from myocardium and opens into the right atrium between the opening of the inferior vena cava and the right atrioventricular orifice. The tributaries of the coronary sinus are the great, middle and small cardiac veins. The great cardiac vein (心大静脉) begins at the cardiac apex, and ascends in the anterior interventricular sulcus to the atrioventricular sulcus, which passes to the left and posteriorly to enter the coronary sinus at its origin. The middle cardiac vein (心中静脉) begins at the cardiac apex and runs posteriorly in the inferior interventricular sulcus to end in the coronary sinus near its atrial termination. The small cardiac vein (心小静脉) lies in the anterior part of the inferior atrioventricular sulcus between the right atrium and ventricle, and opens into the atrial end of the coronary sinus.

The anterior cardiac veins (心前静脉), usually two or three, sometimes five veins, drain the venous blood of anterior part of the right ventricle. They cross the right part of the atrioventricular groove, passing deep or superficial to the right coronary artery, and end in the right atrium.

The smallest cardiac veins (心最小静脉) open directly into all chambers of the heart. Their numbers and sizes are highly variable. They primarily return venous blood from the inner myocardial walls into the right atrium and ventricle and, to a lesser extent, into the left atrium and ventricle.

6.2.8 Pericardium (心包)

The pericardium (Fig. 6-11) contains the heart and the cardiac parts of its great vessels, with a normal combined thickness of 1 mm to 2 mm. Pericardium divides into 2 parts which are the fibrous pericardium and the serous pericardium. Many functions of pericardium are facilitating intrathoracic cardiac stability, reducing friction, limiting cardiac distension and chamber dilation and so preventing hypertrophy.

1. Fibrous Pericardium

The fibrous pericardium (纤维心包) is roughly conical and covers the heart. Superiorly, it is continuous exteriorly with the adventitia of the great vessels. Inferiorly, it is mainly attached to the central tendon of the diaphragm and a small muscular area of its left half.

2. Serous Pericardium

The serous pericardium (浆膜心包) contains 2 layers which are parietal layer (adheres to the heart and forms its epicardium) and visceral layer (adheres to the internal surface of the fibrous pericardium). The serous pericardium produces the lubricating pericardial fluid that allows the heart to beat in a kind of frictionless bath. The potential space between the parietal and visceral layers of serous pericardium is called the pleural cavity (胸膜腔). Normally, the cavity contains a small amount of serous fluid which acts as a lubricant to facilitate movements and shape change of the heart. The points of reflection of the serous pericardium around the great veins (the venae cava and four pulmonary veins) and arteries (the aorta and the pulmonary trunk) of the heart are arranged as two complex pericardial tubes.

3. The Pericardial Sinus

The transverse sinus of pericardium (心包横窦) is posterior to ascending aorta and pulmonary trunk and anterior to superior vena cava and left atrium. Ascending aorta and the pulmonary trunk can be clamped by the sinus to block the blood stream temporarily during the operation of the heart.

The oblique sinus of pericardium (心包斜窦) is culdesac, an inverted J in shape, bounded by pulmonary veins on either side, inferior vena cava, and lies behind the left atrium.

The anterior inferior sinus of pericardium (心包前下窦) is located at the anteroinferior reflection of pericardial cavity between the anterior and inferior portions of serous pericardium. It's the lowest site of pericardial cavity with the upright position.

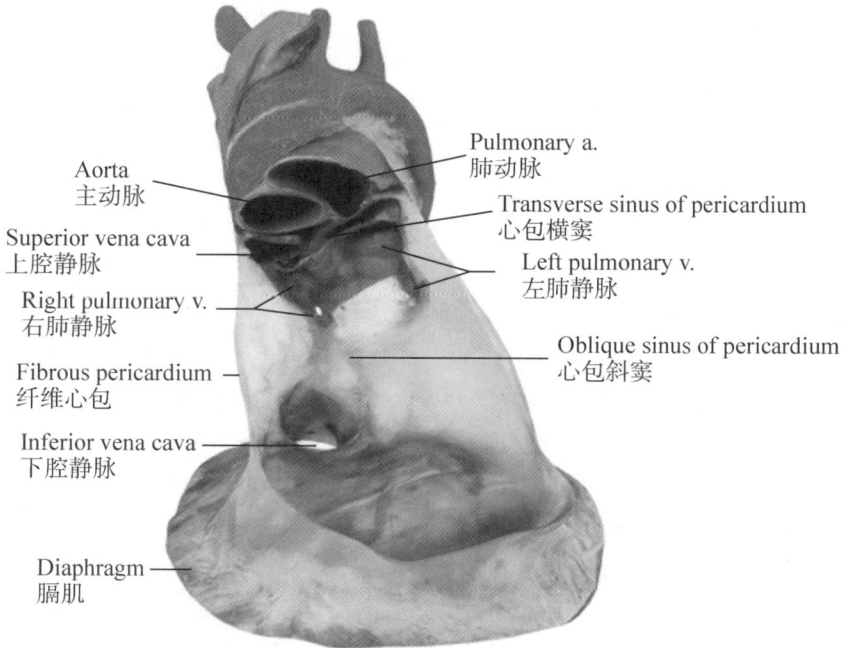

Fig.6-11   Pericardium

（南京医科大学　张永杰）

6.3　Arteries

The contraction of the left ventricle forces oxygenated blood into the arteries of the systemic circulation, and contraction of the right ventricle forces deoxygenated blood into the pulmonary circulation. The distribution of the arteries of the systemic circulation is always symmetry in the body, in the trunk of the body consisting of parietal and visceral branches. Furthermore, they are the shortest possible course and running, in the limbs, along the flexor surface, where they are less exposed to injury. In addition, they usually do not pass directly through muscles, avoiding compression. Arteries often travel alongside veins and nerves within a sheath of fascia, forming a neurovascular bundle.

6.3.1　Arteries of Pulmonary Circulation (肺循环)

1. Pulmonary Trunk

Pulmonary trunk (肺动脉干) conveys the venous blood (deoxygenated blood) from the right ventricle of the heart to the lungs. It is a short, wide vessel, about 5 cm in length and 3 cm in diameter, arising from the conus arteriosus of the right ventricle, superior and to the left of the supraventricular crest. It extends obliquely upward and backward, passing behind the ascending aorta, then splits up into the left and right pulmonary arteries at the level of the body of the T6 to provide blood for oxygenation in the lungs. The pulmonary trunk is connected to the aorta via the arterial ligament (动脉韧带), a remnant of the obliterated ductus arteriosus (ductus Botalli). In the developing fetus, the ductus arteriosus transports blood directly from the pulmonary trunk into the aorta and bypasses the fetal lungs.

(1) **Left pulmonary arteries** (左肺动脉)

The left branch of the pulmonary artery is shorter and smaller than the right. The left pulmonary artery emerges from under the concavity of the aortic arch and descends anterior to the descending thoracic aorta to enter the oblique fissure. The branches of the left pulmonary artery are variable. The first and largest branch is usually given off to the anterior segment of the left superior lobe.

(2) **Right pulmonary arteries** (右肺动脉)

The right branch of the pulmonary artery is longer and larger than the left. It runs horizontally to the right, behind the ascending aorta and the superior vena cava, and in front of the right bronchus, to the root of the right lung, where it divides into two branches. The lower branch goes to the middle and lower lobes of the lung; the upper branch distributes to the upper lobe.

6.3.2　Arteries of Systemic Circulation (体循环)

The aorta is the main arterial trunk of the systemic circulation, which ascends from the left ventricle to a position just above the heart, where it arches to the left, and then descends through the thorax and abdomen. It includes three portions as ascending aorta, aortic arch and descending aorta. Branches of the aorta carry oxygenated blood to all of the cells of the body.

1. Ascending Aorta

The ascending aorta (升主动脉) (Fig. 6-12) lies within the fibrous pericardium, enclosed in a tube of visceral serous pericardium together with the pulmonary trunk. It commences at the upper part of the base of the left ventricle, about 5 cm in length, on a level with the lower border of the third costal cartilage behind the left half of the sternum. It passes obliquely upward, forward, and to the right, in the direction of the heart's axis, as high as the upper border of the second right costal cartilage, describing a slight curve in its course, and being situated. The anatomic dilations of the ascending aorta, which occurs just above the aortic valve. There are three aortic sinuses(主动脉窦): the left, the right and the posterior sinuses. The left and right aortic sinuses give rise to the left and right coronary arteries (左右冠状动脉).

2. Aortic Arch

The aortic arch (主动脉弓), continuing from the ascending aorta, lies mainly within the superior mediastinum. The arch of the aorta begins at the level of the upper border of the second sternocostal articulation of the right side, and runs at the first upward, backward, and to the left in front of the trachea, then, it directs backward on the left side of the trachea and finally passes downward on the left side of the body of T4 vertebra and continuous with the descending aorta. The aortic isthmus is a small stricture at the border of the aortic arch with the descending aorta. The concavity of the aortic arch is most commonly inferior to the sternal plane. From right to left, the brachiocephalic trunk (头臂干), left common carotid artery (左颈总动脉) and left subclavian artery (左锁骨下动脉) arise from the convex aspect of the aortic arch.

The brachiocephalic trunk is the first branch from the aortic arch. It is short and rises superiorly through the mediastinum to a point near the junction of the sternum and the right clavicle, where it branches into the right common carotid artery (右颈总动脉), which extends to the right side of the neck, the head, and the right subclavian artery (右锁骨下动脉), which supplies the right shoulder and the upper limb. The left common carotid artery supplies to the left side of the neck and head, and the left subclavian artery supplies the left shoulder and the upper limb.

3. Descending Aorta

The descending aorta (降主动脉) is contained in the posterior mediastinum. It is continuous with the aortic arch at the level of the lower border of T4 vertebra, further subdivided into thoracic and abdominal aorta by the aortic hiatus of diaphragm in front of the lower border of T12 vertebra. It leaves at its origin, and generally reaches the midline, anterior to the vertebral bodies. It provides visceral branches to the organs in the thoracic and abdominal cavities, and parietal branches to the thoracic and abdominal wall and vertebral column. It finally bifurcates into the left and right common iliac arteries in front of the lower border of L4 vertebra.

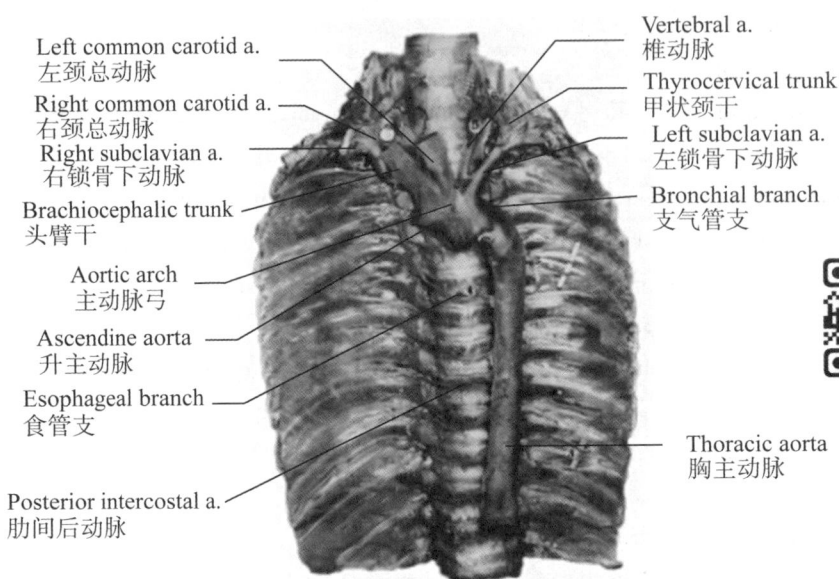

Fig.6-12　The aortic arch

4. Arteries of Head and Neck

(1) Common carotid arteries

The common carotid arteries (颈总动脉) provide the main blood supply to the head and neck region. There is one common carotid artery on either side of the body and these arteries differ in their origin. The left common carotid artery arises from the aortic arch within the superior mediastinum, while the right common carotid artery arises from the brachiocephalic trunk posterior to the right sternoclavicular joint. They ascend in the neck just above the level of the upper border of the thyroid cartilage, and each divides into two branches: the external carotid artery (颈外动脉), which supplies the external head, face and most portion of the neck, and the internal carotid artery (颈内动脉), which supplies the cranial and orbital contents. The common carotid artery has two specialized organs near its bifurcation: the carotid sinus (颈动脉窦) and the carotid glomus (颈动脉小球). The carotid sinus appears as the dilation at the bifurcation of the common carotid artery and the beginning of the international artery, it contains baroreceptors which can monitor changes of blood pressure. The carotid glomus (carotid body) is an oval structure lying posterior to the carotid bifurcation, and contains chemoreceptors which can monitor the changes in blood chemistry, primarily oxygen content.

(2) External carotid arteries

The external carotid arteries (颈外动脉) begins opposite to the upper border of the thyroid cartilage, levels with the intervertebral disc between the third and the fourth cervical vertebrae, taking a slightly curved course, passes upward and forward, and then inclines backward to the space behind the neck of the mandible, where it divides into the superficial temporal artery (颞浅动脉) and the maxillary artery(上颌动脉). A fingertip placed in the carotid triangle (the termination of the common carotid) perceives a powerful arterial pulsation. The principal branches arising from the external carotid artery arc described as follows.

1) The superior thyroid artery (甲状腺上动脉) arises from the anterior surface near the bifurcation, and passes downward and forward to the superior pole of the thyroid gland. It serves the muscles of the hyoid region, the larynx and vocal folds, and the thyroid gland.

2) The lingual artery (舌动脉) arises from the anterior surface of the external carotid artery at the level of hyoid bone, passes deep to the hyoglossus muscle and into the tongue. It supplies the tongue and sublingual gland.

3) The facial artery (面动脉) arise from anterior surface of the external carotid artery just above the lingual artery, passes deep to the stylohoid and posterior belly of the digastrics, and deep between the submandibular gland and mandible, and emerges over the edge of the mandible just anterior to the masseter muscle (pulsations of facial artery can be detected at this point and it's also an important point to control bleeding from the face), then enters the face. It serves the pharyngeal area, palate, chin, lips, and nasal region.

4) The occipital artery (枕动脉) arises from posterior aspect of the external carotid artery, near the level of origin of the facial artery, passes upward and posteriorly deep to the posterior belly of the digastrics, and serves the posterior portion of the scalp.

5) The posterior auricular artery (耳后动脉) arises from posterior aspect of the external carotid artery. It's a small branch and passes upward and posteriorly to serve the auricle of the ear and the scalp over the auricle.

6) The maxillary artery (上颌动脉) is one of the two terminal branches of the external carotid artery. It arises posterior to the neck of mandible, passes through the parotid gland, and goes into the infratemporal fossa just medial to the neck of mandible, and continues into the pterypalatine fossa. The maxillary artery gives off branches to the teeth and gums, the muscles of mastication, the nasal cavity, the eyelids, and the meninges.

7) The middle meningeal artery (脑膜中动脉) branches from the maxillary artery and goes upward to the cranial cavity through the foramen spinosum.

8) The superficial temporal artery (颞浅动脉) is another terminal branch of the external carotid artery. It arises posterior to the neck of mandible and appears as an upward continuation of the external carotid artery. It passes anterior to the ear, crosses the zygomatic process of the temporal bone, and above this point which is divided into anterior and posterior branches. It supplies the parotid gland and to the superficial

structures on the side of the head. Pulsations of the temporal artery can be easily detected in front of the external acoustic pore.

(3) Internal carotid arteries (颈内动脉)

The internal carotid artery ascends toward the base of the skull and passages through the carotid canal (in the petrous part of the temporal bone) to enter the cranial cavity. It gives off no branches in the neck and supplies the anterior part of the brain, the eye and its appendages, and the forehead and nose (Fig.6-13).

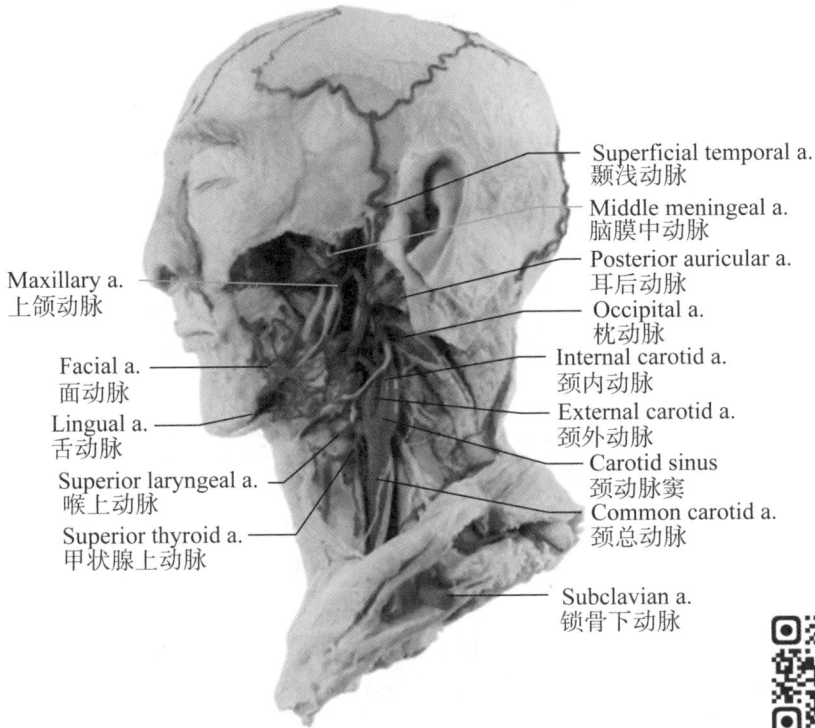

Fig.6-13　Common carotid arteries and branches

5. Arteries of the Upper Limbs

(1) Subclavian arteries

The subclavian arteries (锁骨下动脉) are paired major arteries of the upper thorax. On the right side, the subclavian artery arises from the brachiocephalic trunk behind the right sternoclavicular articulation or immediately superior to it, while on the left side, it springs from the arch of the aorta. It ascends into the neck posterior to sternoclavicular joint, then passes inferolaterally through the scalenus interspace towards the external border of the first rib, where it becomes the axillary artery. The usual branches of each subclavian artery include the vertebral artery (椎动脉), internal thoracic artery (胸廓内动脉), thyrocervical trunk (甲状颈干), costocervical trunk (肋颈干) and dorsal scapular artery (肩胛背动脉). The subclavian artery becomes the axillary artery at the lateral border of the first rib.

1) Vertebral arteries (椎动脉) are the first branches of the subclavian arteries. The vertebral artery ascends through the foramina in the transverse processes of the upper six cervical vertebrae and enters the skull through the foramen magnum, the right and left vertebral arteries converge medially as they ascend to the medulla and unite to form the basilar artery (基底动脉) at the lower border of the pons. Their major branches essentially supply blood to the upper spinal cord, brain stem, cerebellum, and a significant part of the posterior cerebral hemispheres.

2) Internal thoracic arteries (胸廓内动脉) supply the anterior chest wall and the breasts arising inferiorly from the subclavian artery opposite the root of the thyrocervical trunk. It is a paired artery, with one running along each side of the sternum and sending off the anterior intercostal arteries (肋间前动脉), at the level of the sixth intercostal space where it divides into the superior epigastric (腹壁上动脉)and musculophrenic arteries (肌膈动脉).

3) Thyrocervical trunk (甲状颈干) is a short thick trunk, which arises from the front of the subclavian artery, close to the medial border of the scalenus anterior, and divides almost immediately into three branches, the inferior thyroid (甲状腺下动脉), the suprascapular (肩胛上动脉), and the superficial cervical arteries (颈浅动脉).

4) Costocervical trunk (肋颈干) is from the upper and back part of the subclavian artery, behind the scalenus anterior on the right, and medial to the scalenus anterior on the left. It passes backward above the cervical pleura to the neck of the first rib, where it divides into the deep cervical artery (颈深动脉) and the supreme (highest) intercostal artery (肋间最上动脉).

(2) **The axillary artery**

The axillary artery (腋动脉) (Fig.6-14) is the continuation of the subclavian at the outer border of the first rib, and ends at the lower border of the tendon of teres major, where it takes the name of brachial artery (肱动脉). Its direction varies with the position of the limb. At its origin the artery is very deeply situated, but near its termination it is superficial, covered only by the skin and fascia. To facilitate the description of the vessel it divides into three portions: The first part lies above, the second behind, and the third below the pectoralis minor. The branches of the axillary artery include the superior thoracic artery (supreme thoracic artery) (胸上动脉) at the first part, the thoracoacromial (胸肩峰动脉) and lateral thoracic arteries (胸外侧动脉) at the second part, and the subscapular (肩胛上动脉), anterior and posterior humeral circumflex arteries (旋肱前动脉、旋肱后动脉) at the third part.

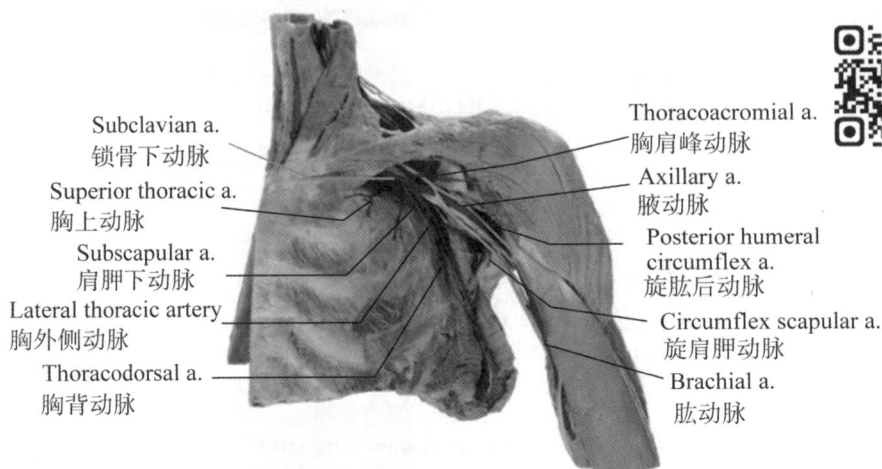

Fig.6-14　Axillary arteries and branches

1) Superior thoracic artery (胸上动脉) is a small branch from the axillary artery near the lower border of the subclavius. It runs anteromedially above the medial border of pectoralis minor, then passes between it and pectoralis major to the thoracic wall to supply these two muscles.

2) Thoracoacromial artery (胸肩峰动脉) is a short branch of the axillary artery. It pierces the clavipectoral fascia and divides into pectoral, acromial, clavicular and deltoid branches.

3) Lateral thoracic artery (胸外侧动脉) descends along the lateral border of pectoralis minor and passes to the deep surface of pectoralis major. It gives off branches to the serratus anterior, pectoral muscles and subscapularis, and breast for female.

4) Subscapular artery (肩胛下动脉) is the largest branch and usually arises from the axillary artery at the inferior border of subscapularis. It is divided into the circumflex scapular (旋肩胛动脉) and thoracodorsal arteries (胸背动脉). The circumflex scapular artery traverses the trilateral space and enters the infraspinous fossa under teres minor. The thoracodorsal artery enters the deep surface of latissimus dorsi, supplies the latissimus dorsi, serratus anterior, teres major and the intercostals.

5) Anterior humeral circumflex artery (旋肱前动脉) arises from the lateral side of the axillary artery at the distal border of subscapularis. It runs horizontally behind coracobrachialis and the short head of biceps, anterior to the surgical neck of humerus. It supplies the humeral head and shoulder joint.

6) Posterior humeral circumflex artery (旋肱后动脉) is larger than the anterior and also arises from the lateral side of the axillary artery at the distal border of subscapularis. It traverses the quadrilateral space curves round the surgical neck of humerus and supplies

the shoulder joint, deltoid, teres major and minor, and triceps brachii (Fig.6-14).

(3) Brachial artery

The brachial artery (肱动脉) is a continuation of the axillary artery, commences at the lower margin of the tendon of teres major, and, passing down the arm, ends about 1 cm below the bend of the elbow at the level of the radial neck, where it divides into the radial and ulnar arteries (桡动脉, 尺动脉). At first, the brachial artery lies medial to the humerus, but as it runs down the arm it gradually spirals in front of the humerus, and at the bend of the elbow it lies midway between its two epicondyles. The other branches of the brachial artery are the profunda brachii, deltoid, superior, middle and inferior ulnar collateral, and muscular arteries.

1) Deep brachial artery (profunda brachii artery)(肱深动脉) is a large vessel which arises from the posteromedial aspect of the brachial artery, distal to the teres major. It curves posteriorly near the radial nerve in the sulcus for radial nerve to supply the triceps brachii muscle, then descends between the brachioradialis and the brachialis to the front of the lateral epicondyle of the humerus, ends by anastomosing with the radial recurrent artery.

2) Superior ulnar collateral artery (尺侧上副动脉) arises from the brachial artery just below the middle of the arm. It accompanies the ulnar nerve and pierces the medial intermuscular septum to descend in the posterior compartment and supply the medial head of triceps brachii. And it ends under the flexor carpi ulnaris by anastomosing with the posterior ulnar recurrent, and inferior ulnar collateral arteries.

3) Inferior ulnar collateral artery (尺侧下副动脉) arises about 5 cm above the elbow. It forms an arch proximal to the olecranon fossa with the middle collateral branch of the profunda brachii artery. Behind the medial epicondyle, it gives off branches anastomose with the superior ulnar collateral and posterior ulnar recurrent arteries around the elbow-joint.

(4) Radial artery

The radial artery (桡动脉) is a direct continuation of the brachial artery, commences at the bifurcation of the brachial, just below the bend of elbow, and passes along the radial side of the forearm to the wrist. Proximally, it is overlapped anteriorly by the belly of brachioradialis, but elsewhere in its course it is covered only by the skin, superficial and deep fasciae. Above the wrist joint, the tendon of flexor carpi radialis is medial to its distal portion. At the wrist, the radial artery crosses the scaphoid bone and passes to the dorsum of hand. In the hand, it passes forward between the two heads of the first interosseous dorsalis, into the palm of the hand, finally, unites with the deep palm branch of the ulnar artery to form the deep palm arch.

1) Radial recurrent artery (桡侧返动脉) arises from the radial artery immediately

below the elbow. It ascends between the branches of the radial nerve, anterior to the supinator and then between the brachioradialis and brachialis. It supplies these muscles and then anastomoses with the radial collateral branch of the profunda brachii artery.

2) Superficial palmar branch (掌浅支) arises from the radial artery just before it passes to the dorsum of hand. It passes through and supplies the thenar muscles, and usually anastomoses with the terminal portion of the ulnar artery to form the superficial palmar arch.

3) Principal artery of thumb (拇主要动脉) arises from the radial artery to the tendon of flexor pollicis longus, and the artery seperates into two branches running along both sides of the thumb, and another branch (arteria radialis indicis) running along the lateral side of the index finger to its tip.

(5) Ulnar artery

The ulnar artery (尺动脉) arises from the brachial artery just distal to the elbow at the level of the radial neck. It descends on the medial side of forearm, initially deep to pronator teres, then between the flexor carpi radialis and flexor digitorum superficialis. At the wrist, it lies superficial to the flexor retinaculum and lateral to the pisiform bone, and enters the hand. In the hand, its terminal branch unites with the superficial palmar branch of the radial artery to form the superficial palm arch.

1) Common interosseous artery (骨间总动脉) is a short branch of the ulnar artery, about 1 cm in length, arises immediately below the tuberosity of the radius, and passes backward to the upper border of the interosseous membrane, then divides into two branches, the anterior and posterior interosseous arteries.

2) Ulnar recurrent artery (尺侧返动脉). The anterior ulnar recurrent artery arises from the ulnar artery distal to the elbow, and the posterior ulnar recurrent artery arises from the ulnar artery distal to the anterior ulnar recurrent artery. The anterior ulnar recurrent artery ascends between brachialis and pronator teres, and anastomoses with the inferior ulnar collateral artery. the posterior ulnar recurrent artery passes dorsomedially between the flexor digitorum profundus and flexor digitorum superficialis, and ascends between the medial epicondyle and olecranon.

3) Deep palmar branch (掌深支) arises from the ulnar artery distal to the pisiform bone. It passes the hypothenar muscles and anastomoses with the terminal branch of the radial artery to the deep palmar arch (Figs.6-15 & 6-16).

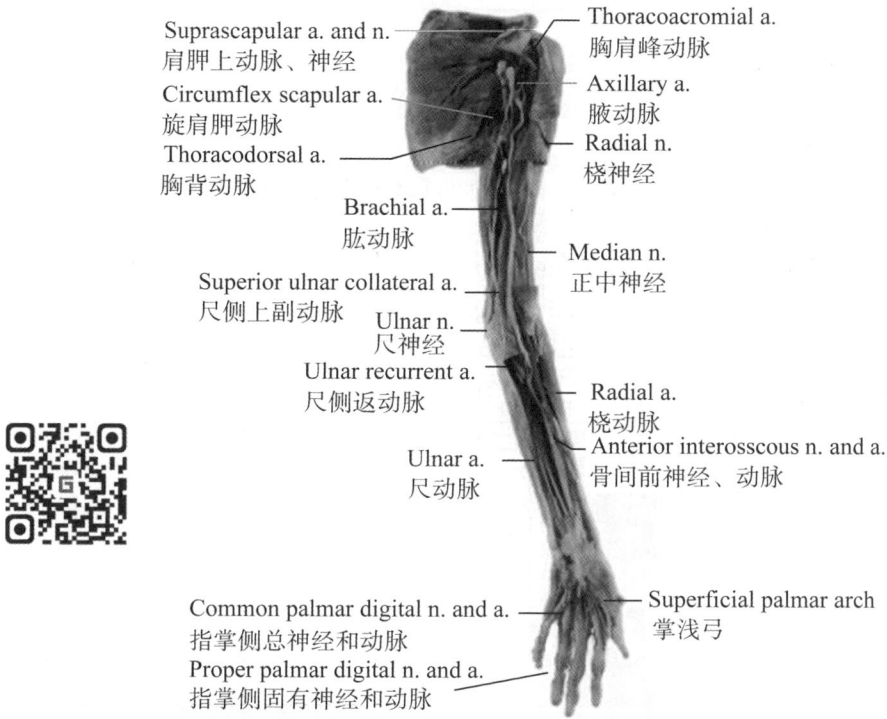

Suprascapular a. and n.
肩胛上动脉、神经

Circumflex scapular a.
旋肩胛动脉

Thoracodorsal a.
胸背动脉

Brachial a.
肱动脉

Superior ulnar collateral a.
尺侧上副动脉

Ulnar n.
尺神经

Ulnar recurrent a.
尺侧返动脉

Ulnar a.
尺动脉

Common palmar digital n. and a.
指掌侧总神经和动脉

Proper palmar digital n. and a.
指掌侧固有神经和动脉

Thoracoacromial a.
胸肩峰动脉

Axillary a.
腋动脉

Radial n.
桡神经

Median n.
正中神经

Radial a.
桡动脉

Anterior interosscous n. and a.
骨间前神经、动脉

Superficial palmar arch
掌浅弓

Fig.6-15   Muscles, blood vessels and nerves of the anterior aspect of the upper limb

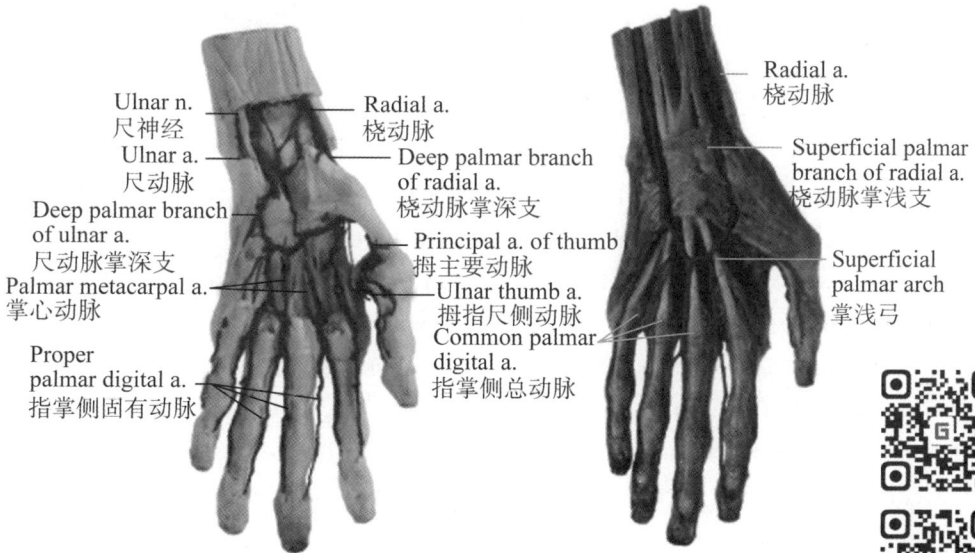

Ulnar n.
尺神经

Ulnar a.
尺动脉

Deep palmar branch of ulnar a.
尺动脉掌深支

Palmar metacarpal a.
掌心动脉

Proper palmar digital a.
指掌侧固有动脉

Radial a.
桡动脉

Deep palmar branch of radial a.
桡动脉掌深支

Principal a. of thumb
拇主要动脉

Ulnar thumb a.
拇指尺侧动脉

Common palmar digital a.
指掌侧总动脉

Radial a.
桡动脉

Superficial palmar branch of radial a.
桡动脉掌浅支

Superficial palmar arch
掌浅弓

Fig.6-16   Arteries of the hand

(6) Superficial palmar arch and deep palmar arch

1）Superficial palmar arch (掌浅弓) is formed mainly by the terminal branch of the ulnar artery and the superficial palmar branch of the radial artery. It lies between the palmar aponeurosis and the tendons of flexor digitorum superficialis, and forms a convex arch level with a transverse line. It gives off three common palmar digital arteries (指掌侧总动脉) and one ulnar artery of little finger (小指尺侧动脉) from its convexity. The common palmar digital arteries pass distally on the second to fourth lumbricals, each joined by a corresponding palmar metacarpal artery from the deep palmar arch, and divide into two proper palmar digital arteries running along the contiguous sides of all four fingers. The ulnar artery of little finger runs along the medial side of the little finger.

2) Deep palmar arch (掌深弓) is formed by deep palmar branch of the ulnar artery and the terminal branch of the radial artery. It lies deep to the tendons of the flexor digitorum profundus and proximal to the superficial parmar arch level with the carpometacarpal joint. It gives off three palmar metacarpal arteries to join the corresponding common palmar digital arteries (Fig.6-16).

6. Arteries of the Thorax

Thoracic Aorta (胸主动脉) is contained in the posterior mediastinum. It is continuous with the aortic arch at the level of the lower border of the fourth thoracic vertebra, and ends in front of the lower border of the twelfth thoracic vertebra at the aortic hiatus of the diaphragm. It leaves the vertebral column at its origin, and generally reaches the midline anterior to the vertebral bodies. It provides visceral branches to the organs in the thoracic cavity, and parietal branches to the thoracic wall and vertebral column.

(1) **Parietal branches of the thoracic aorta**

1) Posterior intercostal arteries (肋间后动脉) are usually nine pairs, arising from the posterior aspect of the descending thoracic aorta, and are distributed to the lower nine intercostal spaces (the third to the eleventh spaces). Each artery runs firstly backward through a space which is bounded above and below by the necks of the ribs, medially by the body of a vertebra, and laterally by an anterior costotransverse ligament, where it gives off a spinal branch entering the vertebral canal through the intervertebral foramen and is distributed to the spinal cord and its membranes and the vertebrae. Each artery crosses its intercostal space and continues forwards in its costal groove, as far as the angle of the rib, anastomoses with an anterior intercostal branch from either the internal thoracic or musculophrenic artery. Each posterior intercostal artery has dorsal, collateral, muscular and cutaneous branches.

2) Subcostal arteries (肋下动脉) constitute the lowest pair of branches derived from the thoracic aorta, and are in series with the intercostal arteries. Each artery runs laterally anterior to the body of the twelfth thoracic vertebra, and then, lies below the twelfth ribs.

3) Superior phrenic arteries (膈上动脉) are usually two to three small branches

arising from the lower part of the thoracic aorta and are distributed posteriorly to the upper surface of the diaphragm, and anastomose with the musculophrenic and pericardiacophrenic arteries.

(2)Visceral branches of the thoracic aorta

1) Bronchial arteries (支气管动脉) always vary from origin, number and size. There is usually only one right bronchial artery, which may arise from the right third posterior intercostal artery, or the superior left bronchial artery, or various right posterior intercostal arteries. The left bronchial arteries are usually two in number, and arise from the thoracic aorta. The bronchial arteries supply the pulmonary areolar tissue, bronchopulmonary lymph nodes, pericardium, visceral pleura and thoracic esophagus.

2) Esophageal arteries (食管动脉) are usually four or five in number, arise from the front or the right side of the thoracic aorta, and pass obliquely downward forming a chain of anastomoses along the esophagus. They anastomose with the esophageal branches of the inferior thyroid arteries above, and with ascending branches from the left inferior phrenic and left gastric arteries below.

3) Pericardial arteries (心包动脉) consist of a few small vessels which are distributed to the posterior surface of the pericardium (Fig.6-17).

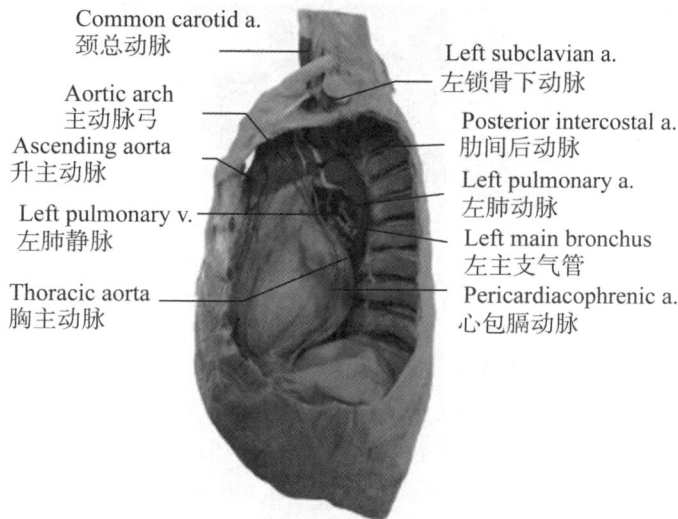

Common carotid a.
颈总动脉
Left subclavian a.
左锁骨下动脉
Aortic arch
主动脉弓
Ascending aorta
升主动脉
Posterior intercostal a.
肋间后动脉
Left pulmonary a.
左肺动脉
Left pulmonary v.
左肺静脉
Left main bronchus
左主支气管
Thoracic aorta
胸主动脉
Pericardiacophrenic a.
心包膈动脉

Fig.6-17   Thoracic aorta and its branches

7. Arteries of the Abdomen: Abdominal Aorta

Abdominal aorta (腹主动脉) begins at the aortic hiatus of the diaphragm in front of the lower border of the body of T12 vertebra. It descends in front of the vertebral column, ends on the body of L4 vertebra, and divides into two common iliac arteries. It provides larger visceral branches to the organs in the abdominal cavity, and parietal branches to the abdominal wall and vertebral column (Fig.6-18).

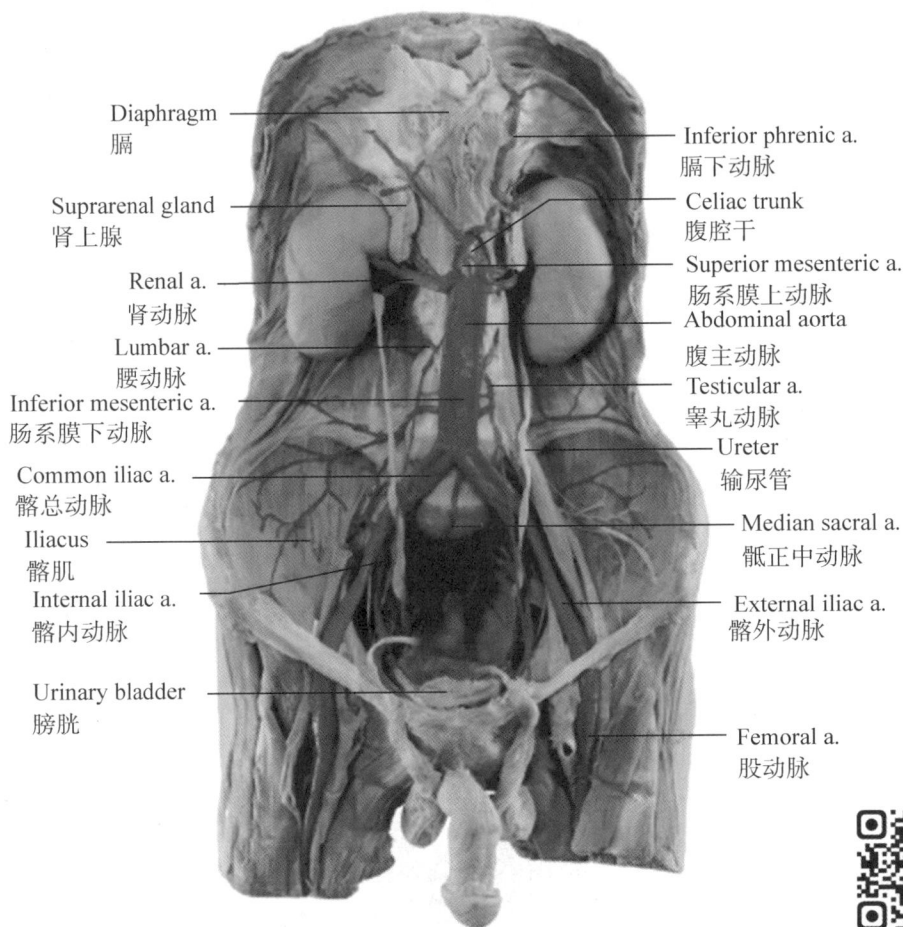

Fig.6-18   Abdominal aorta and its branches

(1) Parietal branches (Fig.6-19)

Inferior phrenic arteries (膈下动脉) are two small vessels, which supply the diaphragm but present varieties in their origin, usually arise from the abdominal aorta superior to the level of the coeliac trunk, or directly from the coeliac trunk, or occasionally from the renal artery. Each inferior phrenic artery gives off two or three small superior suprarenal arteries (肾上腺上动脉).

Lumbar arteries (腰动脉) are usually four in number on either side, and arise from the posterolateral aspect of the abdominal aorta, opposite to the bodies of the upper four lumbar vertebrae. The lumbar arteries anastomose with one another and the lower posterior intercostal, subcostal, iliolumbar, deep circumflex iliac and inferior epigastric arteries. Their branches supply the back muscles, vertebrae and their joints and the skin of the back.

Median sacral artery (骶正中动脉) is a small vessel, which arises from the back of the abdominal aorta above its bifurcation. It descends in the middle line in front of the fourth and fifth lumbar vertebrae, sacrum and coccyx, and ends in the glomus coccygeum. It gives off small branches reaching the pelvic surface of the sacrum, anus and rectum.

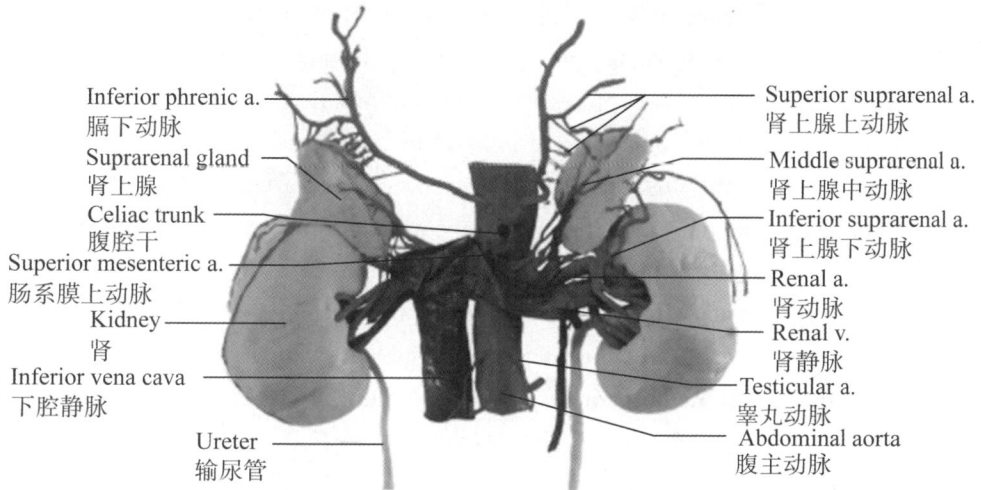

Inferior phrenic a.
膈下动脉
Suprarenal gland
肾上腺
Celiac trunk
腹腔干
Superior mesenteric a.
肠系膜上动脉
Kidney
肾
Inferior vena cava
下腔静脉
Ureter
输尿管

Superior suprarenal a.
肾上腺上动脉
Middle suprarenal a.
肾上腺中动脉
Inferior suprarenal a.
肾上腺下动脉
Renal a.
肾动脉
Renal v.
肾静脉
Testicular a.
睾丸动脉
Abdominal aorta
腹主动脉

Fig.6-19   The parietal branch of abdominal aorta

(2) Paired visceral branches

Middle suprarenal arteries (肾上腺中动脉) are two small vessels which arise from the lateral side of the abdominal aorta at the level of the first lumbar vertebra. They pass lateralward and slightly upward, over the crura of the diaphragm, to the suprarenal glands.

Renal arteries (肾动脉) are two large trunks, which arise from the lateral side of the aorta just below the origin of the superior mesenteric artery. Each is directed across the crus of the diaphragm, so as to form nearly a right angle with the aorta. The right renal artery is longer than the left, and passes behind the inferior vena cava, the right renal vein, head of the pancreas, and descending part of the duodenum. The left renal artery passes behind the left renal vein, the body of the pancreas and the splenic vein. In its extrarenal course, each renal artery gives off one or more inferior suprarenal arteries (肾上腺下动脉), and branches supplying perirenal tissue and the renal pelvis. Near the hilum of the kidney, each artery is divided into an anterior and a posterior branch, and then divide into segmental arteries (segmental, lobar, interlobar, arcuate and interlobular arteries, and afferent and efferent glomerular arterioles) supplying the renal vascular segments. Accessory renal arteries are common (approximately 30%) and usually arise from the abdominal aorta above or below the renal artery and follow it to the hilum, or to the superior or inferior pole. Rarely accessory renal arteries arise from the coeliac trunk, or superior mesenteric arteries, or the common iliac arteries.

The testicular arteries (睾丸动脉) in the male and the ovarian arteries (卵巢动脉) in the female are small paired vessels that arise from the front aspect of the abdominal aorta just below the renal arteries. The testicular arteries are two slender vessels of considerable length, and distribute to the testis. They descend along the psoas major and enter the pelvis anterior to the ureters and external iliac arteries. Both arteries then enter the deep inguinal ring and travel within the spermatic cord in the inguinal canal to the scrotum. Proximally, the testicular artery supplies the upper and middle parts of the ureter. Distally, the testicular artery gives off one or more internal testicular arteries, an inferior testicular artery, and branches supplying the epididymis. The ovarian arteries supply the ovaries. They descend behind the peritoneum, crossing the external iliac vessels to enter the lesser pelvis, then, turn medially in the suspensory ligament of the ovary and spit into several branches to supply the ovary and the lateral portion of the uterine tube. On each side one of its branches passes lateral to the uterus to unite with the uterine artery, and other branches accompany the round ligaments of uterus to the skin of the major labium and the inguinal region.

(3) Unpaired Visceral Branches

1) Celiac trunk (腹腔干) is the first unpaired branch of the abdominal aorta and arises just inferior to the aortic hiatus. It is a short and thick trunk about 1—3 cm long and passes almost horizontally anteriorly and slightly to the right superior to the body of the pancreas and the splenic vein. It is immediately divided into three arteries: the left gastric (胃左动脉), the common hepatic (肝总动脉) and the splenic arteries (脾动脉).

Left gastric artery (胃左动脉) passes upward and adjacent to the cardiac orifice of the stomach, then run along the lesser curvature between the two peritoneal leaves of the lesser omentum with multiple branches to the anterior and posterior surfaces of the stomach, after which it anastomoses with the right gastric artery. At the highest point of its course it gives off oesophageal branches.

Common hepatic artery (肝总动脉) directs anteriorly and laterally to the upper margin of the superior part of the duodenum and enters the hepatoduodenal ligament, where it is subdivided into the proper hepatic artery (肝固有动脉) and the gastroduodenal artery (胃十二指肠动脉). The proper hepatic artery ascends anterior to the hepatic portal vein and medial to the bile duct within the free margin of the hepatoduodenal ligament. Near the porta hepatis, it is divided into the left and right hepatic arteries (肝左动脉、肝右动脉) and enters the left and right lobes of liver respectively. The right hepatic artery branches a cystic artery (胆囊动脉) to the gallbladder before it enters the liver. The proper hepatic artery gives off a relatively small artery as the right gastric artery (胃右动脉). The right gastric artery runs forwards into the lesser omentum just above the superior part of the duodenum, and then it travels within the lesser omentum along the lesser curvature of the stomach, giving off branches to the anterior and posterior surfaces of the stomach to anastomose with the left gastric artery. The gastroduodenal artery descends posterior to the superior part of the duodenum to the inferior border of the pylorus, and divides into the right gastroepiploic artery (胃网膜右动脉) and superior pancreaticoduodenal arteries (胰十二指肠上动脉). The right gastro-omental artery passes inferiorly towards the midline and then runs laterally along the greater curvature between the greater omentum. It gives off gastric branches to the pyloric antrum and distal body of the stomach, omental branches into the greater omentum, and duodenal branches to the inferior aspect of the superior part of the duodenum. It ends by anastomosing with the left gastro-omental artery. The superior pancreaticoduodenal arteries include the posterior and anterior superior pancreaticoduodenal arteries. The posterior superior pancreaticoduodenal artery (胰十二指肠上后动脉) usually arises as the first branch of the gastroduodenal artery, and the anterior superior pancreaticoduodenal artery (胰十二指肠上前动脉) usually arises as a smaller terminal branch of the gastroduodenal artery. They descend respectively posterior or anterior to the head of the pancreas and to the groove between the descending duodenum and head of the pancreas, and supply the descending duodenum and head of the pancreas.

Splenic artery (脾动脉) is the largest branch of the celiac trunk, and is remarkable for the tortuosity of its course. It passes horizontally to the left, behind the stomach and the omental bursa, and along the upper border of the pancreas to the splenic hilum. Along its course, it gives off multiple small branches, including the dorsal pancreatic artery, the great pancreatic artery, and the artery to the tail of the pancreas. These branches often anastomose with the inferior pancreatic artery. Near the splenic hilum, it gives off the short gastric arteries (胃短动脉), the left gastroepiploic artery (胃网膜左动脉) and the posterior gastric artery (胃后动脉). The short gastric arteries vary in number, commonly between five and seven. They pass the gastrosplenic ligament to supply the fundus of the stomach on its greater curvature. The left gastro-omental artery runs anteroinferiorly into the gastrocolic ligament, and often anastomoses with the right gastro-omental artery. It gives off gastric branches to the fundus and body of the stomach, and omental branches to the greater omentum. A posterior gastric artery usually arises from the splenic artery posterior to the body of the stomach and ascends behind the omental bursa towards the fundus to supply the posterior surface of the stomach.

2) Superior mesenteric artery (肠系膜上动脉) is a large vessel which supplies the whole length of the small intestine, except the superior part of the duodenum; it also supplies the cecum, the ascending colon and about one-half of the transverse colon. It

arises from the front aspect of the abdominal aorta about 1 cm to 2 cm below the celiac trunk, at the level of the body of L1 vertebra. It passes steeply downward and forward, anterior to the uncinate process of the pancreas and the inferior part of the duodenum, and descends between the layers of the mesentery to the right iliac fossa. Its terminal branch anastomoses with the termination of the ileocolic artery. The superior mesenteric artery usually gives off the jejunal and ileal arteries (空肠动脉、回肠动脉) from its left side, and the ileocolic arteries (回结肠动脉), the right colic arteries (右结肠动脉), the middle colic arteries (中结肠动脉) and inferior pancreaticoduodenal arteries (胰十二指肠下动脉) from its right side.

Inferior pancreaticoduodenal artery (胰十二指肠下动脉) is given off from the superior mesenteric or from its first intestinal branch opposite the upper border of the inferior part of the duodenum. It divides into the anterior and posterior inferior pancreaticoduodenal arteries, and accordingly anastomoses with the anterior and posterior superior pancreaticoduodenal arteries. They distribute branches to the head of the pancreas and the descending and inferior parts of the duodenum.

Jejunal arteries (空肠动脉) are usually 4 to 6 in number and arise from the left side of the proximal portion of the superior mesenteric artery. They are distributed in the mesentery and to the jejunum via 1 to 3 tiers of arterial arcades. The most distal arterial arcade gives rise to straight arteries reaching the jejunum.

Ileal arteries (回肠动脉) are more numerous (around 8 to 12) and slightly smaller than the jejunal arteries. They arise from the left and anterior aspects of the superior mesenteric artery and run in the mesentery with 2 to 6 arterial arcades before giving rise to multiple straight arteries running directly towards the ileum.

Ileocolic artery (回结肠动脉) is the lowest branch arising from the concavity of the superior mesenteric artery, which is divided into a superior branch and an inferior branch. The superior branch runs up and anastomoses with the right colic artery. The inferior branch separates into the anterior and posterior cecal arteries, the appendicular artery, and an ileal branch that anastomoses with the end of the superior mesenteric artery. The appendicular artery (阑尾动脉) usually arises directly from the ileocolic artery. It descends posterior to the terminal portion of the ileum, and then runs along the free edge of mesoappendix to the terminal portion of appendix.

Right colic artery (右结肠动脉) is relatively small, and arises from the middle of the concavity of the superior mesenteric artery, or from a stem common to it and the ileocolic artery. It passes to the right behind the peritoneum and distributes to the ascending colon. Near the left side of the ascending colon, it is divided into a descending branch and an ascending branch. The descending branch anastomoses with the superior branch of the ileocolic artery, and the ascending branch anastomoses with a branch of the middle colic artery. These anastomoses form the marginal artery at the right colic flexure.

Middle colic artery (中结肠动脉) arises from the superior mesenteric just below the pancreas and passes downward and forward between the layers of the transverse mesocolon. It is usually divided into the right and left branches and distributed to the transverse colon. The right branch anastomoses with the ascending branch of the right colic artery, and the left branch anastomoses with a branch of the left colic artery near the left colic flexure.

3) Inferior mesenteric artery (肠系膜下动脉) is smaller than the superior mesen-teric artery and arises from the abdominal aorta at the level of the body of the L3 vertebra, about 3—4 cm proximal to the aortic bifurcation. It supplies the left half of the transverse colon, the descending colon, the sigmoid colon, and the greater part of the rectum.

Left colic artery (左结肠动脉) usually arises from the inferior mesenteric artery and runs to the left behind the peritoneum and in front of the psoas major. After a short but variable course, it is divided into an ascending branch and a descending branch. The ascending branch crosses in front of the left kidney and ends, between the two layers of the transverse mesocolon, by anastomosing with the middle colic artery. The descending branch anastomoses with branches from the sigmoid artery to form part of the marginal artery. The left colic artery is the dominant arterial supply of the left colic flexure.

Sigmoid arteries (乙状结肠动脉) are 2 to 5 in number, and descend obliquely in the sigmoid mesocolon anterior to the left psoas major. They supply the distal descending colon and sigmoid colon, and anastomose superiorly with the left colic artery and inferiorly with the superior rectal artery.

Superior rectal artery (直肠上动脉) is the continuation of the inferior mesenteric artery. It descends into the pelvis between the layers of the mesentery of the sigmoid colon. At the level of the third sacral vertebra, it is divided into two branches that descend on each side of the rectum and anastomose with the branches of the inferior rectal artery within the rectal submucosa.

The mesenteric artery and its branches can be seen in Fig. 6-20.

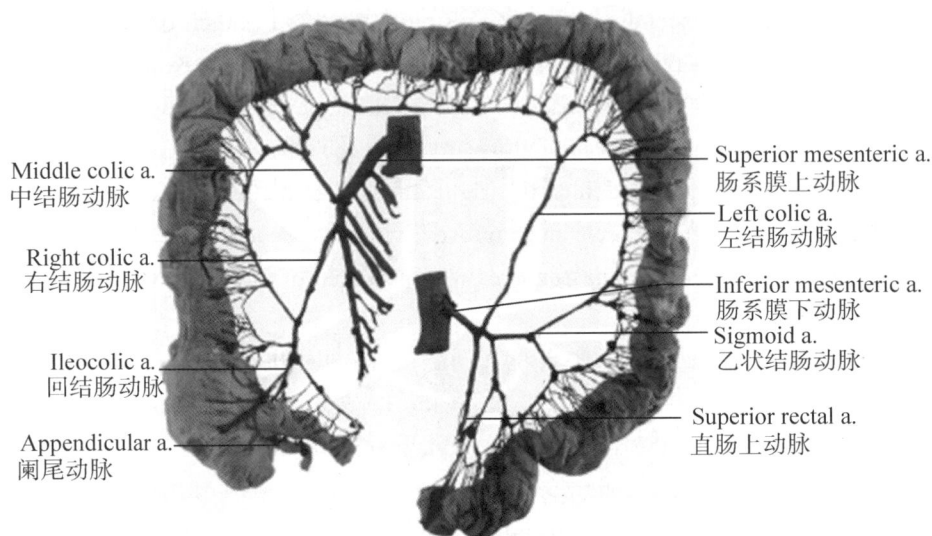

Middle colic a.
中结肠动脉

Right colic a.
右结肠动脉

Ileocolic a.
回结肠动脉

Appendicular a.
阑尾动脉

Superior mesenteric a.
肠系膜上动脉

Left colic a.
左结肠动脉

Inferior mesenteric a.
肠系膜下动脉

Sigmoid a.
乙状结肠动脉

Superior rectal a.
直肠上动脉

Fig.6-20　The mesenteric artery and its branches

8. Arteries of the Pelvis

Common Iliac Arteries

Common iliac arteries (髂总动脉) are two large arteries that originate from the aortic bifurcation at the level of L4 vertebra. They end in front of the sacroiliac joint and bifurcate into the external and internal iliac arteries (髂外动脉、髂内动脉). The distribution of the common iliac arteries is basically in the pelvis and to the lower limbs. Each common iliac artery also gives small branches to the peritoneum, psoas major, ureter, adjacent nerves and surrounding areolar tissue.

1) External iliac arteries (髂外动脉). External iliac arteries are the principal arteries of the lower limbs and have few branches in the pelvis. Each external iliac artery descends laterally along the medial border of psoas major and passes out of the pelvic cavity deep to the midpoint of the inguinal ligament (between the anterior superior iliac spine and the pubic symphysis), and then enters the thigh as the femoral artery. Before it passes beneath the inguinal ligament, it gives off the deep circumflex iliac (旋髂深动脉) and inferior epigastric arteries (腹壁下动脉). The inferior epigastric artery originates from the external iliac artery posterior to the inguinal ligament. It curves forwards and pierces the transversalis fascia to enter the posterior layer of the rectus sheath, then anastomoses with the superior epigastric artery. The deep circumflex iliac artery arises laterally from the external iliac artery opposite to the origin of the inferior epigastric artery. It ascends and runs laterally to the anterior superior iliac spine deep to the inguinal ligament. It gives off branches to the iliac crest and the adjacent abdominal muscles.

2) Internal iliac arteries (髂内动脉). The internal iliac arteries are the main arterial

supply of the walls and viscera of the pelvis, the buttock, the reproductive organs, and the medial compartment of the thigh. Each is approximately 4 cm long, which begins at the common iliac bifurcation, descends posteriorly to the superior margin of the greater sciatic foramen and gives off the vesicular and parietal branches (Fig.6-18).

Parietal branches

Iliolumbar artery (髂腰动脉) ascends laterally anterior to the sacro-iliac joint and reaches the medial border of psoas major, divided into the lumbar and iliac branches to supply the psoas major, quadratus lumborum, iliopsoas, hip bone and the cauda equina.

Lateral sacral arteries (骶外侧动脉) are usually double and descend medially to the anterior sacral foramen. Its branches are distributed to the piriformis, levator ani and sacral canal.

Superior and inferior gluteal arteries (臀上动脉、臀下动脉) pass through the suprapiriform or infrapiriform foramen to reach the gluteal region correspondingly. The inferior gluteal artery runs deep to the gluteus maximus. The superior gluteal artery is divided into the superficial and deep branches; its superior branch enters the deep surface of gluteus maximus, and its deep branch runs to the gluteus medius and minimus. The branches of them mainly serve the muscles of the buttock and the hip joint.

Obturator artery (闭孔动脉) runs anteroinferiorly on the lateral pelvic wall, and leaves the pelvis via the obturator canal. Its branches mainly serve the obturator externus, the upper medial thigh muscles as the pectineus, adductors longus, brevis and magnus and gracilis, and the hip joint (Fig.6-21).

Vesicular branches

Superior vesical artery (膀胱上动脉) lies on the lateral wall of the pelvis, and runs anteroinferiorly. It supplies the fundus of the urinary bladder, the distal end of the ureter, the proximal end of the ductus deferens and the seminal glands. It also gives origin to the umbilical artery (脐动脉) in the fetus, and its distal portion remains a fibrous cord as the medial umbilical ligament (脐内侧韧带) in the adult.

Inferior vesical artery (膀胱下动脉) runs anteromedially. In the male, it supplies the fundus of the urinary bladder, prostate, seminal glands and distal ureter. In the female, it supplies the urinary bladder and the vaginal wall.

Uterine artery (子宫动脉) usually arises inferior to the obturator artery on the lateral wall of the pelvis. It runs inferomedially within the broad ligament of uterus. About 2 cm lateral to the cervix of uterus, it crosses the ureter anteriorly before branching. One major branch ascends the uterus within the broad ligament of uterus until it reaches the ovary, and anastomoses with branches of the ovarian artery. It gives off numerous branches to supply the cervix and body of the uterus, uterine tube and ovary. Another branch descends to supply the cervix of uterus and anastomoses with branches of the vaginal artery.

Inferior rectal arteries (直肠下动脉) are several small branches and distribute in the inferior portion of the rectum. They anastomose with the branches of superior rectal artery and the anal artery in the rectal wall.

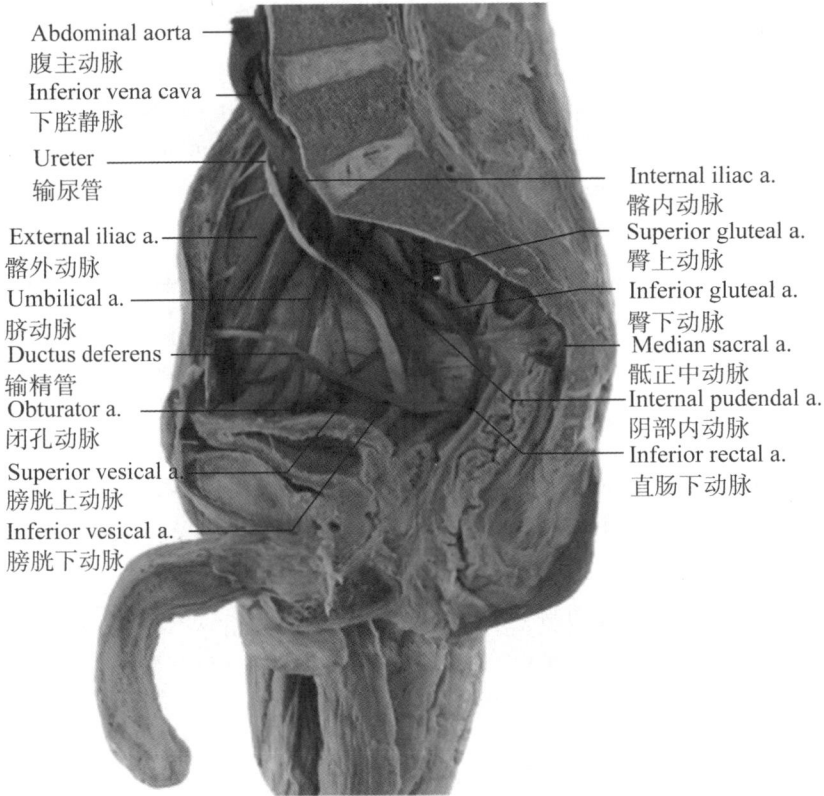

Fig.6-21   Blood vessels of the pelvic cavity (male)

Internal pudendal artery (阴部内动脉) leaves the pelvic cavity by passing through the infrapiriform foramen and reaches the gluteal region, and then it curves around the ischial spine and enters the ischio-anal fossa via the lesser sciatic foramen. It gives off the anal artery (肛动脉), perineal artery (会阴动脉), and dorsal artery of penis (阴茎背动脉) in the male and clitoris artery (阴蒂动脉) in the female to serve the musculature of the perineum and the external genitalia.

9. Arteries of the Lower Limb

(1) Femoral Artery

The femoral artery (股动脉) (Fig.6-22) is the principal arterial supply to the lower limb. It continues from the external iliac artery at the midpoint of inguinal ligament and passes through an opening in the adductor magnus to become the popliteal artery(腘动脉). The femoral artery gives off several branches in the proximal thigh, including the superficial epigastric (腹壁浅动脉), superficial circumflex iliac (旋髂浅动脉), external pudendal (阴部外动脉) and deep femoral arteries (profunda femoris arteries, 股深动脉).

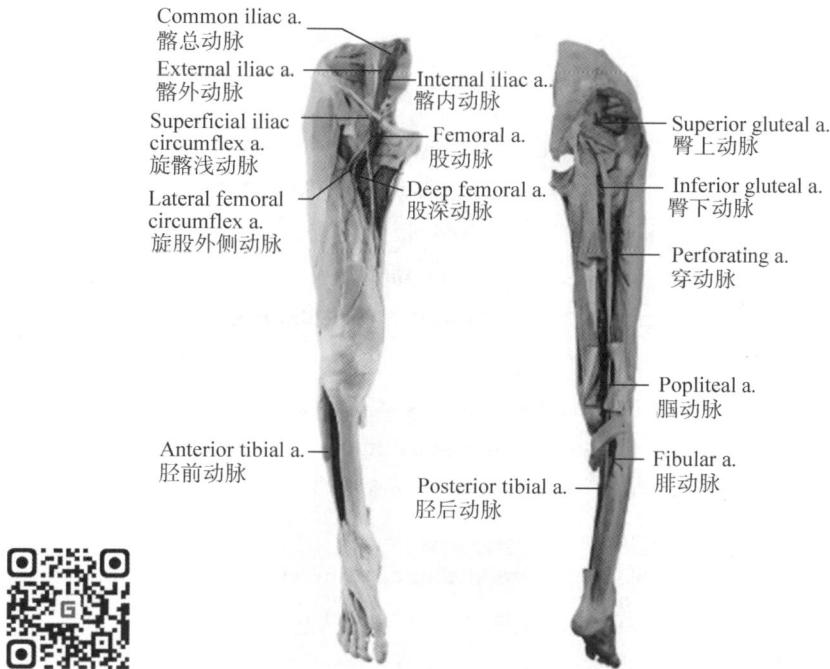

Fig.6-22   Arteries of the lower lib

1) Superficial epigastric artery arises from the front aspect of the femoral artery about 1 cm below the inguinal ligament, and passes through the femoral sheath and the cribriform fascia, then ascends in the abdominal superficial fascia nearly as far as the umbilicus. It anastomoses with branches of the inferior epigastric artery and its contralateral fellow.

2) Superficial iliac circumflex artery arises from the femoral artery near the origin of superficial epigastric artery. It turns laterally distal to the inguinal ligament towards the anterior superior iliac spine, and distributes to the skin, subcutaneous tissue and superficial inguinal lymph nodes, anastomosing with the deep circumflex iliac, superior gluteal and lateral circumflex femoral arteries.

3) External pudendal artery arises from the medial aspect of the femoral artery and distributes to the integument on the lower part of the abdomen, the penis and scrotum in the male, and the labium majus in the female, anastomosing with the branches of internal pudendal artery.

4) Deep femoral artery is the largest branch arising posterolaterally from the femoral artery about 3.5cm distal to the inguinal ligament. It passes between pectineus and adductor longus, then between the adductor longus and adductor brevis, before it descends between adductor longus and adductor magnus. It gives off the medial circumflex femoral

artery (旋股内侧动脉) to the medial group of thigh muscles and hip joint, lateral circumflex femoral arteries (旋股外侧动脉) to the anterior group of thigh muscles and knee joint, three perforating arteries (穿动脉) to the posterior group of thigh muscles and femur.

(2) Popliteal artery

The popliteal artery (腘动脉) is the continuation of the femoral artery and descends laterally from the opening in adductor magnus to the popliteal fossa. It divides into anterior and posterior tibial arteries (胫前动脉 / 胫后动脉) distal to popliteus. It also supplies several small branches to the knee joint including lateral and medial superior genicular, middle genicular, lateral and medial inferior genicular branches.

(3) Posterior tibial artery

The posterior tibial artery (胫后动脉) begins at the lower border of the Popliteus, opposite the interval between the tibia and fibula. It descends medially in the flexor compartment and divides into the medial and lateral plantar arteries under abductor hallucis, midway between the medial malleolus and the calcaneal tubercle. The other branches of the posterior tibial artery are the circumflex, fibular, nutrient, muscular, perforating, communicating, medial malleolar and calcaneal arteries.

(4) Fibular artery

The fibular artery (腓动脉) arises from the posterior tibial artery about 2.5 cm below the lower border of the popliteus. It passes obliquely toward the fibula, and then descends along the medial side of fibula, contained in a fibrous canal. It then runs behind the tibiofibular syndesmosis and divides into lateral calcaneal branches.

(5) Anterior tibial artery

The anterior tibial artery (胫前动脉) commences at the bifurcation of the popliteal artery at the lower border of the popliteus, passes forward between the two heads of the tibialis posterior, and through the aperture above the upper border of the interosseous membrane. It then descends on the anterior surface of the intero-sseous membrane, gradually approaching the tibia, and then on the front of the ankle joint, where it is more superficial, and becomes the dorsalis pedis artery (dorsal artery of foot, 足背动脉) (Fig.6-23). Dorsal artery of foot passes to the proximal end of the first intermetatarsal space and turns into the sole between the heads of the first dorsal interosseous to complete the deep plantar arch, and also provides the first plantar metatarsal artery. Anterior to the ankle joint, its palpation can be felt at the midpoint of the line between the lateral malleolus and the medial malleolus, and lateral to the tendon of extensor hallucis longus.

Superior extensor
retinaculum
伸肌上支持带

Perforating branch of
fibular a.
腓动脉穿支

Dorsal artery of foot
足背动脉

Lateral tarsal a.
跗外侧动脉

Arcuate a.
弓状动脉

Dorsal metatarsal a.
跖背动脉

Dorsal digital a.
趾背动脉

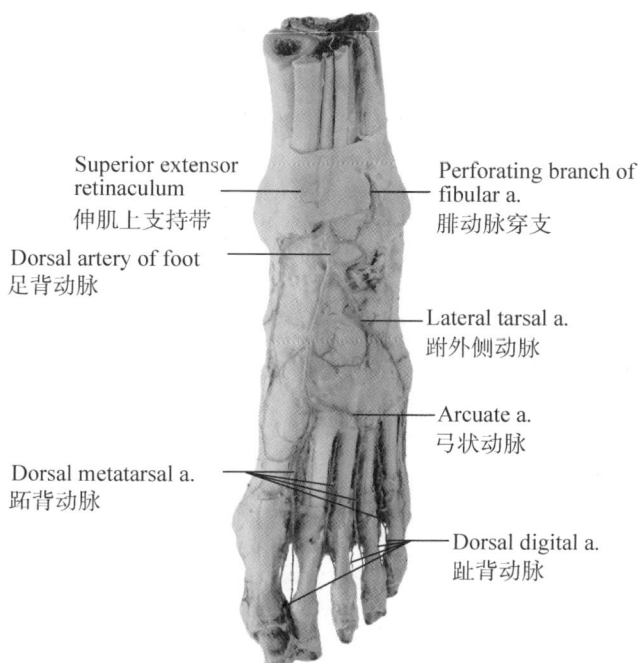

Fig.6-23   Arteries in the dorsal part of the foot

（南京医科大学   张永杰）

6.4   Veins

6.4.1   Introduction

The Veins convey the blood from the capillaries of different parts of the body to the heart. They consist of two distinct sets of vessels, the pulmonary ones and the systemic ones.The pulmonary veins (肺静脉), unlike other veins, contain arterial blood, which they return from the lungs to the left atrium of the heart. The systematic veins (体循环的静脉) return the venous blood from the body generally to the right atrium of the heart. Veins normally accompany arteries and often have similar names. They are always larger than the arteries, sometimes more visible than the arteries because they are closer to the skin's surface. Most veins eventually empty the unoxygenated blood into the vena caves.

1. General Feature of the Veins

The veins have thin walls, larger lumens, venous valves (absent in the thorax and the abdomen), venous plexus, and venous rete. The walls of veins are similar to those of arteries which are composed of three distinct layers. However, the middle layer of the venous wall is poorly developed compared to that of the arterial wall. Consequently, veins have thinner walls that have less smooth muscle and less elastic connective tissue than those of comparable arteries. They also have two sets which are superficial veins and deep veins. The special structures of the veins are sinuses of the dura mater and diploic veins.

2. Composition of the Veins

The pulmonary veins are R. & L. superior & inferior pulmonary veins whose blood flow directly to the left atrium. The systemic veins whose blood flow directly to the right atrium, dividing into superior vena cava system, the inferior vena cava system (the hepatic portal system), and the cardiac vein system.

1) The head, neck, upper limb, and thoracic cavity return blood to the right atrium of the heart via the superior vena cava.

2) The lower limb, abdominal and pelvis cavity return blood to the right atrium of the heart via the inferior vena cava.

3) Veins that drain the abdominal viscera are exceptions. They originate in the capillary networks of the stomach, intestines, pancreas, and spleen, and carry blood from these organs through a hepatic portal vein to the liver. This unique venous pathway is called the hepatic portal system. In the liver, the hepatic portal vein (肝门静脉) branches into smaller venules and finally into capillary beds. In the capillary beds of the liver, nutrients are exchanged for storage and the blood is purified. The capillaries then join into venules that empty into the hepatic vein (肝静脉), which carries blood to the inferior vena cava.

4) The recurrent factors of the blood in veins contain the venous valves, the dilation of the ventricles of the heart, the negative pressure of the thoracic cavity, the movements of the viscera, the impulses of the artery, the continuous blood flow from capillaries.

6.4.2　Pulmonary Veins (肺循环的静脉)

The Pulmonary Veins return the arterialized blood from the lungs to the left atrium of the heart. There are four in number, two from each lung, and are destitute of valves. They originate from capillary networks in the alveolar walls. The four veins are right superior pulmonary vein, right inferior pulmonary vein, left superior pulmonary vein, and left inferior pulmonary vein.

6.4.3　Systematic Veins (体循环的静脉)

The vena cava system includes the superior vena cava system and the inferior vena cava system.

1. Veins of Head and Neck

(1) Facial vein

The facial vein (面静脉) begins at the medial angle of the eye (angular vein) and runs downward and backward through the face, posterior to the facial artery. It passes over the surface of the masseter. It below the angle of the mandible, and joins an anterior branch of the retromandibular vein to form a common facial vein, which drains into the internal jugular vein. Connections with cavernous sinus through the ophthalmic vein, and also through pterygoid venous plexus via the deep facial vein. Its junction with the superior labial vein is often termed the angular vein (Fig. 6-24). "Danger triangle of the face" (危险三角) lies between the root of the nose and two angles of the mouth. In this area, the facial vein has no valves. This area connects with the cavernous sinus and pterygoid venous plexus. These veins carry any infection from this part of the face to the brain through these connecting veins. And the infection of the brain can result in serious conditions like meningitis, cavernous sinus thrombosis, and brain abscess.

(2) The retromandibular vein

The retromandibular vein (下颌后静脉) is a deep vein of the face that is formed by the merger of the superficial temporal vein with the maxillary vein. It runs within the substance of the parotid gland, descending posterior to the ramus of the mandible. At the inferior pole of the parotid gland, the retromandibular vein separates into anterior and posterior branches. The anterior branch anastomoses with the facial vein and forms the common facial vein, while the posterior branch anastomoses with the posterior auricular veins, forming the external jugular vein. The retromandibular vein drains the venous blood from the jaw, the lateral skull, and the parotid gland.

(3) The external jugular vein

The external jugular vein (颈外静脉) mainly drains blood from the scalp, face and superficial regions of the neck, formed behind the angle of the mandible by the union of posterior auricular, the retromandibular and occipital vein. They cross sternocleidomastoid to enter the subclavian vein.

(4) Anterior jugular vein

The anterior jugular vein (颈前静脉) arises from the superficial submandibular veins, drains submandibular and anterior neck regions and descends near the midline, runs posterior to the sternal end of sternocleidomastoid to drain into the external jugular vein or subclavian vein. There are usually two anterior jugular veins, united just above the

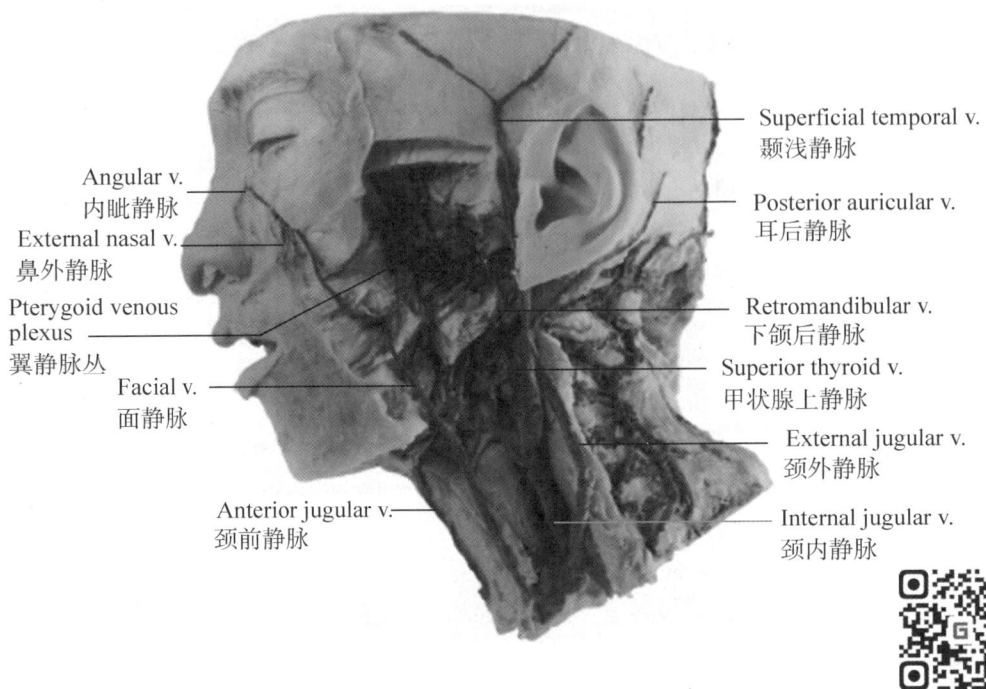

Angular v.
内眦静脉

External nasal v.
鼻外静脉

Pterygoid venous
plexus
翼静脉丛

Facial v.
面静脉

Superficial temporal v.
颞浅静脉

Posterior auricular v.
耳后静脉

Retromandibular v.
下颌后静脉

Superior thyroid v.
甲状腺上静脉

External jugular v.
颈外静脉

Anterior jugular v.
颈前静脉

Internal jugular v.
颈内静脉

Fig.6-24   Veins of head and neck

manubrium by a large transverse jugular arch, receiving the inferior thyroid tributaries.

(5) Internal jugular vein

The internal jugular vein (颈内静脉) begins at the jugular foramen, where it is continuous with the sigmoid sinus, descending to join the subclavian vein to form brachiocephalic vein and lie lateral first to the internal, then to the carotid sheath. Internal jugular vein mainly collects blood from the skull, brain, superficial parts of the face, and much of the neck. They are chief extracranial tributaries and common facial veins. The internal jugular vein contains lingual vein, pharyngeal vein, superior thyroid vein, and middle thyroid vein.

(6) Subclavian vein

The subclavian vein (锁骨下静脉) continues from the axillary vein at the lateral border of the first rib. It Joins the internal jugular vein to form the brachiocephalic vein. The subclavian vein contains the external jugular vein and inferior thyroid vein.

2. Veins of the Upper Limb

Veins of the upper limb are divided into two sets: the superficial veins and the deep veins. The two sets anastomose frequently with each other. The superficial veins are just beneath the skin. The deep veins accompany the arteries, and constitute the venae comitantes of those vessels.

(1) Superficial veins

The superficial veins (Fig.6-25) are the digital, metacarpal, cephalic, basilic, median, cubital vein at the cubital fossa and the dorsal venous network of the hand.

1) Cephalic vein (头静脉) arises from the lateral side of the dorsal venous rete on the back of the hand and winds around the lateral border of the forearm, and then ascends into the cubital fossa and up on the lateral side of the biceps. It continues up in the deltopectoral groove, then pierces the clavipectoral fascia to drain into the axillary vein.

2) Basilic vein (贵要静脉) arises from the medial side of

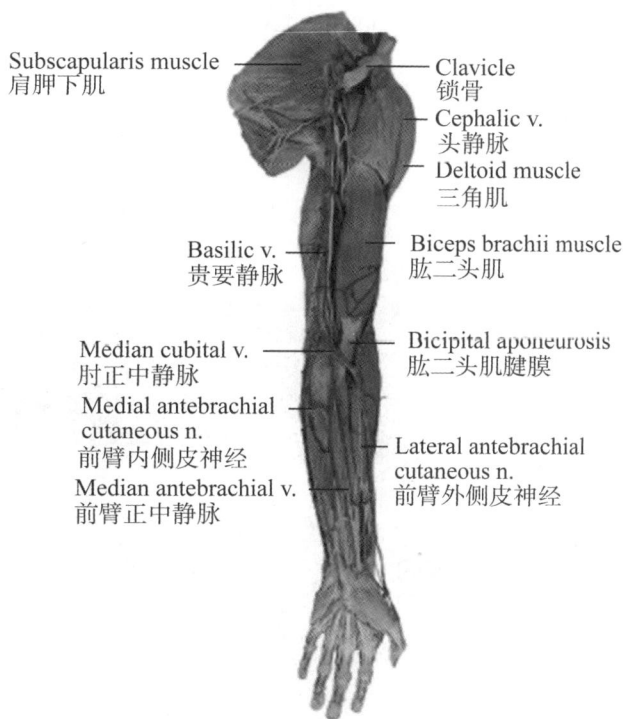

Fig.6-25   Superficial veins of the upper limb
(n.: nerve; v.: vein)

the dorsal venous rete of the hand and winds around the medial border of the forearm; it then ascends into the cubital fossa where it is joined by the median cubital vein, and up on the medial side of the biceps to the middle of the arm where it pierces the deep fascia and joins the brachial vein or axillary vein.

3) Median cubital vein (肘正中静脉) links the cephalic vein and basilic vein in the cubital fossa. It is a frequent site for intravenous injection to remove a sample of blood or add fluid to the blood.

(2) Deep veins

The deep veins follow the course of the arteries, forming their venae comitantes, becoming the axillary vein, and ultimately the subclavian vein. They are generally arranged in pairs, and are situated one on either side of the corresponding artery, and connected at intervals by short transverse branches.

3. Veins of the Thorax

Veins on the internal aspect of the body wall can be seen in Fig.6-26.

(1) The innominate veins

The innominate veins (brachiocephalic veins) (头臂静脉或无名静脉) are two large trunks with one placed on either side of the root of the neck, and formed by the union of the internal jugular and subclavian veins of the corresponding side; they are devoid of valves.

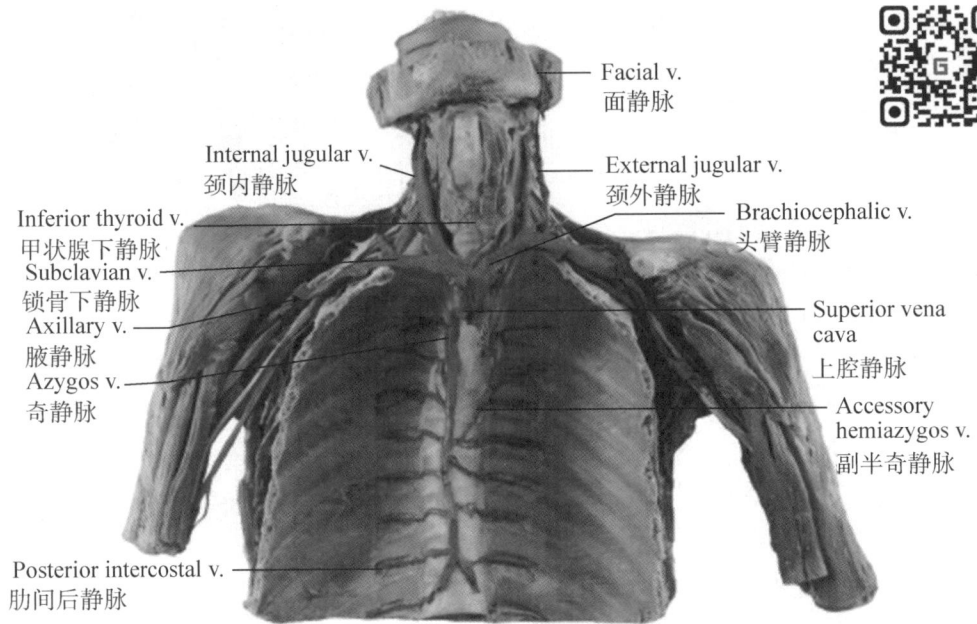

Fig.6-26   Veins on the internal aspect of the body wall

(2) Superior vena cava

The superior vena cava(上腔静脉) is formed by a union of right and left brachiocephalic veins behind the right sternocostal synchondrosis of the first rib and runs vertically down on the right of the ascending aorta. They are joined by the azygos vein at the level of the sternal angle and enter the right atrium at the level of the lower border of the third right sternocostal joint. The superior vena cava collects blood from the head, neck, and the upper half of the body, and also receives blood from the thoracic wall and the oesophagus via the azygos system.

(3) Parietal tributaries anterior wall of the thorax

Parietal tributaries anterior wall of the thorax contains thoracoepigastric vein, anterior intercostal vein (internal thoracic vein & brachiocephalic vein). Posterior intercostal vein (肋间后静脉) drains the blood from intercostal spaces. It usually receives the left bronchial vein, and sometimes the left superior phrenic vein, and communicates below with the accessory hemiazygos vein. The posterior intercostal veins drain directly or indirectly into the azygos vein on the right and the hemiazygos or accessory hemiazygos veins on the left.

(4) **Visceral tributaries**

Visceral tributaries receive the right subcostal and intercostal veins, the upper three or four of these latter opening by a common stem, the highest superior intercostal vein. It receives the hemiazygos veins, several esophageal, mediastinal, and pericardial veins, and, near its termination, the right bronchial vein.

(5) **Azygos vein**

The azygos vein (奇静脉) begins at a continuation of right ascending lumbar vein. It ascends along the right side of the vertebral column and joins the superior vena cava by aching above the right lung root at the level of T4 to T5. It also receives right posterior intercostals and subcostal veins plus some of the bronchial, esophageal and pericardial veins, and hemiazygos vein. Its tributaries contain hemiazygos vein, accessory hemiazygos vein, veins of the vertebral column, external vertebral venous plexus and internal vertebral venous plexus. It receives mediastinal, oesophageal, and the ninth to eleventh left posterior intercostal veins. The hemiazygos vein (半奇静脉) is often connected to the left renal vein. It is formed by the oesophageal and mediastinal tributaries, the common trunk of the left ascending lumbar vein and left subcostal vein, and by the lower three posterior intercostal veins. It ascends anterior to the vertebral column before crossing the column posterior to the aorta, oesophagus and thoracic duct at the level of T8. The accessory hemiazygos vein (副半奇静脉) is formed by veins from the fourth to eighth intercostal spaces and sometimes by the left bronchial veins. It descends to the left of the vertebral column before crossing T7, where it joins with the azygos vein. Sometimes it joins the hemiazygos vein and, in this case, their common trunk drains into the azygos vein.

4. Veins of the Lower Limb

Veins of the lower limb are subdivided, like those of the upper limb, into two sets, the superficial and deep ones; the superficial veins are placed beneath the integument between the two layers of the superficial fascia; the deep veins accompany the arteries. Both sets of the veins are provided with valves, which are more numerous in the deep set than in the superficial set (the valves are also more numerous than in the veins of the upper limb). Within and between some of the lower limb muscles can form venous plexuses.

(1) **The superficial veins** (Fig.6-27)

1) Great saphenous vein (大隐静脉), which is the longest vein in the body, begins at the medial end of the dorsal venous arch of the foot and passes anterior to the medial malleolus, and ascends on the medial side of the leg, then passes behind the knee and curves forward around the medial side of the thigh. In the thigh, the long saphenous vein receives many tributaries. It inclines anteriorly through the thigh to enter the femoral vein

through the saphenous hiatus which lies about 3—4 cm below and lateral to the pubic tubercle. Its tributaries contains superficial medial femoral vein, superficial lateral femoral vein, external pudendal vein, superficial epigastric vein, superficial iliac circumflex vein.

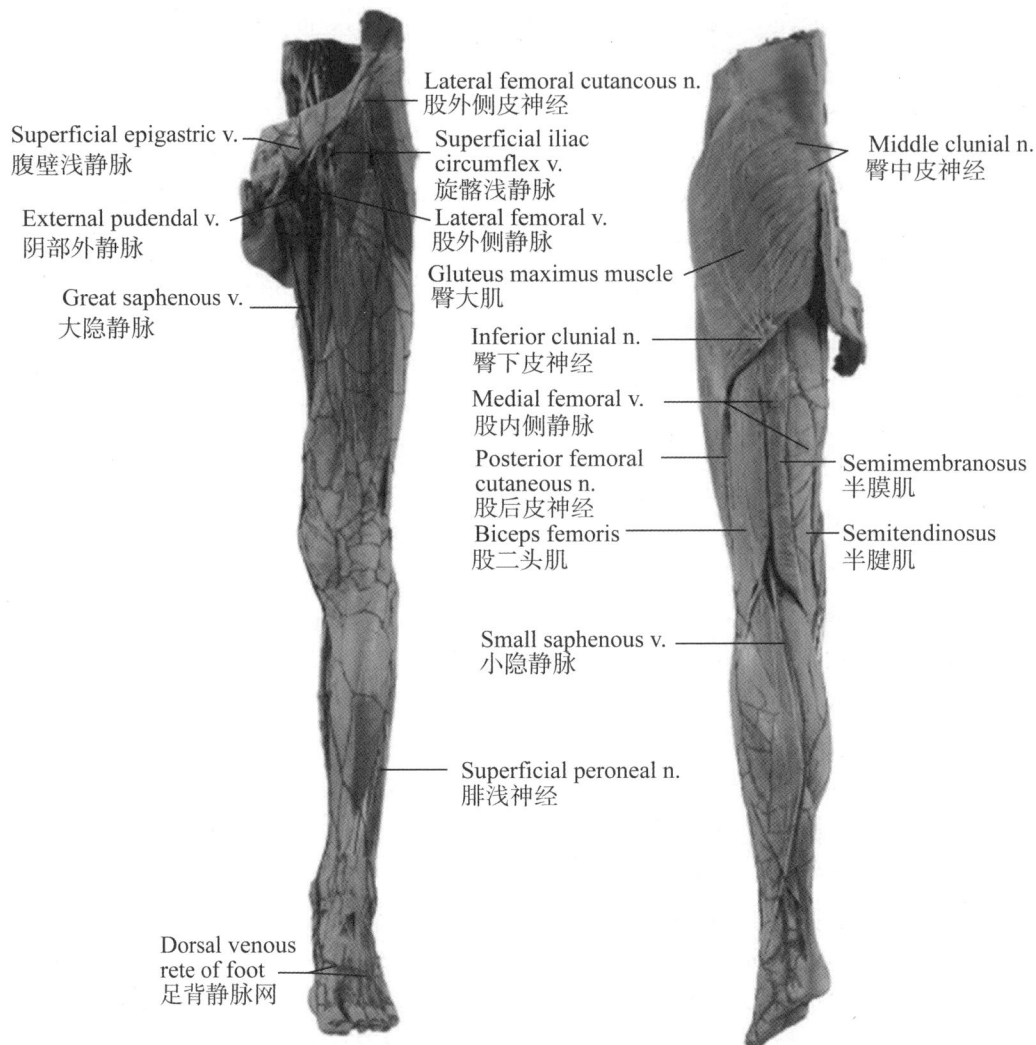

Fig.6-27　Superficial veins of the lower limb

2) Small saphenous vein (小隐静脉) arises from the lateral part of the dorsal venous arch of the foot and ascends behind the lateral malleolus and then runs up the midline of the back of the leg. It pierces the deep fascia and enters the popliteal vein, and drains the lateral side of the foot and ankle and the back of the leg.

(2) **Deep veins**

Deep veins of the lower extremity accompany the arteries and their branches; they possess numerous valves. They contain external iliac vein, femoral vein, popliteal vein, anterior tibial vein, and posterior tibial vein.

5. Veins of the Pelvis

Veins of the pelvis (Fig.6-28) contain the internal iliac vein, the external iliac vein, and the common iliac vein. The internal iliac vein contains parietal tributaries which accompany arteries and visceral tributaries. External iliac veins accompany the artery. Common iliac vein is formed by the union of internal and external iliac veins in front of the sacroiliac joint, ends upon L4－L5 by uniting each other to form inferior vena cava. Parietal tributaries contain superior gluteal vein, inferior gluteal vein, obturator vein, lateral sacral vein. Parietal tributaries of internal iliac vein accompany with arteries. Visceral tributaries contain rectal venous plexus, vesical venous plexus, and uterine venous plexus.

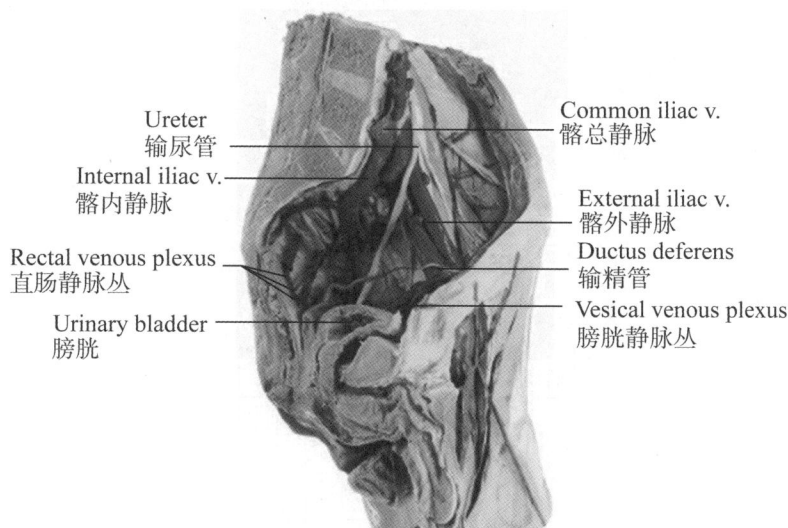

Fig.6-28 Veins of the pelvis

6. Veins of the Abdomen

(1) Inferior vena cava

The inferior Vena Cava (下腔静脉, Fig.6-29) is formed by a union of two common iliac veins anterior and just to the right of L4－L5 and ascends on the right side of the aorta, lies in a deep groove on the posterior surface of the liver, sometimes completely surrounded by liver tissue, pierces vena cava foramen of the diaphragm at the level of T8, and drains into the right atrium. It conveys blood from the whole body below the diaphragm to the right atrium.

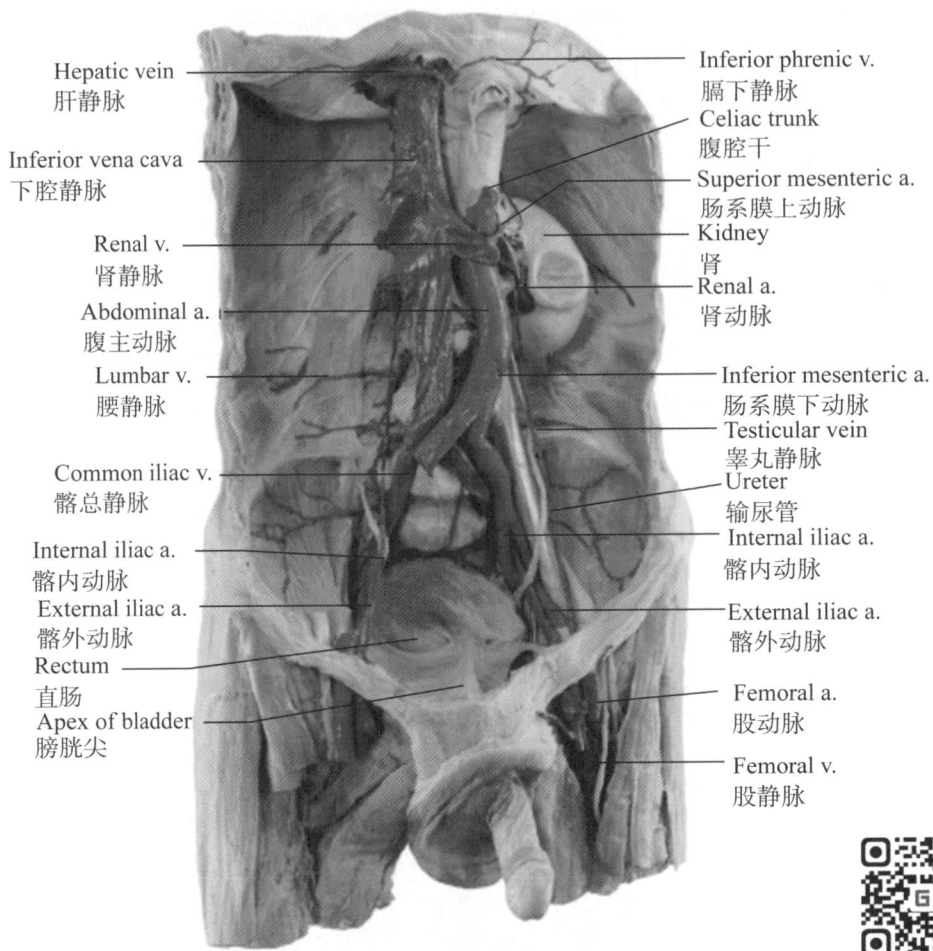

Hepatic vein
肝静脉

Inferior vena cava
下腔静脉

Renal v.
肾静脉

Abdominal a.
腹主动脉

Lumbar v.
腰静脉

Common iliac v.
髂总静脉

Internal iliac a.
髂内动脉

External iliac a.
髂外动脉

Rectum
直肠

Apex of bladder
膀胱尖

Inferior phrenic v.
膈下静脉

Celiac trunk
腹腔干

Superior mesenteric a.
肠系膜上动脉

Kidney
肾

Renal a.
肾动脉

Inferior mesenteric a.
肠系膜下动脉

Testicular vein
睾丸静脉

Ureter
输尿管

Internal iliac a.
髂内动脉

External iliac a.
髂外动脉

Femoral a.
股动脉

Femoral v.
股静脉

Fig.6-29   Veins of the posterior abdominal wall

(2) Hepatic portal vein

The hepatic portal vein (肝门静脉) (Fig. 6-30) is formed behind the neck of the pancreas by the union of the superior mesenteric vein and splenic vein and ascends upwards and to the right, posterior to the first part of the duodenum, and then enters the lesser omentum to the porta hepatis, approximately 8 cm long ascends obliquely to the right, where it divides into right and left branches. There are no functioning valves in the hepatic portal system. It drains blood from the gastrointestinal tract from the lower end of the oesophagus to the upper end of the anal canal, pancreas, gall bladder, bile ducts, and spleen. Tributaries of the hepatic portal vein contain the superior mesenteric vein, inferior mesenteric vein, splenic vein, left gastric vein, right gastric vein, cystic vein and the paraumbilical vein (Fig. 6-30).

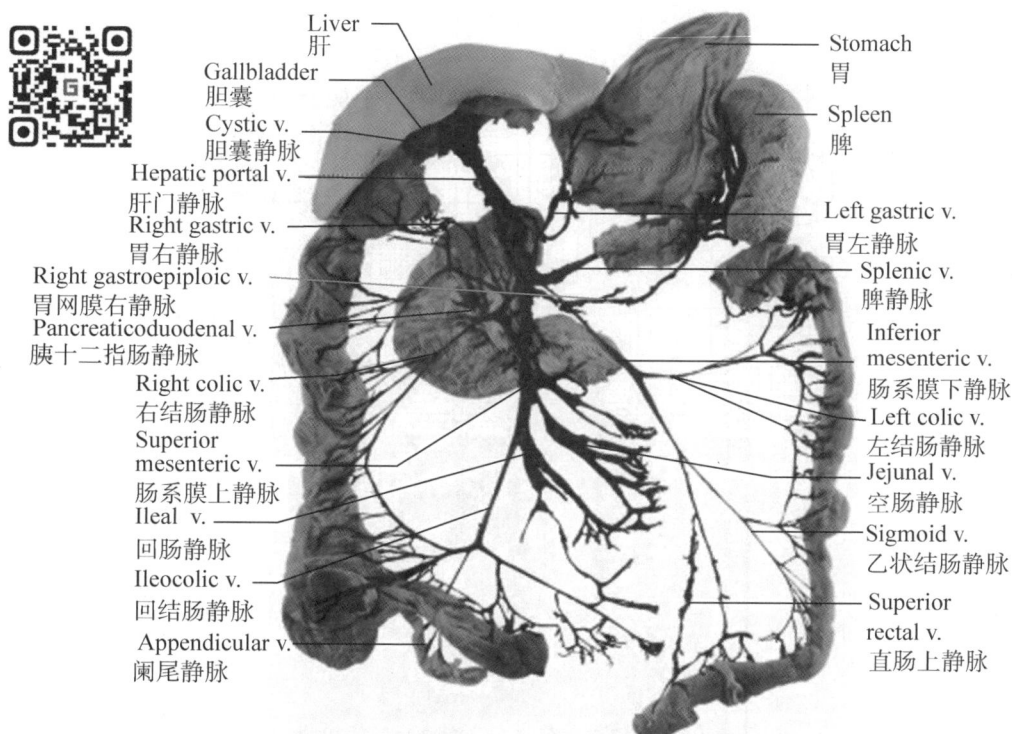

Fig.6-30　The hepatic portal vein and its tributaries

(3) **Portosystemic anastomoses hepatocirrhosis** (Fig.6-31)

1) At the lower end of the oesophagus: hepatic portal vein → left gastric vein → esophageal venous plexus → esophageal vein → azygos vein → superior vena cava.

2) At rectal venous plexus: hepatic portal vein → splenic vein → inferior mesenteric vein → superior rectal vein → rectal venous plexus → inferior rectal and anal veins → internal iliac vein → inferior vena cava.

3) At periumbilical venous rete: hepatic portal vein→paraumbilical vein→periumbilical venous rete→thoracoepigastric and superior epigastric vein → superior vena cava; and periumbilical venous rete→superficial epigastric and inferior epigastric veins → inferior vena cava.

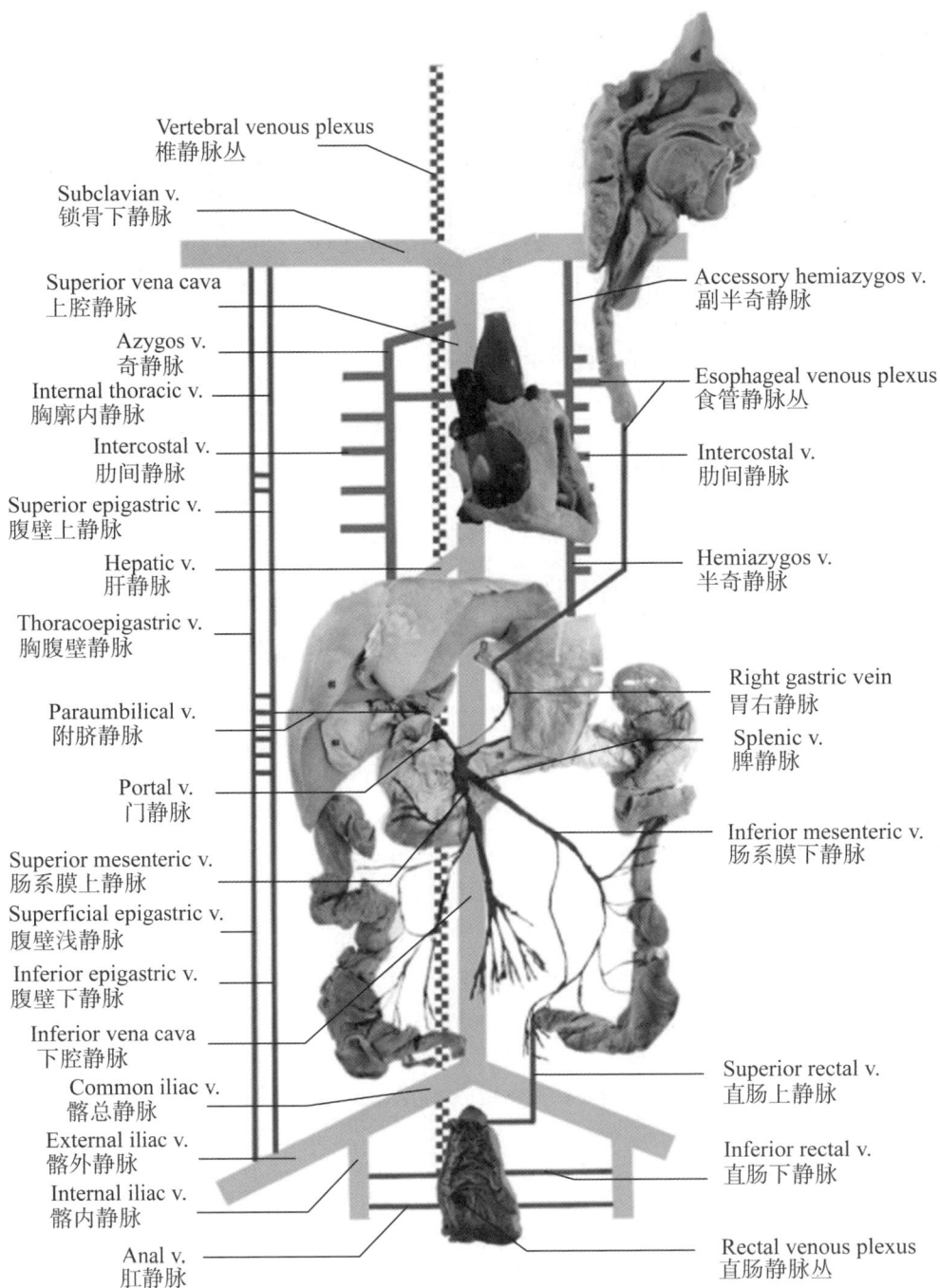

Vertebral venous plexus
椎静脉丛

Subclavian v.
锁骨下静脉

Superior vena cava
上腔静脉

Azygos v.
奇静脉

Internal thoracic v.
胸廓内静脉

Intercostal v.
肋间静脉

Superior epigastric v.
腹壁上静脉

Hepatic v.
肝静脉

Thoracoepigastric v.
胸腹壁静脉

Paraumbilical v.
附脐静脉

Portal v.
门静脉

Superior mesenteric v.
肠系膜上静脉

Superficial epigastric v.
腹壁浅静脉

Inferior epigastric v.
腹壁下静脉

Inferior vena cava
下腔静脉

Common iliac v.
髂总静脉

External iliac v.
髂外静脉

Internal iliac v.
髂内静脉

Anal v.
肛静脉

Accessory hemiazygos v.
副半奇静脉

Esophageal venous plexus
食管静脉丛

Intercostal v.
肋间静脉

Hemiazygos v.
半奇静脉

Right gastric vein
胃右静脉

Splenic v.
脾静脉

Inferior mesenteric v.
肠系膜下静脉

Superior rectal v.
直肠上静脉

Inferior rectal v.
直肠下静脉

Rectal venous plexus
直肠静脉丛

Fig.6-31 Anastomosis of the hepatic portal vein and vena cava

Exercise

1. A 13-year-old boy was hospitalized due to hemiplegia of the right limb. Transesophageal echocardiography (TEE) showed that a gap of about 7 mm in length and 3 mm in width could be seen at the interatrial septum. What is the name of this gap?

(A) Foramen ovale.

(B) Fossa ovalis.

(C) Tricuspid valve.

(D) Pulmonary valve.

(E) Orifice of coronary sinus.

2. A 29-year-old male was admitted to the emergency department after a serious car accident. Ultrasonic examination showed the thyroid was damaged. Which artery was most likely to be damaged?

(A) The common carotid artery.

(B) The external carotid artery.

(C) The facial artery.

(D) The superficial temporal artery.

(E) The superior and inferior thyroid arteries.

3. A 7-year-old girl fell off while sliding in kindergarten. A thin piece of wood inserted into the abdomen. Ultrasonic examination revealed that the body of pancreas was lacerated, the blood vessels around the pancreatic body bled and moved along the upper edge of the pancreas. Which vessel was most likely damaged?

(A) The superior mesenteric artery.

(B) The hepatic portal vein.

(C) The left gastric artery.

(D) The splenic artery.

(E) The left gastro-omental artery.

4. A 57-year-old woman was admitted to hospital with weakness, poor appetite, and abdominal distention. Ultrasonic examination revealed the portal vein circulation of the liver was blocked and spider nevus also appears on the palm. The blood in portal vein was still delivered to the vena cava system through which of the following vein?

(A) The azygos and hemiazygos veins.

(B) The gonadal veins.

(C) The external iliac veins.

(D) The splenic veins.

(E) The vesical venous plexus.

5. The surgeon performed a thoracocentesis. During this procedure, the needle was needed to pass above the rib. The operation is mainly to prevent damage to which of the following structures in the subcostal groove?

(A) Intercostal artery and vein.

(B) Intercostal nerve.

(C) Intercostal nerve and artery.

(D) Intercostal nerve and vein.

(E) Intercostal nerve, artery, and vein.

Answer

1. The correct answer is A.

During fetal period, the foramen ovale exists on atrial septum of the left and right atrium. In the first year after birth, the foramen ovale is usually closed, forming the fossa ovalis. If patent-oval-foramen exists, the blood and thrombus enter the left atrium from the right atrium.

2. The correct answer is E.

The right common carotid artery (Choice A) originates from the brachiocephalic trunk, and the left common carotid artery directly originates from the aortic arch. Both common carotid arteries ascend along the trachea, diverging laterally from behind the sternoclavicular joint, as well as dividing into the internal carotid artery and the external carotid artery (Choice B) at the upper edge of the thyroid cartilage.

The facial artery (Choice C) is an important branch of the external carotid artery which originates from the angle of the mandible, passes obliquely up by the posterior surface of the submandibular gland. Then, the facial artery curves upward over the body of the mandible at the anterior-inferior angle of the masseter to enter the face.

The superficial temporal artery (Choice D) is the terminal branch of the external carotid artery which pierces the lower part of the thyrohyoid membrane to supply the tissues of the upper part of the larynx.

The superior thyroid artery (Choice E) is a branch of the external carotid artery, descending along the larynx and reaching the upper part of the thyroid lobe. The inferior thyroid artery is a branch of the thyroid neck trunk. After separation, the inferior thyroid artery crosses the back of the common carotid artery and descends on longus colli to the lower border of the thyroid gland.

3. The correct answer is D.

The superior mesenteric artery (Choice A) originates from the abdominal aorta at the level of the body of the first lumbar vertebra, as well as descends behind the transition of the pancreatic head and neck. It is not easily lacerated.

The hepatic portal vein (Choice B) starts from the convergence of the superior mesenteric and the splenic veins posterior to the neck of the pancreas at the level of the first lumbar intervertebral disc and enters the liver. It is not damaged in this situation.

The left gastric artery (Choice C) is a branch of the celiac trunk and runs along the superior border of the lesser curvature of the stomach.

The splenic artery (Choice D) is the largest branch of the celiac trunk. It takes a tortuous course to the left along the superior border of the pancreas. It gives off branches to the neck, body, and tail of the pancreas. Therefore, it is easily damaged if pancreas is lacerated.

The left gastro-omental artery (Choice E) is a branch of the splenic artery. It descends along the greater curvature of the stomach and the anastomoses with the right gastro-omental artery.

4. The correct answer is A.

The hepatic portal vein is connected with vena cava system via three venous plexuses, including the esophagus venous plexus, the rectal venous plexus and the paraumbilical venous plexus. Blood in the azygos and hemiazygos veins drains into the superior vena cava which connects to esophagus venous plexus. Therefore, if the portal vein is blocked, portal blood may enter the superior vena cava via the azygos and hemiazygos veins.

The gonadal veins (Choice B), the external iliac vein (Choice C) and the vesical venous plexus (Choice e) are not connected with the portal vessels.

The splenic vein (Choice D) directly drains into the hepatic portal vein.

5. The correct answer is E.

The intercostal nerve, the artery, and the vein lie in the subcostal groove of a rib. Therefore, these structures are easily damaged if the needle directly passes through the inferior border of the rib.

The Lymphatic System

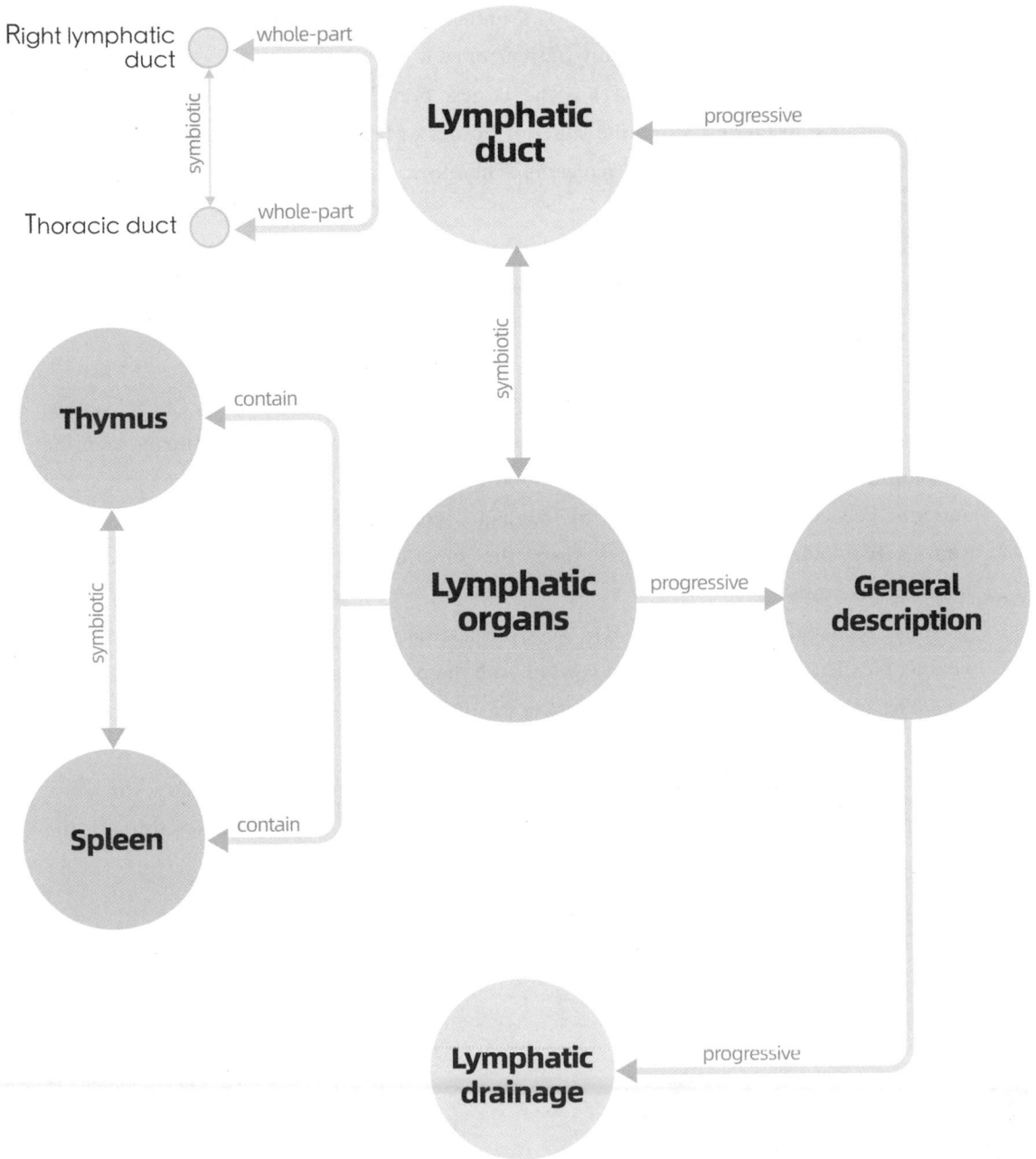

Right lymphatic duct — whole-part → Lymphatic duct

Right lymphatic duct — symbiotic — Thoracic duct

Thoracic duct — whole-part → Lymphatic duct

Lymphatic duct — progressive — General description

Lymphatic duct — symbiotic — Lymphatic organs

Thymus — contain — Lymphatic organs

Thymus — symbiotic — Spleen

Spleen — contain — Lymphatic organs

Lymphatic organs — progressive → General description

General description — progressive → Lymphatic drainage

The Lymphatic System

Chapter 7   Lymphatic System

7.1   General Introduction

The lymphatic system (淋巴系统) (Fig.7-1), consisting of the lymph conducting channels, lymphoid tissues, and lymphoid organs, is part of the immune system, and acts as a secondary (accessory) circulatory system. Lymphatic vessels transport excess fluid away from interstitial spaces in most tissues and return it to the bloodstream. The functions of the lymphatic system are that it removes excess fluids from body tissues, absorbs fatty acid and transports fat to the circulatory system, and produces immune cells (lymphocytes, monocytes, and plasma cells). Moreover blood fluid escapes through the thinwalled capillaries into spaces among the body tissue cells. Lymphatic vessels (淋巴管) which have very thin walls form wide-meshed plexuses in the extracellular matrices of most

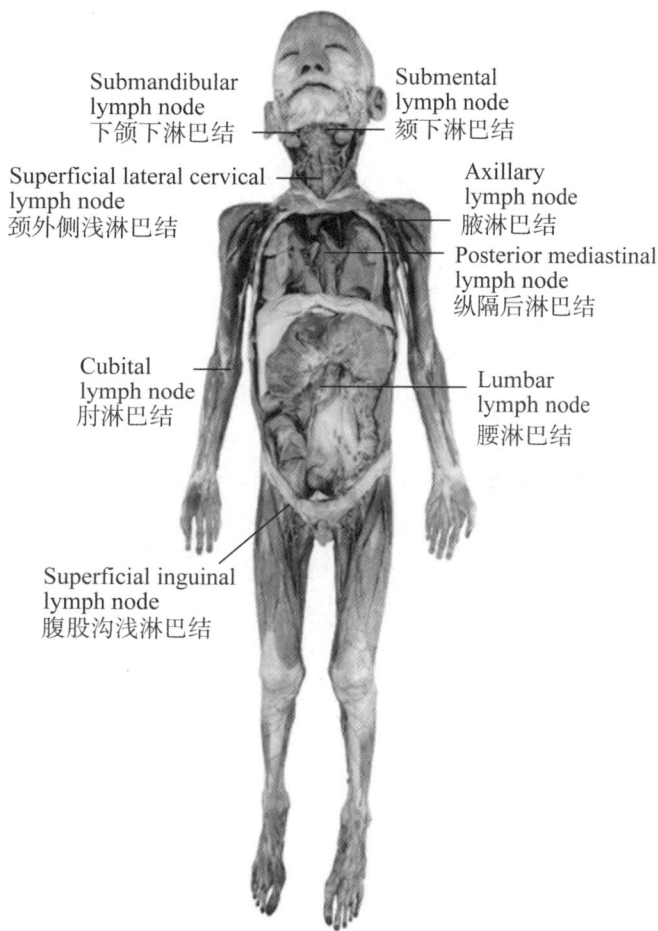

Fig.7-1   Systemic lymphatics and lymph nodes

tissues, picking up these fluids called lymph. The lymphatic system provides an important transport pathway for leukocytes and defends against infection. Cells and biochemicals of the lymphatic system launch both generalized and targeted attacks against "foreign" particles, enabling the body to destroy infectious microorganisms and viruses. This immunity against disease also protects against toxins and cancer cells. When the immune response is abnormal, persistent infection, cancer, autoimmune disorders, and allergies may result.

7.1.1 Composition

1. Lymphatic Vessel

The lymphatic vessel (淋巴管) contains lymphatic capillary, lymphatic vessels which are the superficial and the deep, nine lymphatic trunks, two lymphatic ducts which are the thoracic duct and right lymphatic duct.

2. Lymphatic Organ

The lymphatic organ (淋巴器官) contains the lymphatic nodes, tonsils, spleen, and thymus. Lymphatic tissue includes diffused lymphoid tissues and lymph nodes. They are mainly situated in the wall of the respiratory-alimentary tracts and consist of aggregated lymphocytes and associated cells. Lymphocytes populate lymphoid tissues and are concerned with immune defense.

7.1.2 Tissue Fluid and Its Formation

At the arterial end of a capillary, liquid is forced out as tissue which is similar to plasma in composition except it has no plasma proteins, platelets & RBCs because they are too large to leak out of the capillaries. Tissue fluid transfers across these exchange vessels is driven by the balance between the hydrostatic pressure. The majority of fluid gets reabsorbed back into the blood vessels, while around 10% of the fluid stays in the tissue. That amount of residual fluid in the tissues is called the interstitial fluid. When the interstitial fluid gets absorbed into the lymphatic capillaries, it becomes the lymph.

7.1.3 Lymphatic Capillary and Lymphatic Vessels

1. Lymphatic Capillary

The lymphatic capillary (毛细淋巴管) begins blindly. The wall is composed of a single layer of overlapping endothelial cells, basal laminae are incomplete or absent and they lack associated pericytes, and are generally quite permeable to much larger molecules. They are numerous and form complex networks. The brain, spinal cord, bone marrow, parenchyma of the spleen and eyeball lack lymphatic capillaries.

2. Lymphatic Vessels (淋巴管)

The walls of lymphatic vessels are similar to those of veins, but thinner. Like veins, lymphatic vessels have flap-like valves that help prevent the backflow of lymph. The larger lymphatic vessels lead to specialized organs called lymph nodes. After leaving the nodes, the vessels merge to form lymphatic trunks. The lymphatic trunks are named according to the region of the body that they drain the lymph from. There are four pairs of trunks: the lumbar, bronchomediastinal, subclavian and jugular. There is also one unpaired intestinal lymph trunk that drains lymph from the majority of organs of the gastrointestinal tract. The lymphatic trunks then converge into the two lymphatic ducts, the right lymph duct and the thoracic duct.

7.1.4   Lymphatic Ducts (淋巴导管)

1. Right Lymphatic Duct

The right lymphatic duct (右淋巴导管) receives lymph from the right side of the head and neck, the right upper limb, and the right thorax (right bronchomediastinal trunk, right subclavian trunk and right jugular trunk), and empties into the right subclavian vein near the junction of the right jugular vein. It drains lymph from the the right side of the thorax, and right side of the head, neck, and upper limb.

2. Thoracic Duct

The thoracic duct (胸导管) is commonly 36—45 cm in length, begins in front of L1 as a dilated sac, the cisterna chyli, which is formed by the joining of left and right lumbar trunks and intestinal trunk. The thoracic duct passes through the aortic hiatus and enters the posterior mediastinum, lying to the right of the midline, between the aorta and the azygos vein. It travels upward to the left at the level of T5. At the roof of the neck, it turns laterally and arches forwards to enter the left venous angle. Just before termination, it receives the left jugular, subclavian, and broncho-mediastinal trunks, a bicuspid valve at its termination may prevent the backflow of blood. It drains lymph from the lower limbs, pelvic cavity, abdominal cavity, the left side of the thorax, and left side of the head, neck, and left upper limb.

7.1.5   Lymph Node (淋巴结)

The lymph hode has a small oval or bean-shaped body, 0.1—2.5 cm long.

Afferent vessels enter the node on its convex surface, and efferent vessels leave the node at its concave surface—the hilum. They are arranged in groups along the blood vessels.

Regional lymph nodes (局部淋巴结) are the lymph node where the lymph of the organ or part of the body drains first.

Lymph nodes filter foreign substances, such as bacteria and cancer cells, from the lymph before it is re-entered into the blood system through the larger veins.Lymph nodes, which are scattered among the lymph vessels, act as the body's first defense against infection.

Lymph nodes produce the following cells: Lymphocytes (淋巴细胞) are a type of white blood cells, located in many sites in the body, most obviously at strategic sites that are liable to infection. All lymphocytes arise from pluripotent haemopoietic stem cells in the bone marrow. Monocytes (单核细胞) are leukocytes that protect against blood-borne pathogens, and plasma cells produce antibodies. Each lymph node has its blood supply and venous drainage. The lymph nodes usually have names that are related to their location in the body. When a specific location gets infected, the lymph nodes in that area will enlarge to fight the infection.

7.2 Lymphatic Drainage

7.2.1 Lymphatic Drainage of Head and Neck

The lymph nodes of the head are located at the junction of the head and the neck. They consist of occipital lymph nodes, mastoid lymph nodes, and parotid lymph nodes. Submandibular lymph nodes lie near the submandibular gland, and receive lymphatic vessels from the face, nose, and mouth, and submental lymph nodes drain into deep cervical lymph nodes (Fig.7-2).

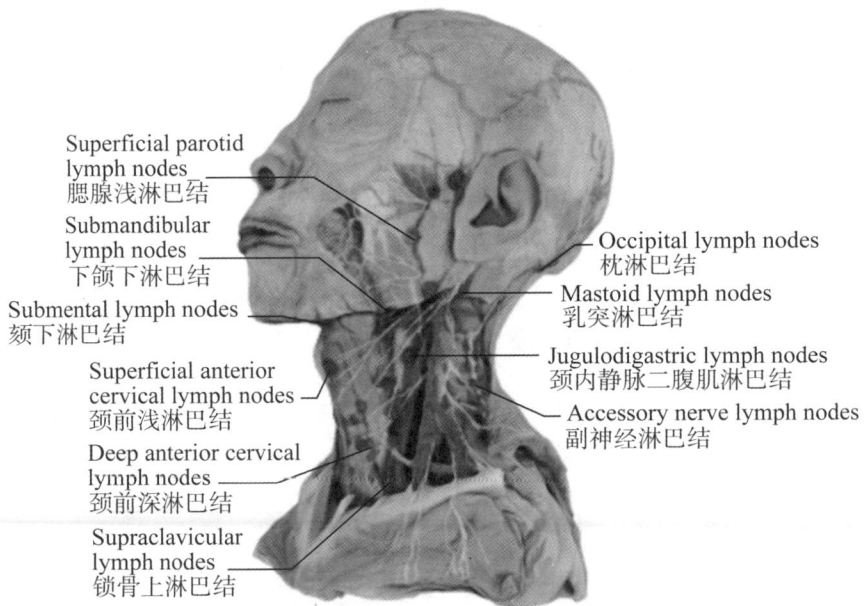

Fig.7-2　Lymphatic vessels and lymph nodes of the head and the neck

The lymph nodes of the neck can be seen in Fig.7-2. The cervical lymph nodes can be subdivided into two major groups. Those superficial to the sternocleido-mastoid muscle are known as the superficial cervical nodes, then subdivided into the pre-auricular or parotid nodes (anterior to the external ear), mastoid nodes (posterior to the external ear), and the occipital nodes. The deep cervical nodes are located in relation to the internal jugular vein, deep to the sternocleidomastoid muscle, and then are subdivided into the superior deep cervical nodes (the upper part of the internal jugular vein) and the inferior deep cervical nodes (the lower part of the internal vein).

7.2.2   Lymphatic Drainage of the Upper Limb

The lymph glands of the upper extremity are divided into two sets, the superficial glands and the deep glands.

Cubital lymph node (肘淋巴结) lies above the medial epicondyle of the humerus and receives lymph vessels from the forearm.

Axillary lymph nodes (腋淋巴结, Fig.7-3) vary in size from a pin-head to a large bean, about 20 mm to 30 mm and found in the axillary region (armpit) of the upper limb. The axillary lymph nodes have a particular clinical relevance due to their arrangement and drainage areas. This is particularly evident in breast cancer, where axillary lymph node status defines the treatment algorithm and approach. They are arranged in five groups.

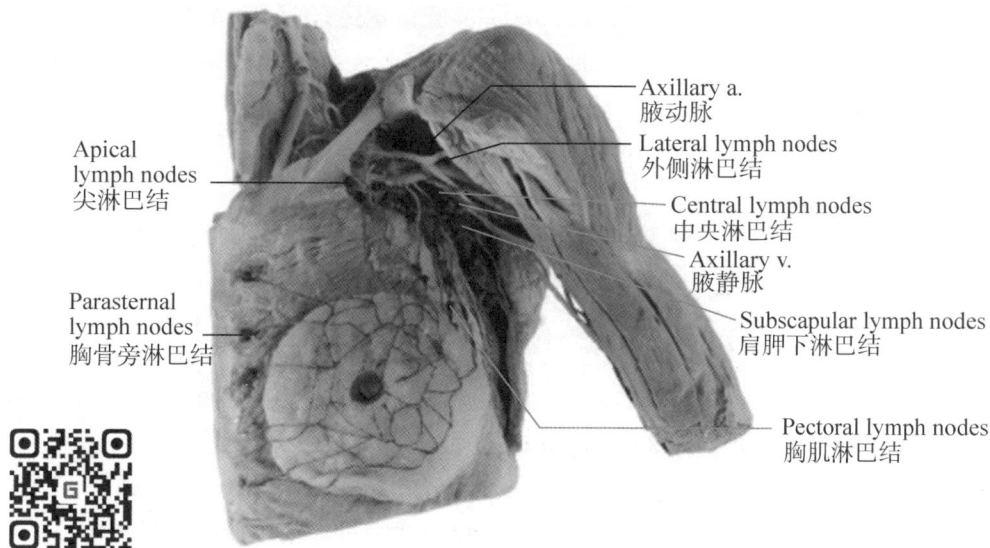

Fig.7-3   Lymphatic vessels of the mammary gland and axillary lymph nodes

Pectoral lymph nodes (胸肌淋巴结), about four or five nodes, lie along the lower border of pectoralis minor behind the pectoralis major and receive lymph vessels from the lateral quadrants of the breast and superficial vessels from the anterolateral abdominal wall above the level of the umbilicus.

Lateral lymph nodes (外侧淋巴结), about four to six nodes, are along the medial side distal part of the axillary vein. They receive lymph from the upper limb, except the vessels that accompany the cephalic vein. Efferent vessels partly to the inferior deep cervical nodes.

Subscapular lymph nodes (肩胛下淋巴结), about six or seven nodes, lie along subscapular vessels, in front of the subscapularis. They receive superficial lymph vessels from the back, down as far as the level of the iliac crests. The efferent of the above three groups passes to the central lymph node and the apical axillary nodes.

Central lymph nodes (中央淋巴结), about three or four large nodes, lie in the center of the axilla in the axillary fat. They receive lymph from the above three nodes. Efferents pass to the apical lymph node.

Apical lymph nodes (尖淋巴结) (infraclavicular lymph nodes), about six to twelve nodes, lie at the apex of the axilla at the lateral border of the first rib. They receive lymph of the efferent lymph vessels from all the other axillary nodes. The efferent of the apical nodes forms the subclavian trunk, the right subclavian trunk joins the right lymphatic duct; the left usually drains directly into the thoracic duct.

7.2.3　Lymphatic Drainage of the Thorax

About three-quarters of the lymphatic drainage is to the axillary nodes.

(I) Lymphatics pass around the edge of the pectoralis major and reach the pectoral group of axillary nodes.

(II) Routes through or between the pectoral muscles may lead directly to the apical nodes of the axilla.

(III) Lymphatics follow the blood vessels through the pectoralis major and enter the parasternal (internal thoracic) nodes.

(IV) Connections may lead across the median plane and hence to the contra-lateral breast.

(V) Lymphatics may reach the sheath of the rectus abdominis and the subperi-toneal and subhepatic plexuses. It should be noted that free communication exists between nodes below and above the clavicle and between the axillary and cervical nodes. Those superficial to the trapezius and latissimus dorsi end in the subscapular nodes. Lymph from the deeper tissues of the thoracic walls drains mainly to the parasternal, intercostal, or diaphragmatic nodes (Fig.7-4).

Pulmonary lymph nodes (肺淋巴结) lie in the angles of bifurcation of branching lobar bronchi. Bronchopulmonary hilar lymph nodes lie in the hilum of the lung. Tracheobronchial lymph nodes are situated above or below the bifurcation of the trachea.

Paratracheal lymph nodes are along each side of the trachea. Pulmonary nodes within the lung parenchyma are continuous with the bronchopulmonary node groups, subsegmental nodes, segmental nodes, lobar nodes, interlobar and hilar nodes.

Anterior mediastinal lymph nodes (纵隔前淋巴结) lie anterior to the large blood vessels of thoracic cavity and pericardium. The efferents unite with those of paratracheal lymph nodes and parasternal lymph nodes to form the right and left bronchomediastinal trunks. The left bronchomediastinal trunk terminates in the thoracic duct, and the right in the right lymphatic duct.

Posterior mediastinal lymph nodes (纵隔后淋巴结) lie along the esophagus and thoracic aorta.

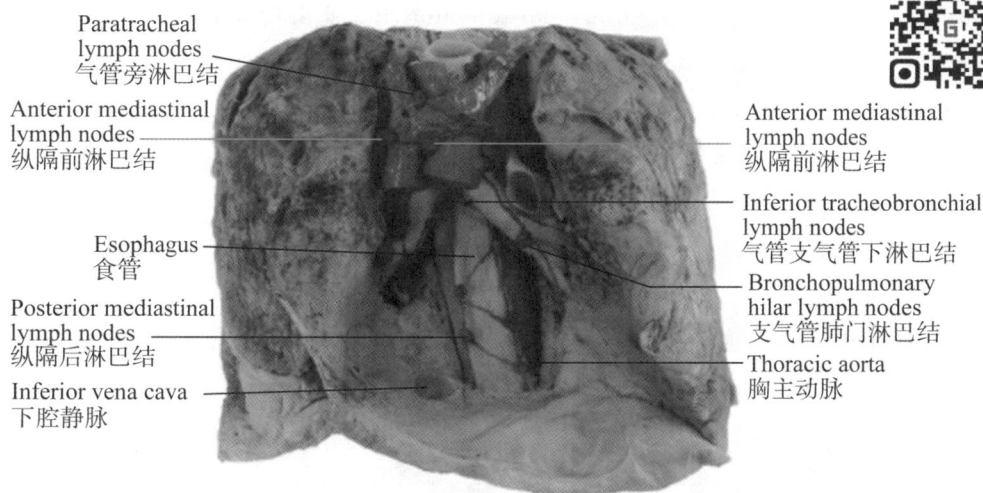

Fig.7-4   Lymphatic vessels and lymph nodes of the trachea, bronchi and lungs

7.2.4   Lymph Nodes of the Abdomen

Lymphatic drainage of the abdominal wall may be divided into two sets, the superficial vessels and the deep vessels. The superficial vessels follow the course of the superficial blood vessels and converge to the superficial inguinal nodes; those derived from the integument of the front of the abdomen below the umbilicus follow the course of the superficial epigastric vessels, and those from the sides of the lumbar part of the abdominal wall pass along the crest of the ilium, with the superficial iliac circumflex vessels. The deep vessels run alongside the principal blood vessels, and drain to the lumbar lymph nodes.

1. Lymphatic Drainage of Abdominal Viscera

Lumbar lymph nodes (腰淋巴结) lie on the posterior abdominal wall, along the abdominal aorta and inferior vena cava. They receive lymph from kidneys, suprarenal glands, testes, ovaries, the fundus of the uterus, uterine tubes, and common iliac nodes. The right and left lumbar trunks are formed by efferent vessels. Paired viscera drain to the lumbar lymph nodes.

Right and left gastric lymph nodes (胃右淋巴结和胃左淋巴结) can be seen in Fig. 7-5. The stomach has a rich network of lymphatics that connect with lymphatics draining other viscera within the proximal abdomen, lying along the same vessels, and finally to the celiac lymph nodes. The right and left gastroomental lymph nodes lie along the same vessels, while the former drain into subpyloric lymph nodes, and the latter drain into splenic lymph nodes. Suprapyloric and subpyloric lymph nodes receive lymphatics from the pyloric part and finally to the celiac lymph nodes. Splenic lymph nodes receive lymphatics from the fundus and leave 1/3 of the stomach, and finally to the celiac lymph nodes. Celiac lymph nodes are situated around the celiac trunk.

Superior mesenteric lymph node (肠系膜上淋巴结) is situated around the superior mesenteric artery.

Inferior mesenteric lymph node (肠系膜下淋巴结) is situated around the inferior mesenteric artery.

Intestinal trunk (肠干) is formed by the efferent vessels of celiac, superior, and inferior lymph nodes.

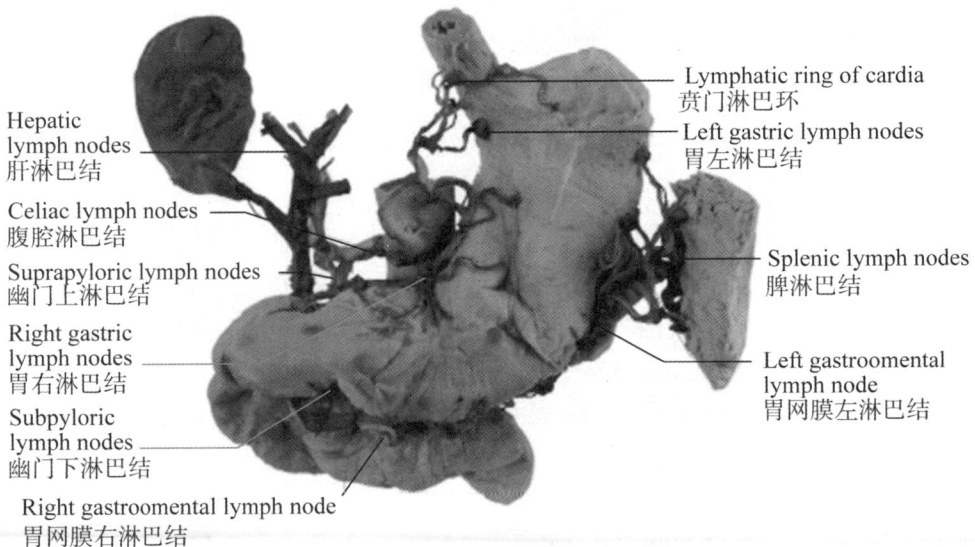

Fig.7-5　Lymph nodes of the stomach

7.2.5   Lymph Nodes of Pelvis

Internal iliac lymph nodes (髂内淋巴结) surround internal iliac vessels and receive afferents from the pelvic viscera, perineum, buttock, and back of the thigh, and drain to the common iliac lymph nodes. When they get close to the anterior and posterior midlines, the right and left groups of the viscera lymph nodes are frequent connections.

External iliac lymph nodes (髂外淋巴结) lie along the external iliac artery and receive afferents from the lower limb and some parts of the pelvic viscera. The efferent vessels drain into the common iliac nodes.

Sacral lymph node (骶淋巴结) is located along the middle sacral artery and lateral sacral artery, and receives lymph from the posterior pelvic wall, rectum, prostate or uterus.

Common iliac lymph nodes (髂总淋巴结) lie along the common iliac artery and receive afferents from all the above nodes, receiving the entire lymphatic drainage of the lower limb. The efferent one passes to the lumbar lymph nodes (Fig. 7-6).

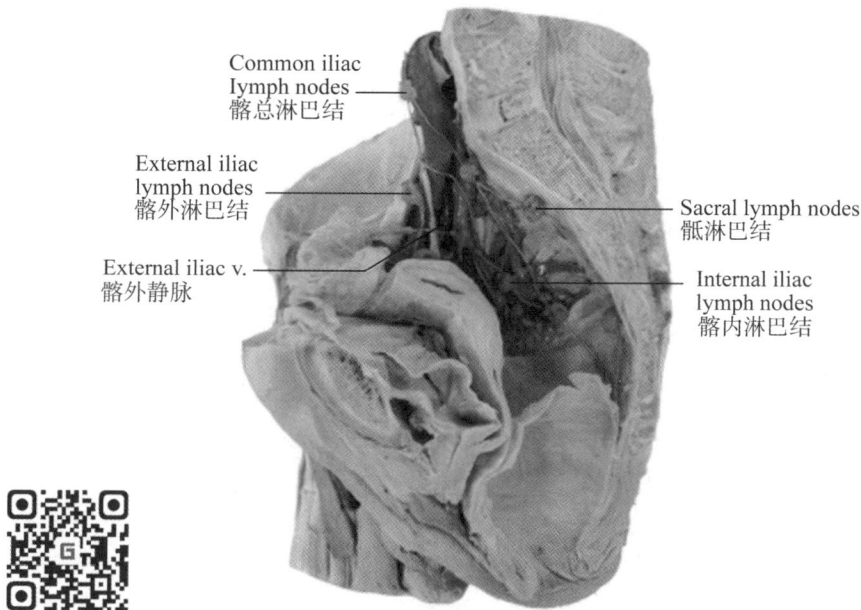

Fig.7-6   Lymph nodes of the pelvic cavity

7.2.6   Lymph Nodes of the Lower Limb

The lymph nodes of the lower extremity consist of the anterior tibial and popliteal and inguinal.

The anterior tibial lymph nodes (胫前淋巴结) are small and inconstant. It lies on the interosseous membrane in relation to the upper part of the anterior tibial vessels, and constitutes a substation in the course of the anterior tibial lymphatic trunks.

Popliteal lymph nodes (腘淋巴结) are embedded in the fatty connective tissue of the popliteal fossa. It receives superficial lymphatic vessels from the posterolateral part of the calf, and deep lymphatic vessels accompanying the anterior and posterior tibia. The efferent one passes to the deep inguinal lymph nodes.

Superficial inguinal lymph nodes (腹股沟浅淋巴结) consist of the superior group, inferior group, and deep inguinal lymph nodes.

Superior group (上群) lies just distal to the inguinal ligament, and it receives lymph vessels from the anterior abdominal wall below the umbilicus, gluteal region, perineal region, and external genital organs.

Inferior group (下群) lies vertically along the terminal great saphenous vein, and it receives all superficial lymph vessels of the lower limb, except for those from the posterolateral part of the calf. The efferent vessels drain into the deep inguinal lymph nodes or external iliac lymph nodes.

Deep inguinal lymph nodes (腹股沟深淋巴结) lie medial to the femoral vein. They receive deep lymph vessels of the lower limb, perineal region, and efferent vessels from the superficial inguinal lymph nodes and drain into the external iliac lymph nodes.

7.3 Thymus and Spleen

7.3.1 Thymus (胸腺)

The thymus is an encapsulated soft organ partly in the neck and partly in the thorax. The greater part of the thymus lies in the anterior mediastinum and the anterior part of the superior mediastinum: Its inferior aspect reaches the level of the fourth costal cartilage. It comprises one to three lobes, each of which consists of numerous lobules containing lymphocytes, which are important in the development and maintenance of the immune system. The organ has a profuse blood supply and lymphatic drainage. The thymus reaches its greatest size at puberty and then begins to regress. Much of its substance is replaced by fat and fibrous tissue, but thymic tissue never disappears completely. The thymus is an essential component of our immune systems. It functions as the initial site of T cell immune maturation through positive and negative selection processes.

7.3.2 Spleen (脾)

The spleen (Fig. 7-7) is an intraperitoneal organ and the largest single mass of lymphoid tissue in the body. It is reddish. The spleen lies in the left hypochondriac region (between the stomach and the diaphragm) deep to the ninth to the eleventh rib. Its long axis corresponds roughly to the tenth rib. Its lower pole extends forward only as far as the midline and cannot be palpated on clinical examination. Its network of the trabeculae, blood vessels and lymphoid tissue provides an environment in which white blood cells (lymphocytes) proliferate while old damaged red blood cells (erythrocytes) are recycled. Although it may seem dispensable as it is possible to live without it, the function of the spleen is erythrocyte storage, phagocytosis, cytopoiesis, and immune responses.

Two surfaces are diaphragmatic which is smooth and convex and visceral which is concave and the hilum of the spleen, the site through which the splenic artery and vein pass.

Two extremities are the anterior extremity which is wider and the posterior extremity which is rounder.

Three borders are superior, inferior, and anterior. The superior border bounds the gastric area, the inferior border bounds the renal area and the anterior border bounds the colic area. The superior border has 2—3 splenic notch, which serves as a landmark on palpation when it is enlarged; normally it is not palpable. The inferior border is more rounded and blunt.

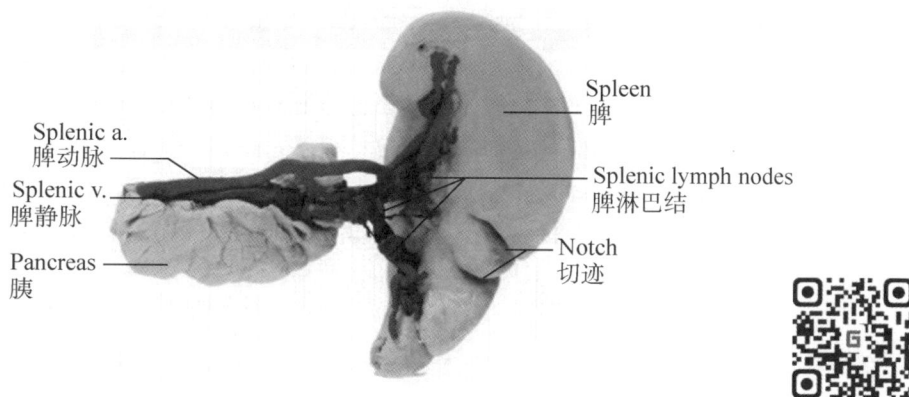

Fig.7-7 Lymphatic vessels and lymph nodes of the spleen

(杭州师范大学医学院　赵建军)

Exercise

1. A 11-year-old girl was admitted to endocrine department due to a lump in the neck. She also complained poor memory in these days. This lump moved up and down with

Systematic Anatomy (2nd Edition)

swallowing. Which of the following structure was most likely affected?

(A)The thymus.

(B) The lingual tonsil.

(C) The parathyroid gland.

(D) The submandibular gland.

(E) The thyroid gland.

2. A 43-year-old man was diagnosed with thyroid cancer. He required a surgery to move the thyroid gland. Which of the following organ would cut during this surgery?

(A) The thymus.

(B) The lingual tonsil.

(C) The parathyroid gland.

(D) The submandibular gland.

(E) The hypophysis.

Answer

1. The correct answer is E.

This is a typical symptom of hypothyroidism. The thyroid gland is located below the thyroid cartilage in the neck, on both sides of the trachea which can be touched when swallowing. The thymus (Choice A) is located behind the sternal stalk which consists of lymphocytes. Lingual tonsil (Choice B) is located at the root of the tongue and participate in the immune function of the body. The parathyroid gland (Choice C) is located at the back of the thyroid gland and regulates the metabolism of calcium and phosphorus. The submandibular gland (Choice D) is located at the lower edge of the mandible and can secrete saliva. These structures cannot be touched.

2. The correct answer is C.

The parathyroid gland (Choice C) is located on the back of the right and left lobes of the thyroid gland and it is inadvertently removed during surgical removal of the thyroid gland.

220

The Sensory Organ

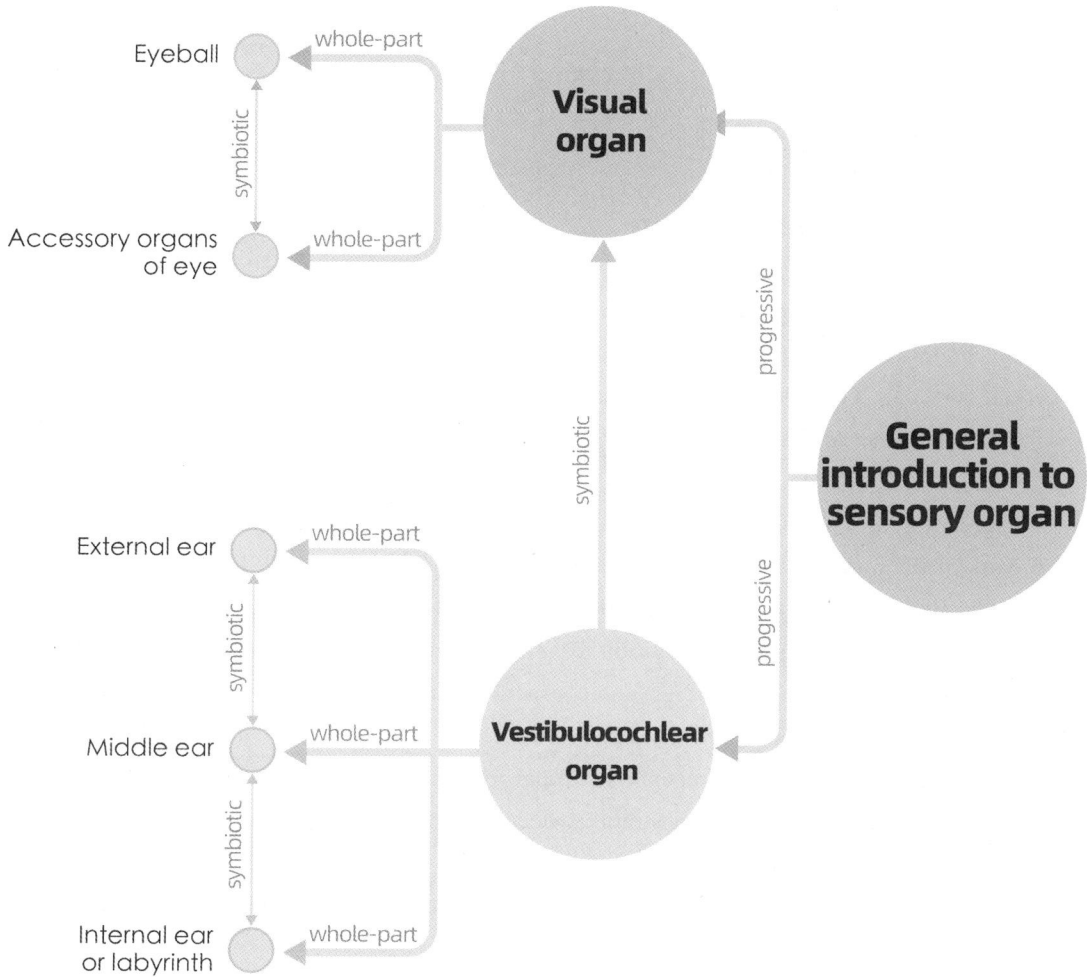

Eyeball — whole-part → **Visual organ**

Accessory organs of eye — whole-part → **Visual organ**

Eyeball — symbiotic — Accessory organs of eye

General introduction to sensory organ — progressive → **Visual organ**

General introduction to sensory organ — progressive → **Vestibulocochlear organ**

Visual organ — symbiotic — **Vestibulocochlear organ**

External ear — whole-part → **Vestibulocochlear organ**

Middle ear — whole-part → **Vestibulocochlear organ**

Internal ear or labyrinth — whole-part → **Vestibulocochlear organ**

External ear — symbiotic — Middle ear

Middle ear — symbiotic — Internal ear or labyrinth

Chapter 8   Sensory Organs

8.1   General Introduction

The sensory organs comprise the receptors, the neural connections and their associated structures. Human beings have sense organs and each sense organ responds to a certain stimulus. For example, the eye senses and sees light. Receptors are the initial part of the sensory nerve that receive the external and internal stimuli from the surroundings like light, touch, sound, smell and taste.

Receptors (感受器) are the terminal devices of sensory nerves, widely distributed in all parts of the body, with different functions and complex structures. Some structures are very simple, only the free endings of sensory nerves, such as pain receptors; some structures are more complex, in addition to nerve endings, there is a capsule of connective tissue outside, such as tactile bodies; some structures are more complex, which is an organ composed of receptors and their subsidiary structures, called sensory organs (感觉器官). Activation of these sensory receptors results in graded potentials that trigger nerve impulses and the interpretation of stimulus occurs in the brain and thus a response to the stimulus is initiated.

Depending on the location of the receptors and the origin of the stimuli, the receptors can be divided into three types.

1. Exteroceptors (外感受器)

Exteroceptors respond to tactile sensations or stimuli that arise outside the body, thus they are located on the surface of the body. These receptors are sensitive to external stimuli like touch, pressure, pain, temperature, light, sound, etc. They are distributed in the skin, mucous membranes, visual and auditory organs.

2. Interoceptors (内感受器)

Interoceptors respond to stimuli arising in internal viscera and blood vessels. These types of receptors are sensitive to chemical changes inside the body, tissue stretch deep within the body and core temperature changes. Thus, they are distributed in the viscera and the internal organs.

3. Proprioceptors (本体感受器)

Proprioceptors refer to receptors that are sensitive to changes in the body position and equilibrium. They respond to stretching in skeletal muscles, tendons, joints, ligaments and connective tissue coverings of bones and muscle.

8.2　Visual Organ

The visual organ (视器, Fig.8-1), commonly known as the eye, is a highly specialized sensory organ responsible for vision located within the bony orbit. It consists of two parts, the eyeball and the accessory organs of eyeball. The main function of the eye is to detect the light rays (photoreception) and to convey the gathered information to the visual cortex in the brain via the optic nerve (CN Ⅱ).

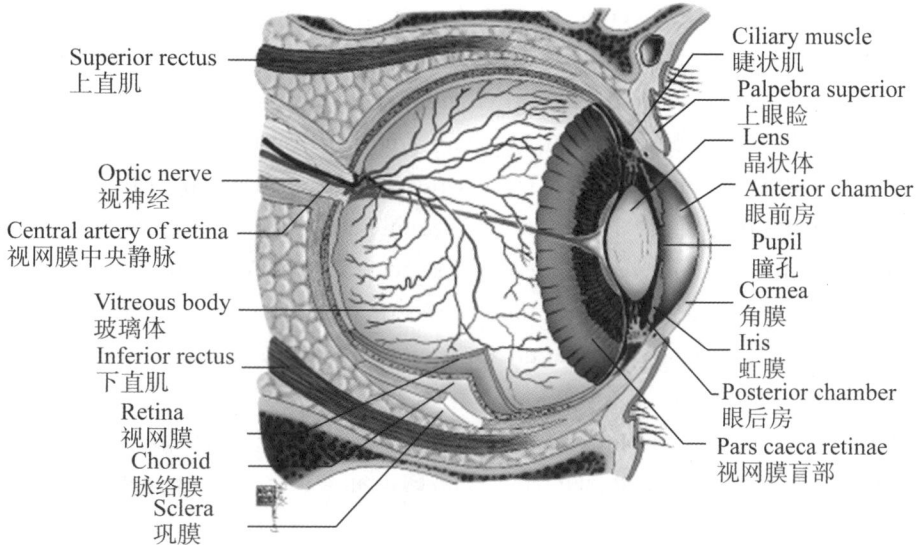

Fig.8-1　Visual organ

8.2.1　Eyeball

The eyeball (眼球) with extraocular muscles and the associated neurovascular structures are located in a bony socket called orbit. The eyeball is attached to the orbit through the extraocular muscles. The central point of the cornea on the anterior surface of the eyeball is called the anterior pole (前极), and the central point of the sclera on the posterior surface of the eyeball is called the posterior pole (后极). The straight line connecting the anterior and posterior poles is called the axis of eyeball (眼轴). The circular line of points at the same distance from the anterior and posterior poles is called the equator (赤道). The line from the center of the pupil to the fovea centralis of the macula lutea is called the optic axis (视轴).

1. Tunica of Eyeball

The eyeball consists of three distinct layers. From superficial to deep, they include: fibrous membrane (纤维膜), vascular tunic (血管膜), and retina (视网膜).

(1) Fibrous membrane (纤维膜)

The fibrous membrane is composed of tough and dense connective tissue. This outermost layer comprises of cornea and sclera, the layer that protects the inner structures of the eyeball.

1) The cornea (角膜) occupies the anterior one sixth of the fibrous membrane and is a convex part of the eye that covers the front portion of the eye. It is transparent and avascular. It is colourless, elastic, and has refractive effect; the cornea is rich in sensory nerves, so it is sensitive. The cornea is the thickest at its periphery, entirely composed of proteins and cells organized in five layers. The nutrition of the cornea depends on the supply of aqueous humor, tear and limbal vascular exudate.

2) Sclera (巩膜) accounts for the posterior 5/6 of the fibrous membrane. It is opaque and milky white in colour because of the irregularly thickened collagen fibers which also prevents the light rays to pass through them. The thickness of the sclera varies and it is the thickest around the optic nerve and the thinnest posterior to the insertion of recti muscle. The aqueous humor enters the vein though the ring-shaped tube called scleral venous sinus (巩膜静脉窦) is located deep at the junction of the sclera and the cornea.

(2) Vascular tunic (血管膜)

The middle layer is rich in blood vessels, so it is called vascular tunic (血管膜), which contains the pigmented cells that make it appear brown in colour. This layer nourishes the eyeball and also helps in absorbing the light rays. It has three parts going from the anterior to posterior as iris, ciliary body and choroid.

1) Iris (虹膜) is the most anterior part of the vascular membrane, located between the cornea and the lens, in the shape of a disc with a round hole in the center called the pupil (瞳孔) (Fig. 8-2). There are two kinds of smooth muscles running in different directions in the iris. One is the sphincter pupillae (瞳孔括约肌), which surrounds the pupil near the edge of the pupil, and can make the pupil narrow when it contracts. It is innervated by the parasympathetic fibers from the oculomotor nerve (CN Ⅲ). The other is the dilator pupillae (瞳孔开大肌), whose muscle fibers are arranged radially from the periphery of the iris to the pupil. When contracting, it pulls the edge of the pupil to make the pupil open. It is innervated by the sympathetic fibers from the superior cervical ganglion. The acute angle formed by the root of iris and the cornea is called the iridocorneal angle

(filtration angle). This angle contains the trabecular meshwork that facilitates the drainage of the aqueous humor into the Schlemm's canal, and as such is an important point in the pathway of the aqueous humor. An injury of the iris can squeeze the iridocorneal angle and obstruct the aqueous humor outflow, which leads to closed-angle glaucoma.

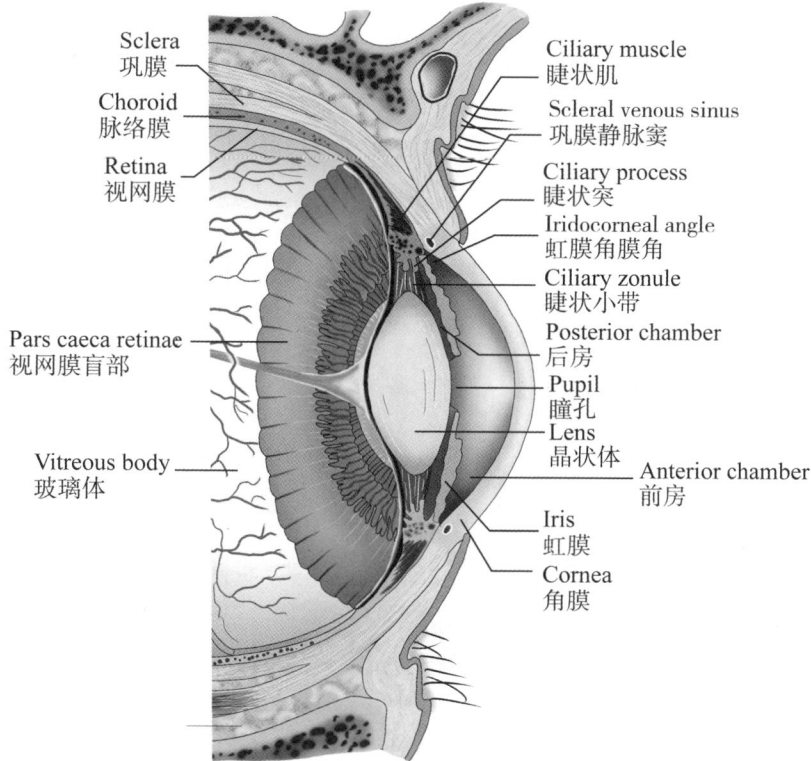

Fig.8-2　Iridocorneal angle

2) Ciliary body (睫状体) is located at the inner surface of the transitional portion of the cornea and the sclera. The ciliary body forms a complete ring around the iris with thicker (the anterior end) and gradually thinner (the posterior side). The ciliary body is triangular in shape. Thus, it looks triangular in shape on the cross-section of the eye. The smooth muscle in the ciliary body is called the ciliary muscle (睫状肌). The ciliary zonule (睫状小带) is the thread-like structure connecting the ciliary body and the lens, also known as the suspensory ligament of lens (晶状体悬韧带). When the ciliary muscle contracts, the ciliary body moves forward and inward, resulting in relaxation of the ciliary zonule, which increases the curvature of the lens and the refractive ability and plays an important role in the process of accommodation. Epithelial cells on the surface of the ciliary body secrete aqueous humor.

3) Choroid (脉络膜) occupies the posterior 2/3 of the vascular membrane, which

adjoins the sclera on the outside and connects to the retina from inside. It is a loose connective tissue rich in blood vessels and pigmented cells thus have a nourishing effect on the eyeball and also absorbs the light rays and prevents light from getting reflected by the interference of various objects.

(3) Retina

The retina (视网膜) is the innermost layer of the eyeball that extends from the site of exit of the optic nerve to the internal surface of the iris. The main function of retina is to record the image acting as a film and then send it to the visual cortex via the optic nerve (Fig. 8-3).

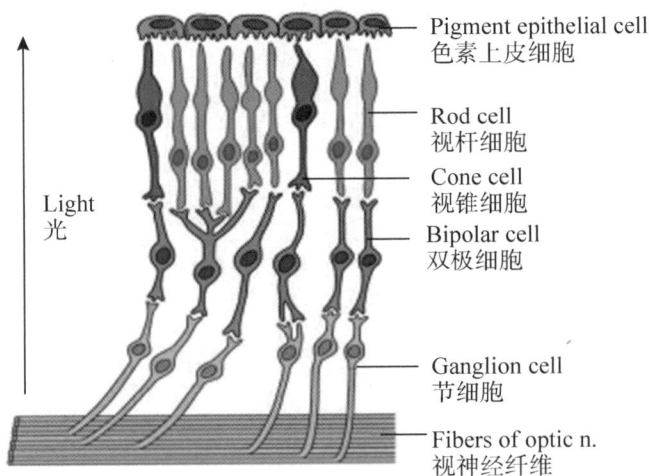

Fig.8-3   Schematic diagram of nerve of retina

Retina is transparent in colour and has three parts. The part of retina that lines the inner surface of the iris and ciliary body has no light sensitive function and is called the pars caeca retinae (视网膜盲部); while the portion that lines the inner surface of the choroid has a light-sensitive function, it is called the pars optica retinae (视网膜视部). The ora serrata (锯状缘) is the serrated edge between the pars optica retinae and the pars caeca retinae. The optic disc (视神经盘) or optic papilla (视神经乳头), commonly known as the blind spot (盲点), is the first part of the optic nerve, and it is the point where the optic nerve, the central artery and the vein of retina leave the eyeball. There are no rods and cones present at this point and thus no vision is recorded at this point. At about 3.5 mm on the temporal side of the optic disc, there is a yellow small area called the macula lutea (黄斑); the central depression of macula lutea is called fovea centralis (中央凹), which consists of maximum concentration of cone cells thereby providing the sharpest resolution and is the area most sensitive to light. The structure of the optic part of the retina is divided into two layers, the outer pigment cell layer and the inner nerve layer.

The pigment cell layer is a single layer of pigment cells, which can absorb light and protect the visual cells from strong light stimulation; while the nerve layer is composed of three layers of cells and from outside to inside are cone and rod cell layer, bipolar cell layer, and ganglion cell layer. Cone and rod cells (视锥和视杆细胞) are photoreceptors cells, which act as the receptors for vision. The three layers of nerve cells communicate with each other through various synapses. The axons of the ganglion cells gather at the back of the eye to form the optic disc, and pass through the sclera to form the optic nerve.

2. Contents of Eyeball

The contents of the eyeball include the aqueous humor, lens, and vitreous body. They are all transparent structures without blood vessels, which have a refractive effect on light and form the dioptric system (屈光系统) of the eye together with the cornea.

(1) Eye chamber and aqueous humor

1) Chamber of eye (眼房) is an irregular cavity among the cornea, the lens, the ciliary body, and the ciliary zonule, and is divided into an anterior chamber and a posterior chamber by the iris. The anterior chamber of the eye (眼前房) is between the cornea and the iris. In the peripheral part of the anterior chamber, the angular part where iris and cornea meet is termed as the iridocorneal angle (虹膜角膜角), also known as the angle of anterior chamber (前房角). The posterior chamber of the eye (眼后房) is the space bounded by the iris, ciliary body, ciliary zonule and lens. The two chambers communicate with each other through the pupil.

2) Aqueous humor (房水) is produced by the ciliary body, a transparent fluid with a relatively low refractive index that fills the chamber of the eye. Its circulation route is as follows: Ciliary body secretes it in the posterior chamber, then reaches the anterior chamber via pupil. It enters the scleral venous sinus (巩膜静脉窦) through the iridocorneal angle, and drains into the ophthalmic vein (眼静脉) through the anterior ciliary vein (睫前静脉).

In addition to its refractive effect, aqueous humor also nourishes the cornea and lens and maintains normal intraocular pressure. If the circulation of aqueous humor is blocked, it will cause the intraocular pressure to increase and compress the optic nerve, leading to vision loss or blindness, which is called glaucoma (青光眼).

(2) Lens

Lens (晶状体) is a circular biconvex structure found anterior to the vitreous body and posterior to the iris. It is transparent and elastic, without blood vessels and nerves. The anterior surface of lens is less convex compared to the posterior surface. The light rays that enter the eye is converged onto the retina using the refractive power of the lens. The periphery of the lens is connected to the ciliary body by the ciliary zonule, the contraction and relaxation of the ciliary muscles can relax or tense the ciliary zonule, thereby adjusting the curvature of the lens. While looking at nearby objects, the ciliary muscles are contracted to tense the ciliary zonule, and then curvature of the lens increases thereby increasing the refractive power. With age, the elasticity of the lens decreases, when looking at nearby objects, the curvature of the lens cannot be increased accordingly, resulting in blurred vision, which is called presbyopia (老花眼). A cataract (白内障) is referred to as the condition of opacification of lens or when the lens is obscured.

(3)Vitreous body

The colourless, transparent jelly-like substance filled between the lens and the retina, and surrounded by a hyaloid membrane is the vitreous body (玻璃体). It is the largest structure of the eyeball, occupying the four-fifths of the entire eye. In addition to its refractive function, the vitreous also supports the retina and stabilizes the metabolism inside the eye.

8.2.2 Accessory Organs of Eyes

1. Eyelids and Conjunctiva

(1) Eyelids

Eyelids (眼睑) are thin soft tissue structures that are movable folds of muscle and skin, cover and protect the anterior surface of the eyeball. The free edges of the eyelids are called the lid margin (睑缘). The gap between the upper and lower palpe-bral margins is called the palpebral fissure (睑裂), and the medial and lateral corners of the palpebral fissure are called the medial and lateral angle of eye (内眦和外眦), respectively. Eyelashes grow on the palpebral margins. Near the medial angle of the eye there is a slightly concave space between the upper and lower eyelids called the lacrimal lacus (泪湖), and the small red protrusion in the lacrimal lake is called the lacrimal caruncle (泪阜), which are small channels within each eyelid, via the lacrimal puncta.

The eyelids are composed of the following five layers from shallow to deep: skin, superficial fascia, muscular layer, tarsus and conjunctiva. The skin of the eyelids is thin and the subcutaneous fascia is loose. The muscle layer of the eyelid is mainly the orbicularis oculi (眼轮匝肌), and there is also a levator palpebrae superioris (上睑提肌) on the deep side of the orbicularis oculi of the upper eyelid. The levator palpe-brae superioris helps in elevation of upper eyelid while orbicularis oculi helps in closure of eyelid. The tarsal plate (睑板), which is composed of dense connective tissue, which is the support of the eyelid. There are tarsal gland (睑板腺) inside, whose ducts open at the palpebral margins and secrete fatty liquid, which has the function of lubricating the eyelid margins. Blockage of the tarsal gland ducts may form a cyst, also known as a chalazion (睑板腺囊肿).

(2) Conjunctiva

The conjunctiva (结膜) is a layer of transparent mucosa rich in blood vessels and lines both the inner surface of the eyelids and the anterior surface of the eyeball (except the cornea). It allows the eyelid and eye to move smoothly and freely with keeping it moist and protecting it from contact injury. Conjunctiva is divided into three parts. The bulbar conjunctiva (球结膜) covering the front of the sclera, the palpebral conjunctiva (睑结膜) covering the back of the eyelids, and the cup-shaped depression formed by the reflected parts of the conjunctiva are called the superior and inferior conjunctival fornix (结膜上穹和结膜下穹). All the conjunctiva surrounds a sac-like cavity called the conjunctival sac (结膜囊).

2. The Lacrimal Apparatus

The lacrimal apparatus (泪器) (Fig.8-4) consists of the lacrimal gland and the lacrimal passage.

(1) The lacrimal gland

The lacrimal gland (泪腺) is located in the lacrimal fossa of anterolateral part of the upper wall of the orbit, and its excretory duct opens in the superior conjun-ctival fornix; after blinking, the tear crosses the front of the eyeball and finally enters the lacrimal lacus. Tears can moisten, protect and provide nutrients to the conjunctiva and cornea.

(2) The lacrimal passage

The lacrimal passage (泪道) includes the lacrimal punctum, lacrimal ductule, lacrimal sac and nasolacrimal duct.

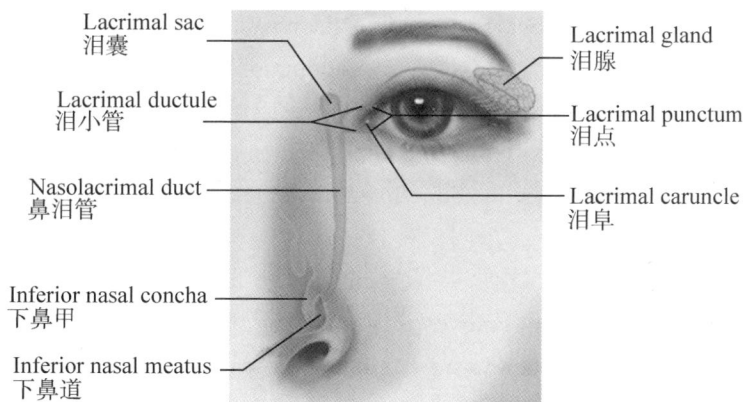

Fig.8-4　Lacrimal apparatus

1) Lacrimal puncta (泪乳头) are two small protrusions found on the inner side of the medial end of the upper and lower eyelid's margin, the small holes at the top of the lacrimal papillae are called lacrimal punctum (泪点), which are the opening of lacrimal ductule. Lacrimal puncta face back to the lacrimal lacus to receive the tears.

2) Lacrimal ductule (canaliculi) (泪小管) starts from the lacrimal puncta on the inner side of the upper and lower eyelid margins and drain into the lacrimal sac inward.

3) Lacrimal sac (泪囊) is the upper dilated end of the nasolacrimal duct in the fossa for lacrimal sac on the medial wall of the orbit.

4) Nasolacrimal duct (鼻泪管) connects to the lacrimal sac and opens downward to the inferior nasal meatus.

3. Extraocular Muscles

There are seven extraocular muscles (眼球外肌). The levator palpebrae superioris is the muscle that can lift the upper eyelid, and the other six muscles are the muscles that can move the eyeball, including four rectus muscles and two oblique muscles.

(1) The levator palpebrae superioris

The levator palpebrae superioris (上睑提肌) is located between the superior rectus muscle and the superior orbital wall. It starts at the back of the superior orbital wall and ends at the superior tarsus and the skin of upper eyelid with elevating and retracting the upper eyelid and allowing unhindered upward gaze. It receives somatic motor innervation from the superior division of oculomotor nerve (CN III).

(2) Straight muscles

They arise from the common tendinous ring (总腱环) and are named as the superior rectus (上直肌), inferior rectus (下直肌), medial rectus (内直肌) and lateral rectus (外直肌). The rectus muscles attach to the sclera of eyeball in front of the equator, the superior and inferior rectus muscles are located above and below the eyeball, the angle of superior rectus and inferior rectus is located lateral to the visual axis, so the superior rectus is responsible for elevation, incyclotorsion and adduction (inward, rotational movement) while inferior rectus is responsible for depression, extorsion (inward, rotational movement) and adduction. The medial and lateral rectus muscles are located at the medial and lateral sides of the eyeball, with adduction and abduction respectively.

(3) Oblique muscles

The superior obliquus (上斜肌) is the thinnest and longest extraocular muscle, arises from the common tendinous ring, moves forward along the medial wall of the orbit above the medial rectus muscle, and then forms a thin tendon, passes through the trochlea formed by the U-shaped fibrocartilage attaching the front and upper part of medial wall of the orbit, and then turns backward and outside, inserted into the sclera behind the equator below the superior rectus muscle. The inferior obliquus (下斜肌) is the only muscle which arises from the anterior part of the orbit. It starts from the anteromedial side of the infraorbital wall and runs backward and outward, and is inserted into the sclera behind the equator under the inferior rectus muscle.

The oblique muscles are angled medially to the visual axis. Thus, the function of the superior obliquus is to turn the eyeball outward and downward, and the function of the inferior obliquus is to turn the eyeball outward and upward when contracted.

8.3   Vestibulocochlear Organ

The ear is the vestibulocochlear organ (前庭蜗器) (Fig. 8-5) that serves the purpose of hearing and posture balancing by transforming information from the external environment into electrical impulses that the brain can comprehend. The vestibular organ (前庭器) senses the changes in position whereas the auditory apparatus (听器) receives sounds waves. The ear is located in the temporal bone of the cranium except the auricle and cartilaginous part of external acoustic meatus. The outer ear along with the middle ear helps to transmit the sound waves while the positional and auditory receptors are located in the inner ear. The ear is anatomically divided into three portions: the external ear, the middle ear and the internal ear.

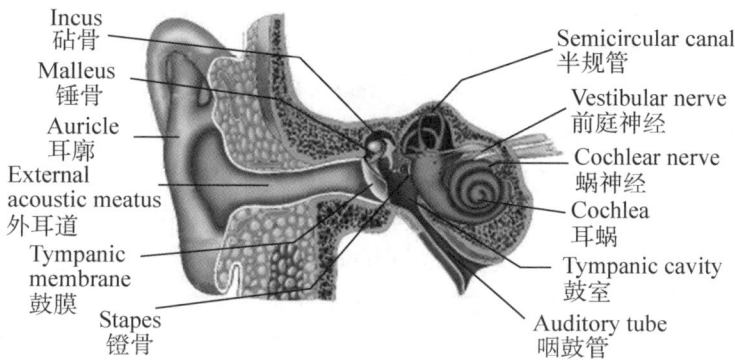

Incus
砧骨
Malleus
锤骨
Auricle
耳廓
External
acoustic meatus
外耳道
Tympanic
membrane
鼓膜
Stapes
镫骨

Semicircular canal
半规管
Vestibular nerve
前庭神经
Cochlear nerve
蜗神经
Cochlea
耳蜗
Tympanic cavity
鼓室
Auditory tube
咽鼓管

Fig.8-5   Vestibulocochlear organ

1. The External Ear

The external ear (外耳) serves to conduct sound to the middle ear, and consists of three parts: the auricle, the external acoustic meatus and the tympanic membrane.

(1) **The auricle**

The auricle (pinna) (耳廓) is composed of elastic cartilage for support and covered with skin. The auricle is attached to the side of the lateral part of the head by the intrinsic and extrinsic muscles and ligaments. The auricle serves as the protection for the delicate inner parts of the ear. The shape of the auricle also helps detect where sounds are coming from in the vertical plane. The auricle has multiple folds, ridges and depressions. The outermost largest rim on the anterolateral surface is the helix (耳轮). It starts from the crus of helix (耳轮脚) and takes a turn as a curve and ends in the fatty soft tissue part called auricular lobule. The auricular lobule (耳垂) is located at the lower part and has no cartilage.

The triangular protrusion in front of the external acoustic pore is called tragus (耳屏). The projection opposite to the tragus is called antitragus (对耳屏). The curved eminence in front of and parallel to the helix is the antihelix (对耳轮). Auricular concha (耳甲) is a depression in front of the antihelix. Auricular concha is divided into two depressions by crus of helix, the upper depression is called the cymba of auricular concha (耳甲艇), and the lower depression is called the cavity of auricular concha (耳甲腔).

(2) **The external acoustic meatus**

The external acoustic meatus (外耳道) is a curved, bony-cartilaginous canal that projects from the auricle to the middle ear that is separated by the tympanic membrane (eardrum). It collects sounds and directs it towards the tympanic membrane. The lateral one third of it is surrounded by the cartilage and the medial two thirds is covered by bone. It is an S-shaped tube and is obliquely placed. The junction of the two parts is narrow. The adult tympanic membrane is easily observed by pulling the auricle backwards and upwards which straightens the cartilaginous part of the external acoustic meatus.

(3) **Tympanic membrane** (鼓膜)

The tympanic membrane is a semi-transparent concave oval membrane located between the floor of the external acoustic meatus and the tympanic cavity of the middle ear. It is divided into two parts: pars flaccida (flaccid part), also called Shrapnell's membrane, and Pars tensa (tense part). The anterior and upper one fourth of the tympanic membrane is the flaccid part (松弛部) which is light red in the biopsy while the lower three fourths is the tense part (紧张部) and is greyish in the biopsy. The triangular reflective area at the anteroinferior portion of the tense part is called cone of light (光锥). The attachment of the lower end and the handle of the malleus on the medial side of the tympanic membrane create the concavity on the lateral side that is called the umbo of the tympanic membrane (鼓膜脐). The tympanic membrane vibrates in response to sound. Sound wave enters the external acoustic meatus and strikes the tympanic membrane setting it in motion. The adult tympanic membrane forms an angle of 45° to 50° with the bottom of the external acoustic meatus.

2. The Middle Ear

The Middle ear (中耳) consists of three parts: the tympanic cavity, the auditory tube, the mastoid antrum and the mastoid cells.

(1) **Tympanic cavity**

The tympanic cavity is an irregular air-filled cavity lined by mucosal membrane, located in the temporal bone situated between the tympanic membranes and the lateral wall of inner ear. It contains three bones or the auditory ossicles, two muscles and one nerve. The tympanic cavity has six walls as follows.

1) The superior wall is the tegmental wall (盖壁) or tegmen tympani (鼓室盖). It is adjacent to the middle cranial fossa by a thin plate of petrous part of temporal bone.

2) The inferior wall is the jugular wall (颈静脉壁), and it is adjacent to the internal jugular vein in jugular fossa through a thin bone plate.

3) The lateral wall is also called membranous wall (鼓膜壁). Most are composed of the tympanic membrane, while a small portion above the tympanic membrane is composed of squamous part of temporal bone.

4) The medial wall is the labyrinthine wall (迷路壁) where the bony labyrinth of the inner ear is located. It also serves as the lateral wall of the inner ear. There is a small bulge called as promontory (岬) present at the middle of the medial wall. Pos-terosuperiorly there is an oval hole called fenestra vestibuli (前庭窗) or oval window (卵圆窗) that is closed by the base of the stapes and annular ligament. There is a round window called as the fenestra cochleae (蜗窗) or round window (圆窗) pos-teroinferiorly that is closed by the secondary tympanic membrane (第二鼓膜). There is an arcuate protuberance posterior and superior to the oval window commonly called as the prominence of facial canal (面神经管凸) through which the facial nerve passes.

5) The posterior wall is the mastoid wall (乳突壁). The upper part of this wall has a large irregular aperture called the opening of the mastoid antrum, which leads into the mastoid antrum. There is a cone-shaped protuberance under this aperture called the pyramidal eminence (锥隆起) containing stapedius muscle.

6) The anterior wall is the carotid wall (颈动脉壁) which is adjacent to the internal carotid artery. At the upper part of this wall, there is a musculotubal canal (肌咽鼓管) leading into the tympanic cavity. This tube is divided by the thin bony septum into two bone tubes: The small upper tube is called semicanal for tensor tympani (鼓膜张肌半管) and the large lower tube is called semicanal for auditory tube (咽鼓管半管). The semicanal for tensor tympani contains the tensor tympani muscle, and the semicanal for auditory tube is the bony part of the auditory tube.

(2) **Auditory ossicles**

The tympanic cavity contains three auditory ossicles (听小骨) arranged from outside to inside as malleus (锤骨), incus (砧骨) and stapes (镫骨). The handle of the malleus is attached to the tympanic membrane and the base of the stapes, also known as the stapes foot plate, sits loosely in the fenestra vestibuli, held in place by the annular ligament. The tympanic membrane moves the malleus, which in turn moves the incus, and then stapes, the footplate of which moves in and out of the oval window and transfers the energy to the endolymph fluid in the internal ear.

(3) **Muscles of the tympanic cavity**

The muscles in the tympanic cavity include the tensor tympani (鼓膜张肌), and the stapedius (镫骨肌). The tensor tympani arises from the cartilaginous part of the auditory tube and the greater wing of the sphenoid bone, then turns outward and downward at a right angle, and attaches to the handle of the malleus to make the tympanic membrane tense to prevent it from being broken. The stapedius is located in the pyramidal eminence. The tendon goes forward through the small hole at the apex of the pyramidal eminence and terminates at the neck of the stapes to make the base of the stapes leave the fenestra vestibuli, so as to reduce the pressure of the inner ear and prevent damage to the inner ear.

(4) **The auditory tube**

The auditory tube (咽鼓管, Fig.8-5) is the tube that connects the pharyngeal cavity and the tympanic cavity. It is composed of the posterolateral bony part (1/3) and the anteromedial cartilaginous part (2/3). The auditory tube passes forward through the pharyngeal opening of the auditory tube (咽鼓管咽口) to the naso-pharynx and backward through the tympanic opening of the auditory tube (咽鼓管鼓室口) to the tympanic cavity. The auditory tube is usually closed but it opens up while swallowing or yawning. Air enters the tympanic cavity through the auditory tube to ventilate the middle ear and also helps in maintaining the middle ear pressure. The auditory tube in young children is short, wide, and relatively horizontal, so when the pharyngeal cavity is infected, the inflammation can spread through the auditory tube to the tympanic cavity causing otitis media (中耳炎).

(5) **Mastoid antrum and mastoid cells**

The mastoid antrum (乳突窦) is an air space in the petrous part of the temporal bone that connects to the tympanic cavity anteriorly and the mastoid cells posteriorly. The mastoid cell (乳突小房) is enclosed spaces filled with air within the mastoid process of the temporal bone. Both the mastoid antrum and the mastoid cells are lined with mucous membrane, which is continuous with the mucosa of the tympanic cavity. Therefore, otitis media can spread through the mastoid sinus to the mastoid chamber and cause mastoiditis (乳突炎).

3. The Internal Ear or Labyrinth

The internal ear (内耳) or labyrinth (迷路) is a complex structure located in the petrous part of the temporal bone, between the tympanic cavity and the internal acoustic meatus. The labyrinth can be divided into membranous labyrinth and bony labyrinth. The membranous labyrinth consists of membranous tubules and the membranous sacs, which is composed of the epithelium and the connective tissue. The bony labyrinth is an osseous tunnel in the temporal bone which encloses the membranous labyrinth, thus both of them are structurally similar. The membranous labyrinth is a closed duct or sac that contains endolymph (内淋巴). The space between the bony labyrinth and the membranous labyrinth contains the perilymph (外淋巴). Endolymph and perilymph do not communicate with each other. Inner ear receives mechanical or vibratory signals from the stapes bone through the oval window.

(1) **Bony labyrinth**

The bony labyrinth (骨迷路) consists of a series of intercommunicating bony cavities which lie within the petrous part of the temporal bone. The bony labyrinth consists of three parts from anteromedial to posterolateral: the cochlea, the vestibule and the three bony semicircular canals.

1) The cochlea (耳蜗). It is located in the front of the bony labyrinth, shaped like a snail shell. Its apex faces anterolateral, which is called the cupula of cochlea (蜗顶). Its base facing the fundus of the internal acoustic meatus is called the base of cochlea (蜗底), and the cochlear nerve passes through the base of the cochlea and enters the cochlea. The cochlea consists of a cochlear spiral canal and a modiolus. The cochlear spiral canal (蜗螺旋管) is arranged spirally around the modiolus and makes two and half turns. The osseous spiral lamina (骨螺旋板) is a spiral bony ridge which projects out from the modiolus like the thread of a screw. The free edge of the lamina splits into the upper and lower lips. The vestibular membrane extends from the upper lip of the lamina till the outer wall of the cochlea, while the basilar membrane extends from the lower lip of the lamina till the outer cochlear wall. This divides the cochlear spiral canal into three parts: the upper vestibular scale (前庭阶), the middle cochlear duct and the lower tympanic scale (鼓阶). The osseous spiral lamina leaves the modiolus at the cupula of the cochlear to form a sickle-shaped thin bone slice, called the hamulus of spiral lamina (螺旋板钩). A hole is formed between the hamulus of spiral lamina and the modiolus, which is called the helicotrema (蜗孔).The Scala vestibuli and Scala tympani communicate with each other at the cupula of the cochlea through the helicotrema. The scala vestibuli starts from the vestibule to the helicotrema, while the scala tympani starts from the helicotrema to the fenestra cochleae.

2) Vestibule (前庭). It is an irregular cavity in the middle of the bony labyrinth. The vestibule lies between the cochlea in the front and the three bony semicircular canals behind. The lateral wall of the vestibule is the medial wall of the tympanic cavity, with a fenestra vestibule and a fenestra cochleae. The posterior vestibular wall has five openings for the three bony semicircular canals.

3) Bony semicircular canals. There are three bony semicircular canals (骨半规管) as follows: the anterior semicircular canal, the lateral semicircular canal and the posterior semicircular canal. These semicircular canals are situated in three planes at the right angle to each other. Each canal has two ends which are called two bony crura (骨脚). One is simple bony crus (单骨脚) and the other is ampullar bony crus (壶腹骨脚). The enlarged part of the ampullary bony crus is called the bony ampulla (骨壶腹). The simple bony crura of the anterior and posterior bony semicircular canals are combined into one common bony crus (总骨脚). Thus, these three semicircular canals open into the vestibule

by five openings.

(2) Membranous labyrinth

The membranous labyrinth (膜迷路) is a closed system of intercommunicating membranous sacs and ducts which lie within the bony labyrinth. It is filled with endolymph and presented with a cochlear duct, saccule, utricle and three semicircular ducts. The membranous labyrinth has two distinct portions, the vestibular portion concerned with balance and the auditory portion or the cochlea duct which is concerned with the hearing.

1) Utricle and saccule. The saccule (球囊) is a small globular membranous sac which lies in the anteroinferior part of the vestibule and the inner surface of the saccule is the sensory tissue called saccular macula (球囊斑) that responds to linear accelera-tion. The utricle (椭圆囊) is an elliptical membranous sac larger than the saccule and it lies in the posterosuperior part of the vestibule. The inner surface of the utricle is covered with sensory tissue for balance called the macula utriculi (椭圆囊斑) that responds to both centrifugal and linear acceleration.

2) The membranous semicircular canal (膜半规管). It is sheathed inside the bony semicircular ducts. In the bony ampullae, the three semicircular ducts also expand to form three membranous ampullae (膜壶腹), and there is a transverse bulge in each ampulla called the ampullary crest (壶腹嵴), which is formed by the thickening of the mucous membrane on one side of the ampulla protruding into the cavity. The ampullary crests are also position receptors, which can feel the stimulation of head rotation and variable speed movement.

3) The cochlear duct (蜗管). It is the spiral anterior part of the membranous labyrinth. It lies within the bony cochlea between the scala vestibuli and scala tympani and contains endolymph. This is a triangular shaped membranous duct that wraps around the modiolus two and a half times, following the quilling of both the spiral canal of the cochlea and the osseous spiral lamina. On the basilar membrane inside this duct is the spiral organ (螺旋器) or organ of Corti (科蒂器), which is the organ of hearing. This structure contains mechanoreceptors called hair cells which moves during oscillations of the endolymph. Each time a sound wave is transmitted, and then hair cells generate electrical impulses that transmit through the cochlear nerve to the auditory cerebral cortex in the brain.

4. Sound Conduction

There are two ways of sound conduction: air conduction and bone conduction. Under normal circumstances, air conduction is the primary method.

(1) Air conduction

Under normal circumstances, the sound waves cause fluctua-tions in the air, and the sound wave enters the external acoustic meatus. It then passes through the tympanic membrane, along the auditory ossicle chain, until the stapes impacts the fenestra vestibuli. This impact causes the perilymph in the scala vestibuli to fluctuate, leading to the protrusion or invagination of the second tympanic membrane. The perilymph fluctuations then cause the endolymph to fluctuate, stimulating the spiral organ. This stimulation is converted into a cochlear nerve impulse, which is transmitted to the cerebral auditory cortex, producing hearing.

(2) Bone conduction

Bone conduction directly stimulates the inner ear. The sound waves cause vibrations in the skull. These vibrations are transmitted directly to the cochlea in the inner ear, causing the perilymph and endolymph fluids to fluctuate, stimulating the spiral organ, which then converts the mechanical vibrations into a cochlear nerve impulses, which is transmitted to the cerebral auditory cortex, producing hearing.

5. The Internal Acoustic Meatus

The internal acoustic meatus (内耳道) is a short bony tube in the petrous part of the temporal bone, starting from the internal acoustic pore and ending at the floor of the internal acoustic meatus. There are many small holes in the fundus of the internal acoustic meatus through which the vestibulocochlear and facial nerves pass through.

（山东大学　扈燕来）

Exercise

1. A 58-year-old man complained small black spots in front of his eyes about five years ago, which floated with the rotation of his eyes. Recently, he had visual fatigue with eye swelling and blurred vision. Which of the following abnormal structure was most likely to be affected?

(A) The aqueous.

(B) The lens.

(C) The vitreous body.

(D) The retina.

(E) The sclera.

2. A 60-year-old woman complained frequent dizziness in the last three days, which was lasting for several seconds to one minute at each attack. When the dizziness occurred, she felt that surrounding objects were moving. When the dizziness was relieved, she walked unstably accompanied by tinnitus. Which of the following structures was most likely affected?

(A) The tympanic membrane.

(B) The tympanic cavity.

(C) The mastoid cells.

(D) The pharyngotympanic tube.

(E) The labyrinth.

Answer

1. The correct answer is C.

The vitreous body is composed of transparent gelatinous substances which is located between the lens and the retina. It plays an important role in refracting and supporting the retina. If the vitreous body is turbid, it is clinically called muscae volitantes.

2. The correct answer is E.

This is a typical symptom of Meniere's disease. The main pathological change of the disease is the hydrops of the membranous labyrinthine which is a part of labyrinth (Choice E). The clinical manifestations of Meniere's disease are recurrent rotational vertigo, fluctuating hearing loss, and tinnitus.

The Nervous System

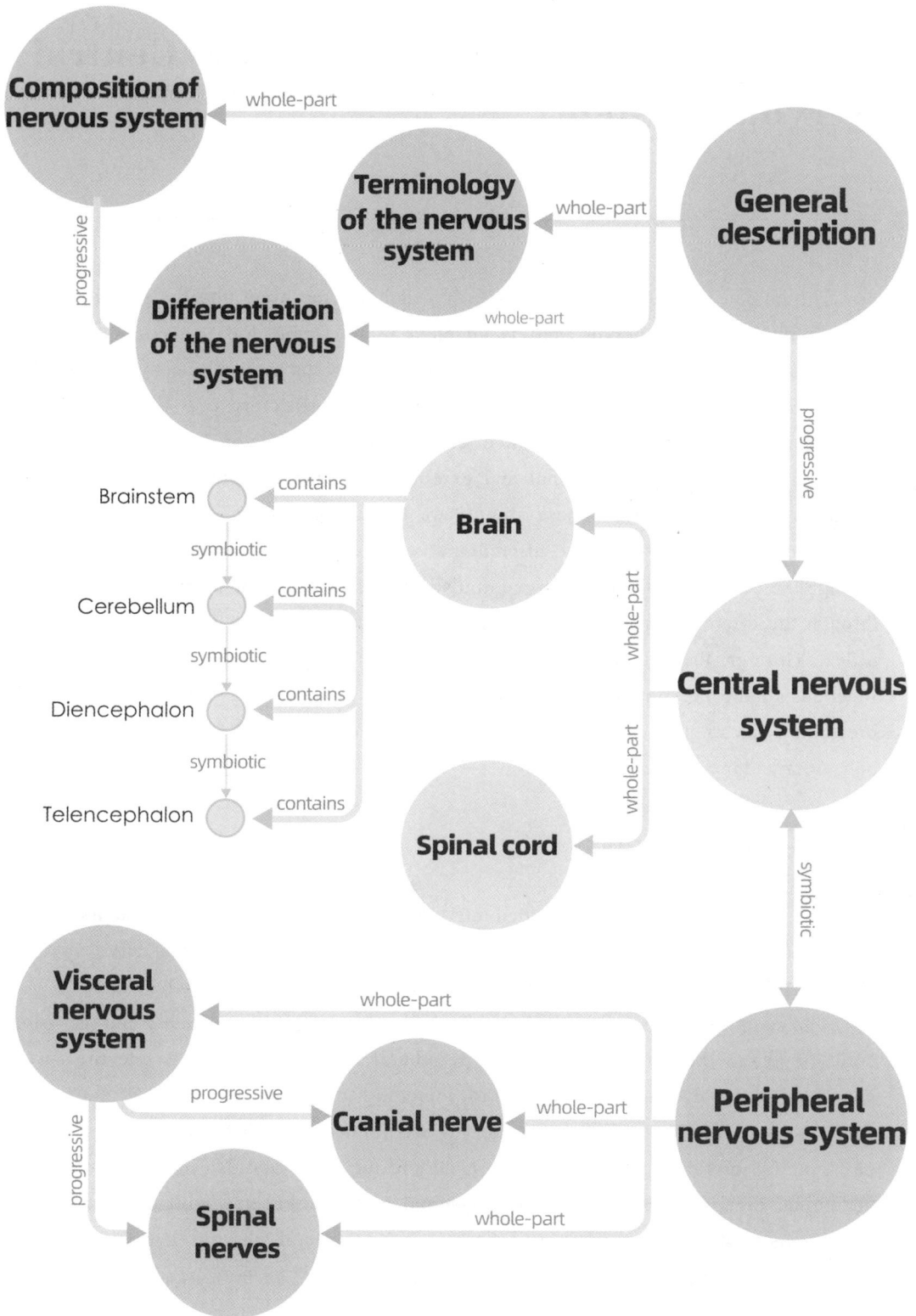

Chapter 9   Nervous System and Central Nervous System

The human nervous system (神经系统) includes the brain and the spinal cord, as well as the peripheral nerves, and is attached to the brain and the spinal cord, and distributed throughout the body. The basic mode of nervous system activity is reflex (反射), and the structural basis for completing reflex is reflex arc (反射弧), including receptor, afferent nerve, nerve center, efferent nerve and effector. The nervous system receives various stimuli of internal and external environment changes through various receptors connected with it. These stimuli are transmitted to the spinal cord and brain centers at all levels through the afferent nerve. The afferent information is integrated through the center, and then the nerve impulse is transmitted to the corresponding effector through the efferent nerve, producing various adaptive responses. This process is called reflex. Through the role of the nervous system, it properly enables many important functions of the nervous system, such as regulation of vital body functions (heartbeat, breathing, digestion), sensation, body movements, even our consciousness, cognition, behaviour and memories.

9.1   Differentiation

The nervous system can be divided into two parts: the central nervous system (中枢神经系统) (the integration and command center of the body) and the peripheral nervous system (周围神经系统) that represents the conduit between the CNS and the body (Fig.9-1).

The central nervous system includes the brain (脑) in the cranial cavity and the spinal cord (脊髓) in the vertebral canal. The peripheral nervous system refers to the nerves connected to the brain and the spinal cord, including the cranial nerves (脑神经) and the spinal nerves (脊神经). The cranial nerves are connected with the brain, a total of 12 pairs, mainly distributed not only in the head and the neck, but also in the chest and the abdominal organs. There are 31 pairs of spinal nerves connected with the spinal cord, mainly distributed in the trunk and limbs. The peripheral nervous system is further subdivided into the somatic nervous system (SNS, 躯体神经系统) and the autonomic

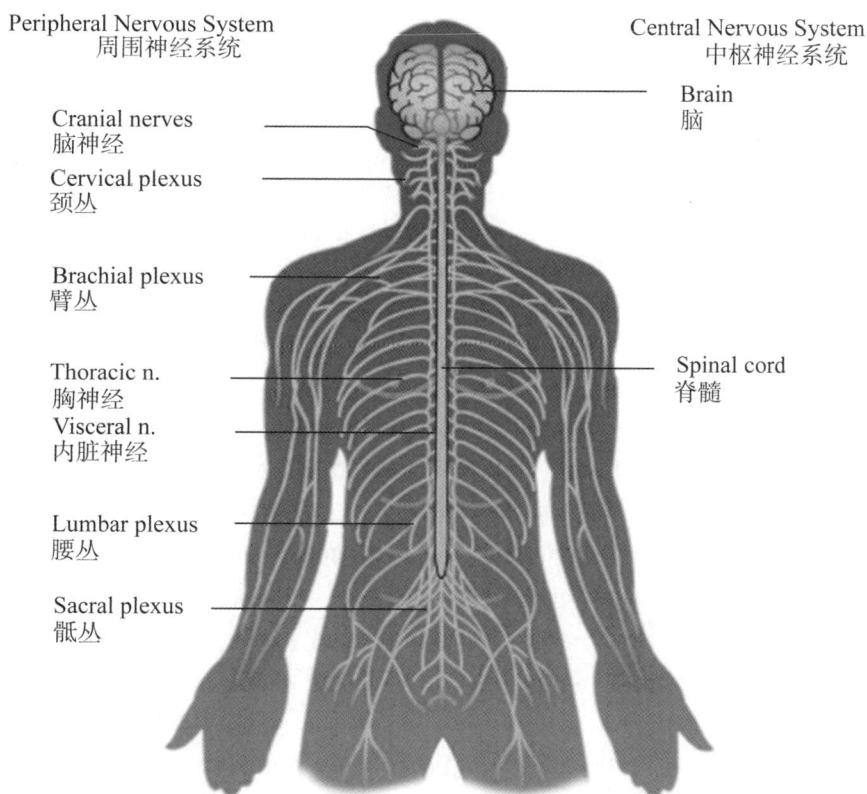

Peripheral Nervous System
周围神经系统

Central Nervous System
中枢神经系统

Cranial nerves
脑神经

Cervical plexus
颈丛

Brachial plexus
臂丛

Thoracic n.
胸神经

Visceral n.
内脏神经

Lumbar plexus
腰丛

Sacral plexus
骶丛

Brain
脑

Spinal cord
脊髓

Fig.9-1   Differentiation of the nervous system

nervous system (ANS,内脏神经系统) according to their distribution. The somatic nerves are distributed on the body surface, bone, joint and skeletal muscle through the cranial nerves and spinal nerves. The visceral nerves are connected to the brain and the spinal cord through the cranial and spinal nerves, and distributed in the viscera, cardiovascular, smooth muscle and glands along with the cranial and spinal nerves.

In the peripheral nervous system, both the somatic nerves and the visceral nerves have sensory and motor fiber components, which are called sensory nerves (感觉神经) and motor nerves (运 动 神 经) respectively. The sensory nerves transmit the nerve impulses from the receptors to the central part, so they are also called the afferent nerves (传 入 神 经). The motor nerves transmit the nerve impulses from the central part to the surrounding effectors, so they are also called efferent nerves (传 出 神 经). The visceral motor nerves can be divided into the sympathetic nerves (交 感 神 经) and the parasympathetic nerves (副交感神经).

9.2　Composition

Two basic types of cells in the nervous system are neurons (神经元) and neuroglia (神经胶质).

1. Neurons

The neurons (神经元), also known as neurocytes (神经细胞), are highly differentiated cells, which are the structural and functional units of the nervous system, and have the functions of receiving stimulation and conducting nerve impulses.

(1) Structure of neurons

The human nervous system contains up to 10^{11} neurons of different shapes. Each neuron consists of two parts: cell body and processes. The cell body is the metabolic center of neurons, except for the basic structure of general cells such as nucleus, cytoplasm, organelles and cell membrane. It also contains its unique Nissl bodies (尼氏体) and neurofibrils (神经原纤维) (Fig.9-2). The chemical essence of Nissl body is ribosomes, which is the site of protein synthesis. Neurofibrils are related to the transport of substances in neurons and have a supporting effect on neurons. There are two kinds of processes from the neuron body: dendrites (树突) and axon (轴突). The dendrites of neurons are devices that receive incoming information from other neurons or receptors. Usually, there are many, short dendrites extending outward from the cell body. There is usually only one axon from the neuronal cell body, but it can emit collateral branches. The length and thickness of the axon are different, with a diameter of $0.2-20.0$ μm. The length can reach more than 1 m. The axon is the main conduction device of neurons, which transmits nerve impulses from the beginning of the axon to the end. The process of synthesis and assembly of macromolecules into organelles is completed in the cell body, and there is one-way or two-way flow between the cell body and the axon. This phenomenon is called axonal transport (轴浆运输). If the cell body of the neuron is damaged, the axon will collapse and even die.

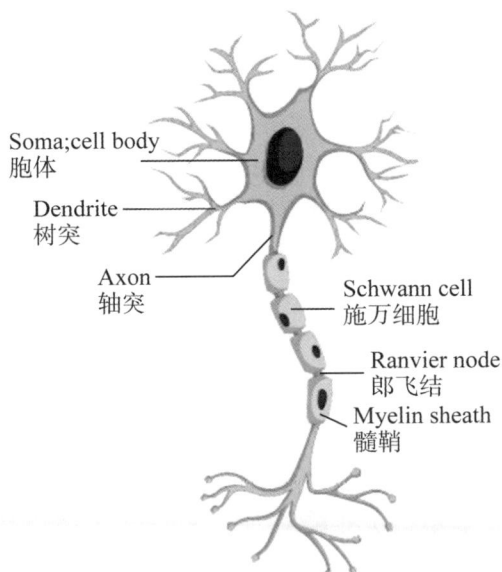

Soma;cell body 胞体
Dendrite 树突
Axon 轴突
Schwann cell 施万细胞
Ranvier node 郎飞结
Myelin sheath 髓鞘

Fig.9-2　Nissl bodies and neurofibrils

(2) **Classification of neurons**

According to the number of neuronal processes, neurons are divided into three categories (Fig.9-3).

1) Pseudounipolar neurons (假单极神经元), which emit a short process from the cell body, and then are divided into two branches in a "T" shape. One branch is distributed in the surrounding tissue, called the peripheral process (周围突), and the other branch enters the brain or the spinal cord, called the central process (中枢突). The primary sensory neurons in the cerebral and spinal ganglia belong to this class.

2) Bipolar neurons (双极神经元), which emit a process from both ends of the cell body to the receptor (peripheral process) or enter the central part (central process), such as bipolar cells in the retina and sensory neurons in the vestibular ganglion.

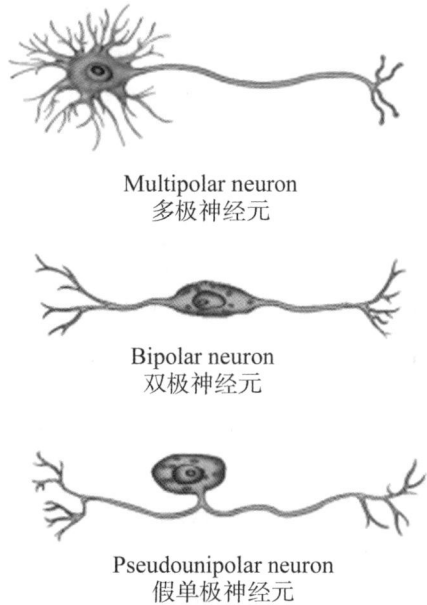

Multipolar neuron
多极神经元

Bipolar neuron
双极神经元

Pseudounipolar neuron
假单极神经元

Fig.9-3　Various types of neurons

3) Multipolar neurons (多极神经元), with multiple dendrites and one axon, the neurons in the central nervous system mostly belong to this category.

According to the function of neurons and the conduction direction of nerve excitation, neurons can also be divided into three categories.

1) sensory neurons (感觉神经元), which transmit various stimuli of internal and external environment changes to the central part, so they are also called afferent neurons (传入神经元), and bipolar neurons as well as pseudounipolar neurons.

2) Motor neuron (运动神经元), located in the central part, is a multipolar neuron, which transmits impulses from the central part to the surrounding parts, so it is also called efferent neuron (传出神经元), which controls the activities of skclctal muscle, myocardium, glands and smooth muscle.

3) Association neuron (联络神经元), or interneuron (中间神经元), is located between sensory neurons and motor neurons in the central nervous system. It is a multipolar neuron in morphology, accounting for 99% of the total number of neurons.

(3) **Neural stem cells** (神经干细胞)

They exist in the nervous system and can proliferate and differentiate into neurons and glial cells. They have the basic characteristics of stem cells: self-renewal ability and multidirectional differentiation potential.

(4) **Nerve fibers** (神经纤维)

The longer processes of neurons and the structures surrounding them are called nerve fibers. According to the myelin sheath, nerve fibers are divided into myelinated fibers (有髓纤维) and unmyelinated fibers (无髓纤维) (Fig. 9-4). The surface of nerve fibers is surrounded by a thin layer of connective tissue called endoneurium (神经内膜). Several nerve fibers are gathered into bundles by loose connective tissue and surrounded by a fine layer of the connective tissue, which is called perineurium (神经束膜). The nerve is composed of nerve tracts of different thickness, which are surrounded by dense connective tissue, called epineurium (神经外膜). The epineurium is a dense layer of collagen fibers, connected with the dura mater at the central end of the cranial and spinal nerves.

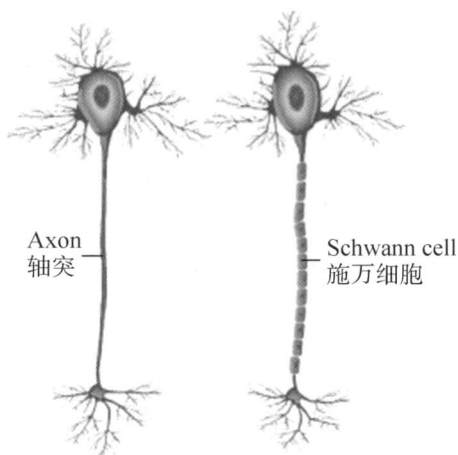

Fig.9-4　Medullated and unmedullated fibers

(5) **Synapse** (突触)

The specialized contact area between neurons or between neurons and effectors is called synapse (Fig.9-5). One neuron must be able to influence the activity of another neuron or effector through synapse. Most synapses need the action of chemical transmitters to complete the transmission of impulses, called chemical synapses (化学突触). Typical chemical synapses include presynaptic membrane (突触前膜), synaptic cleft (突触间隙) and postsynaptic membrane (突触后膜). In addition, there are electrical synapses (电突触) in a few parts of the body, and the synaptic gap is very small, so that the electrical changes of one neuron can directly lead to the electrical changes of another neuron. Most synapses are axonal endings of one neuron that contact with dendrites or cell

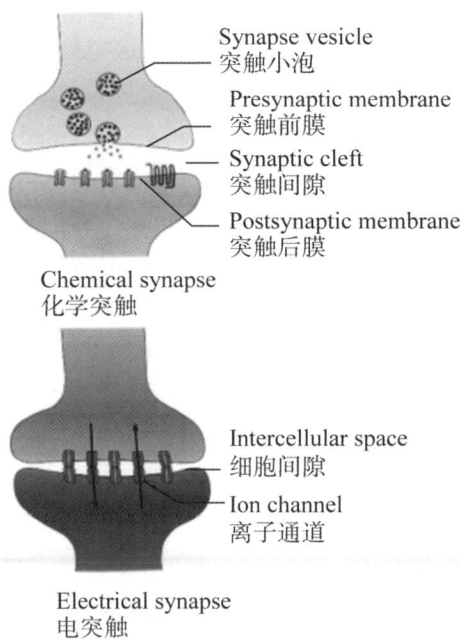

Fig.9-5　Different contact sites of synapses

bodies of another neuron, called axo-tree or axo-body synapses. But there are also axle-axis, tree-tree or body-body synapses.

2. Neuroglia Cells

Neuroglia cells (神经胶质细胞) is also known as glia or glial cells. In the central nervous system, glial cells include oligodendrocytes, astrocytes, ependymal cells and microglia. In the peripheral nervous system, glial cells include Schwann cells and satellite cells. Neuroglia plays a supporting, protective and nutritional role in nerve tissue.

（1）Astrocytes

Astrocytes (星形胶质细胞) are the largest glial cells with the largest number, distributed between the neuronal cell body and its processes. In the past, it was believed that astrocytes only support and nourish neurons, but recent studies have shown that astrocytes have a variety of functions: regulating neuronal metabolism and ionic environment; synthesis and secretion of neurotrophic factors and other active substances; participating in brain immune reaction; guiding neuronal migration.

（2）Microglias

Microglias (小胶质细胞) are actually macrophages in the nervous system, distributed in gray matter and white matter, but more in gray matter. They may originate from monocytes in the blood, enter the developing central nervous system, transform into amebic microglial cells with phagocytosis, phagocytose some remnants of natural degeneration in the development, and proliferate at the same time. After the development of the central nervous system, they will turn into microglia in a static state. When the central nervous system is injured, microglias in a static state are activated, become macrophages and proliferate, phagocytosis and clearing of cell debris and degenerated substances.

（3）Oligodendrocytes

Oligodendrocytes (少突胶质细胞) are distributed around the blood vessels of the central nervous system (CNS), between the fiber bundles of the white matter of the brain and the spinal cord, and around the neurons of the gray matter. The function of oligodendrocyte is to form myelin sheath with myelinated fibers in CNS.

（4）Ependymal cells

Ependymal cells (室管膜细胞) are a layer of cuboidal, columnar or flat epithelial cells that cover the ventricles and the central canal of the spinal cord, called the ependymal. Ependymal cells participate in the material exchange between nerve tissue and cerebrospinal fluid.

9.3　Common Terms

1. Gray Matter (灰质)

In the central nervous system, the place where the cell bodies and dendrites of neurons gather is called gray matter. Because it is rich in blood vessels, it is dark in color on fresh specimens, it is called gray matter. The gray matter distributed on the surface of the brain is called cortex (皮质), such as the cerebral and cerebellar cortex.

2. White Matter (白质)

In the central nervous system, the place where nerve fibers gather in the central nervous system is called white matter. It is named for the myelin sheath contains lipids and is bright and white, such as the white matter of the spinal cord. The white matter located in the deep side of the cerebral and cerebellar is called medulla (髓质).

3. Nucleus (神经核)

In addition to the cortex, the cell bodies of neurons with similar morphology and functions gather into clusters or columns in the central nervous system, which is called nucleus.

4. Ganglion (神经节)

The place where the cell bodies of neurons gather in the peripheral nervous system is called ganglion (pl. ganglia). It includes sensory ganglia and visceral motor ganglia. The former is formed by the aggregation of cell bodies of sensory neurons such as pseudounipolar or bipolar neurons. The latter is formed by the aggregation of the cell bodies of efferent neurons, and controls the activities of cardiovascular, gland and smooth muscle.

5. Fasciculus (纤维束)

In the central nervous system, nerve fibers gather together with basically the same starting and ending, course and functions, which is called fasciculus (or named tract).

6. Nerves (神经)

Nerve fibers gather in the peripheral nervous system to form nerves of different thickness.

7. Reticular Formation (网状结构)

In some central nervous systems, nerve fibers interweave into a network, with scattered neuronal bodies of different sizes, which is called reticular formation, such as brainstem reticular formation.

9.4 Spinal Cord

The central nervous system (CNS, 中枢神经系统) includes the spinal cord and the brain. The brain can be divided into six parts: medulla oblongata, pons, midbrain, cerebellum, diencephalon and telencephalon. The medulla oblongata, pons and midbrain are collectively called brainstem. The sensory information is transmitted to the advanced center through the fasciculus, and the motor information is transmitted to the motor cells of the anterior horn of the spinal cord and the cranial nerve motor nuclei of the brain stem.

1. Position and Shape of the Spinal Cord

The spinal cord (脊髓, Fig.9-6) is located in the vertebral canal, and continues to be the medulla oblongata at the upper part of the foramen magnum of the occipital bone. The end becomes thinner and is called the conus medullaris (脊髓圆锥). In adults, at the lower edge of the L1 vertebra, it continues to be filum terminate (终丝) without nerve tissue. The latter terminates at the back of the coccyx and anchors the spinal cord in place. The spinal cord is in a cylindrical shape, with a total length of 42−45 cm and different thickness. It has two enlargements: cervical enlargement (颈膨大) from the fifth cervical spinal segment to the first thoracic spinal segment; lumbosacral enlargement (腰骶膨大) extends from the second lumbar spinal segment to the third sacral spinal segment. The appearance of these two enlargements is due to the relatively large number of neurons, which is related to the innervation of the upper and lower limbs.

The surface of the spinal cord is divided into symmetrical left and right halves by two longitudinal grooves located in the middle of the spinal cord. The anterior longitudinal groove is deep, called anterior median fissure (前正中裂); the posterior longitudinal sulcus is shallow, called the posterior median sulcus (后正中沟). In addition, there are two external grooves on the surface of the spinal cord, namely, the anterolateral groove and the posterolateral groove, which are respectively attached by the neurofilaments of the anterior and posterior roots of the spinal nerve.

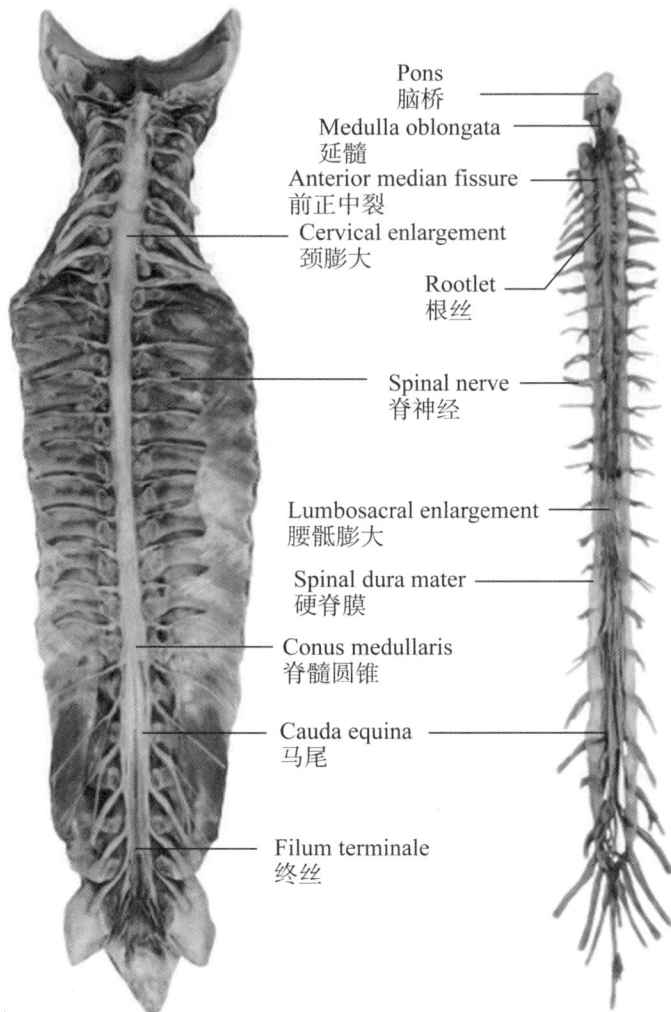

Pons
脑桥

Medulla oblongata
延髓

Anterior median fissure
前正中裂

Cervical enlargement
颈膨大

Rootlet
根丝

Spinal nerve
脊神经

Lumbosacral enlargement
腰骶膨大

Spinal dura mater
硬脊膜

Conus medullaris
脊髓圆锥

Cauda equina
马尾

Filum terminale
终丝

Fig.9-6　The spinal cord

The spinal cord is obviously segmental. The range of the root filaments that make up the anterior and posterior roots of each pair of spinal nerves attached to the spinal cord is called a segments of spinal cord (脊髓节段). There are 31 pairs of spinal nerves. The spinal cord is also divided into 31 corresponding segments: 8 cervical spinal segments (C1 C8), 12 thoracic spinal segments (T1—T12), 5 lumbar spinal segments (L1—L5), 5 sacral spinal segments (S1—S5) and 1 caudal spinal segment (Co1).

Understanding the corresponding relationship between the spinal cord segments and the number of the vertebrae (Fig.9-7) is of great significance to the judgment of the spinal cord disease and the anesthesia level. In adults, the calculation method is as follows: the upper cervical spinal segment (C1—C4) roughly corresponds to the vertebrae of the same ordinal number; the lower cervical spinal cord segment (C5—C8) and the upper thoracic spinal segment (T1—T4) roughly align with the upper vertebral body of the same ordinal number; the middle thoracic spinal segment (T5—T8) roughly aligns with the upper 2 vertebral bodies of the same ordinal number; the lower thoracic spinal segment (T9—T12) roughly aligns with the upper 3 vertebral bodies of the same ordinal number; and the lumbar spinal segment roughly aligns with the 10—12 thoracic vertebrae; the sacral and caudal spinal cords are approximately equal to the first lumbar vertebra. Therefore, the anterior and posterior root filaments of the lumbar, sacral and caudal spinal nerves descend a certain distance in the subarachnoid space of the spinal cord and then exit the corresponding intervertebral foramen. These root filaments of the spinal nerves form the cauda equina (马尾). In clinical practice, the needle is often inserted between the L3—L4 or L4—L5 lumbar spinous processes for subarachnoid puncture to extract cerebrospinal fluid or inject anesthetic to avoid spinal cord injury.

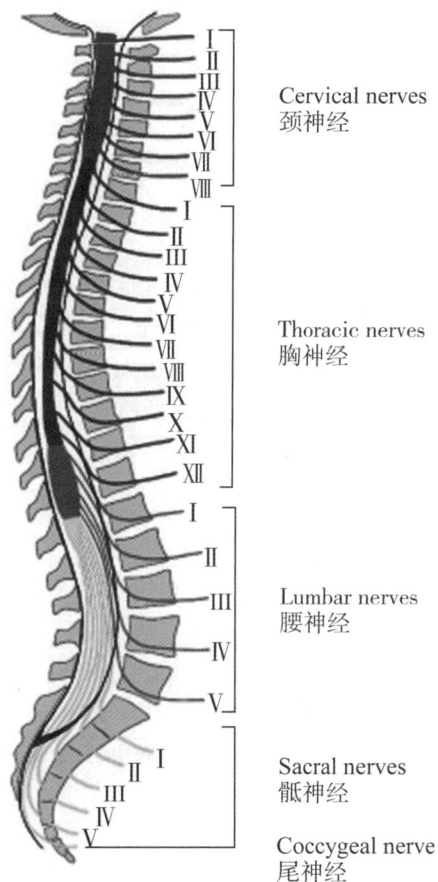

Fig.9-7 Relationship between the spinal cord segments and the number of vertebrae

2. Internal Structure of the Spinal Cord

On the transverse section of the spinal cord, "H" shaped or butterfly shaped gray matter (灰质) is in the middle and white matter (白质) around the gray matter, and the central canal (中央管) with narrow lumen is in the center, which runs through the whole length of the spinal cord, contains cerebrospinal fluid, passes through the fourth ventricle upward, and expands into the terminal ventricle downward at the conus medullaris. The anterior part of the gray matter on each side is enlarged into the anterior horn (前角), and the posterior part is narrower and thinner into the posterior horn (后角). The area between the anterior horn and the posterior horn is called the intermediate zone (中间带). The intermediate zone often extends out of the lateral horn (侧角) to the lateral side, which is located in the T1—L3 lumbar cord segments. The gray matter in the anterior and posterior parts of the central canal is the gray commissure (灰质连合). The white matter is divided into three cords by three longitudinal grooves on the surface of the spinal cord: The anterior funiculus (前索) is between the anterior median fissure and the anterior lateral sulcus; the posterior funiculus (后索) is between the posterolateral sulcus and the posterior median sulcus, and the lateral funiculus (外侧索) is between the anterolateral and posterolateral sulcuses. In front of the anterior commissure of gray matter, there are left and right lateral transverse fibers called anterior white commissure (白质前连合); between the white matter and the lateral side of the base of the posterior horn, gray and white matter are mixed and interwoven, called reticular formation (网状结构), which is most obvious in the cervical cord.

(1) Gray matter of the spinal cord

It is a butterfly-shaped structure made up of neuronal cell bodies, glial cells and neuropile (unmyelinated axons, dendrites and glial cell processes). The gray matter can be functionally divided into three main regions: The anterior horn is responsible for motor function; the lateral (intermediate) horn is responsible for autonomic functions; the posterior horn is mainly responsible for sensory functions. According to the research of Rexed et al. (1950s) on the cellular architecture of the gray matter of the spinal cord, there are ten laminae in total and they are numbered sequentially (I — X) from dorsal to ventral (Fig.9-8).

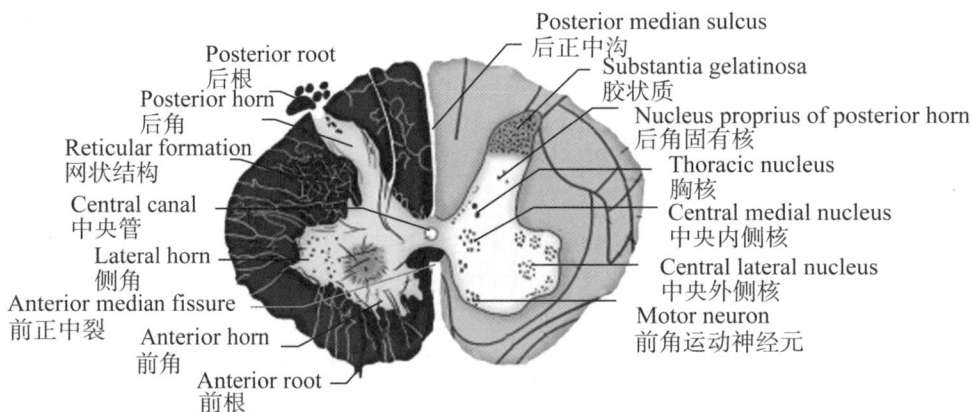

Fig.9-8　Main nuclei of the gray matter of the spinal cord and
the Rexed layered pattern

Lamina I contains the posteromarginal nucleus (后角边缘核). Lamina II is equivalent to the substantia gelatinosa (胶状质). Lamina III and IV contain nucleus proprius of posterior horn (后角固有核). Layers I — IV are equivalent to the head of the posterior horn, and is the main receiving area of the afferent fibers of the skin to feel external pain, temperature, touch, pressure and other stimuli. Lamina Ⅴ is located in the neck of the posterior horn, and the outer part of layer Ⅴ participates in the reticular formation (网状结构). Lamina Ⅵ is located at the base of the posterior horn, and is most obvious at the cervical and lumbosacral enlargements. The Ⅴ－Ⅵ layers receive the proprioception of the posterior root and some primary afferent fibers of the skin. Lamina Ⅶ occupies the majority of the intermediate zone and contains some obvious nuclei: the intermediolateral nucleus (中间外侧核) is located in the lateral horn of T1－L2 or L3 spinal segments, and is the location of the sympathetic preganglionic neuron body, that is, the lower center of the sympathetic nerve. The intermediomedial nucleus (中间内侧核) is located on the lateral side of layer Ⅹ and runs through the entire length of the spinal cord. It receives the afferent from the visceral sensory fibers of the posterior root. The sacral parasympathetic nucleus (骶副交感核), located at the lateral part of the Lamina Ⅶ of the S2－S4 spinal segments, is the location of the cell body of the parasympathetic preganglionic neurons innervating the pelvic organs, that is, the lower center of the parasympathetic nerve. Lamina Ⅷ is located in the anterior horn and consists of intermediate neurons. It receives a large number of descending fibers from the brain and sends out fibers to the anterior horn motor neurons of layer Ⅸ. Lamina Ⅸ is located at the ventral end of the anterior horn and consists of motor neurons in the anterior horn. According to the morphological characteristics, the anterior horn motor neurons include α-motor neuron (α-运动神经元) and γ- motor neuron (γ-运动神经元). The α- motor neuron innervates the extraspindle muscle fibers across the joint, causing joint movement. The γ-motor neuron innervates skeletal muscle fibers in the spindle and regulate muscle tension. The damage to the cell body or axon of the anterior horn motor neuron can cause paralysis and atrophy of the skeletal muscle it controls, decrease in muscle tension, and decrease or disappearance of tendon reflex, which is called flaccid paralysis (such as poliomyelitis). Layer Ⅹ (Lamina Ⅹ) is the anterior and posterior commissure of gray matter, and some posterior root afferent fibers terminate in this layer.

(2) **White matter of the spinal cord**

The fasciculus in the white matter of the spinal cord includes long ascending and descending fasciculus and short fasciculus proprius (固有束) (Fig. 9-9). The long ascending fasciculus transmits various sensory information to the dorsal thalamus and cerebellum. The long descending fasciculus transmits the motor information of the brain to the spinal cord, and the short fasciculus proprius completes the connection between the segments of the spinal cord.

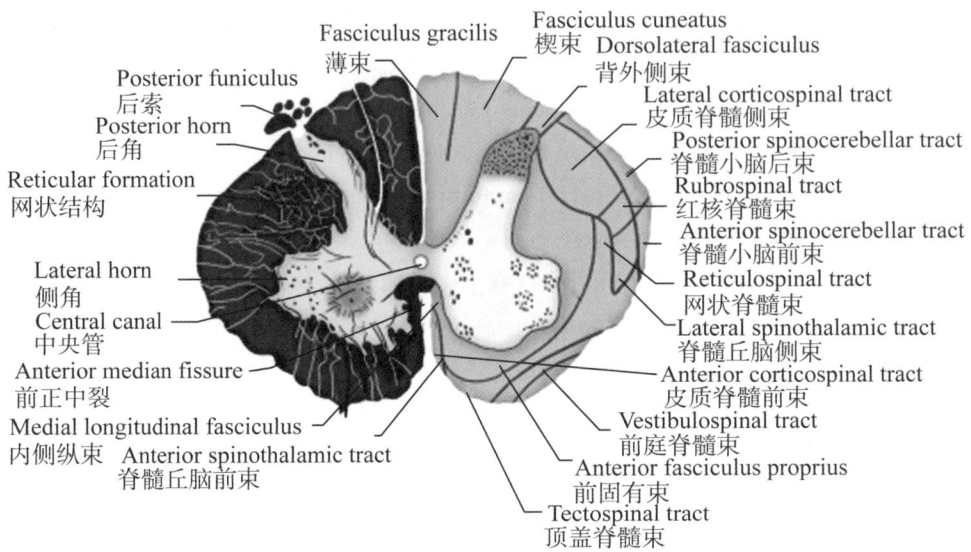

Fig.9-9   Distribution pattern of the ascending and descending fasciculus
in the white matter of the spinal cord

1) Ascending fasciculus (sensory fasciculus)

Fasciculus gracilis (薄束) and *fasciculus cuneatus* (楔束). Located in the posterior funiculus, they are the direct continuation of the coarse fibers in the medial part of the posterior root of the ipsilateral spinal nerve. The fasciculus gracilis starts from the central process of spinal ganglion cells below T5 on the same side. The fasciculus cuneatus rises from the central process of spinal ganglion cells above T4 on the same side. The peripheral processes of these spinal ganglion cells are distributed in proprioceptive receptors such as muscles, tendons, and joints distributed in the trunk and limbs, and fine tactile receptors of skin. The central process enters the spinal cord through the medial part of the posterior root, forming a fasciculus gracilis and a fasciculus cuneatus ascending, and ends at the gracile nucleus and the cuneate nucleus of the medulla oblongata respectively. The fasciculus gracilis and fasciculus cuneatus transmit the conscious proprioception (position sense, motion sense and vibration sense of muscles, tendons and joints) and fine touch sense (such as distinguishing the distance between two points and the texture thickness of objects) from the same side of the body. When the posterior funiculus of the spinal cord is pathological changed or damaged, the proprioception and fine touch information cannot be uploaded to the cerebral cortex, and the proprioception and fine touch loss below the injury plane of the injured side of the patient.

The spinothalamic tract (脊髓丘脑束). It divides into the lateral spinothalamic tract (脊髓丘脑侧束) (located in the anterior half of the lateral funiculus) and the anterior spinothalamic tract (脊髓丘脑前束) (located in the anterior funiculus). The central process of the spinal ganglion cells enters the spinal cord through the posterior root, and the fibers of the lateral part of the spinal ganglion cells rise 1—2 spinal segments in the spinal cord, and terminate in the cells of layer I and layers Ⅳ — Ⅷ. The fibers from the latter cross to the opposite side through the anterior commissure of white matter and rise 1—2 spinal segments (that is, cross and rise at the same time) to form the spinothalamic tract.

The spinothalamic tract transmits the pain, temperature and rough touch of the opposite half of the trunk and limbs. The fibers of the tract have a clear positioning relationship, that is, from the internal to the external, the fibers of the cervical, thoracic, lumbar and sacral spinal segments are in turn. One side of the spinothalamic tract was injured, and the pain and temperature decreased or disappeared in the area below 1—2 spinal segments at the contralateral injury level.

The spinocerebellar tract (脊髓小脑束). The spinocerebellar tract includes the anterior spinocerebellar tract, the posterior spinocerebellar tract, the rostral spinocerebellar tract, etc. i) The anterior spinocerebellar tract (脊髓小脑前束): Located in the front of the periphery of the lateral funiculus, it starts from the layers Ⅴ to Ⅸ below the lumbar spinal segments on both sides (mainly on the opposite side), and enters the cerebellar cortex through the superior cerebellar peduncle. ii) The posterior spinocerebellar tract (脊髓小脑后束): Located at the back of the periphery of the lateral funiculus, it starts from the dorsal nucleus above L2 spinal segments on the same side and ends at the cerebellar cortex through the inferior cerebellar peduncle. These two tracts transmit the unconscious proprioception information of the lower body to the cerebellum, and participate in the process of adjusting the lower limb muscle tension and intermuscular coordination. iii) The rostral spinocere-bellar tract (脊髓小脑吻束): Located around the lateral funiculus of the cervical spinal cord, starts from layers Ⅴ — Ⅷ of the ipsilateral cervical enlargement, and partially overlaps with the anterior and posterior tracts of the spinocerebellar. The fibers enter the cerebellar cortex through the superior and inferior cerebellar peduncles, and transmit the proprioception from the upper limbs and the skin tactile pressure information.

2) Descending fasciculus (motor fasciculus)

The corticospinal tract (皮质脊髓束). This tract starts from the middle and upper parts of the central anterior gyrus of the cerebral cortex and the anterior part of the paracentral lobule, and descends to the pyramid of the lower part of the medulla oblongata. Most of the fibers cross to the opposite side and descend at the back of the lateral funiculus of the spinal cord, forming the lateral corticospinal tract (皮质脊髓侧束). The fibers from this tract directly or indirectly terminate at the anterior horn of the gray matter on the same side of the spinal cord to control the voluntary movement of the upper and lower limb skeletal muscles. A few corticospinal tract fibers directly descend to the innermost part of the anterior funiculus of the spinal cord without crossing in the medulla oblongata to form the anterior corticospinal tract (皮质脊髓前束), which directly or indirectly terminates at the motor neurons of the anterior horn on both sides and dominates the voluntary movement of the bilateral trunk muscles. Therefore, the motor cells of the anterior horn of the spinal cord that control the voluntary movement of the upper and lower limb skeletal muscles only accept the fibers of the contralateral cerebral cortex motor center, while the motor neurons of the anterior horn that control the voluntary movement of the trunk muscles are controlled by the motor centers of the bilateral cerebral cortex. When the corticospinal tract on the injured side of the spinal cord is injured, it only shows paralysis of the limbs below the injured side of the injury plane, while the trunk muscle is not paralyzed. Unlike the paralysis (flaccid paralysis) caused by the injury of motor neurons in the anterior horn of the spinal cord, when the corticospinal tract is injured, the limb muscle tension of the injured side increased, the tendon reflex is hyperreflexed, and pathological reflex occurs, with no obvious muscle atrophy, which is called spastic paralysis.

The rubrospinal tract (红核脊髓束). This tract is located in front of the lateral corticospinal tract of the lateral funiculus, and there is no obvious boundary between them. The tract starts from the red nucleus of the midbrain, crosses to the opposite side and descends in the lateral funiculus of the spinal cord, and terminates at the Ⅴ − Ⅶ layers of the upper cervical spinal cord. This tract has a strong excitatory effect on the motor neurons of the anterior horn of the spinal cord innervating the flexor muscle, and together with the corticospinal tract, it plays an important role in the movement of the distal limb muscles.

The vestibulospinal tract (前庭脊髓束). This tract starts from the lateral nucleus of the vestibular nerve, goes down to the lateral part of the ipsilateral anterior funiculus, and ends at Lamina Ⅷ and part of Lamina Ⅶ. It mainly excites trunk muscles and extensor muscles of limbs and plays an important role in regulating body balance.

The reticulospinal tract (网状脊髓束). This tract starts from the reticular formation of the pons and medulla oblongata. Most of the fibers descend in the anterior funiculus and anteromedial part of the lateral funiculus on the same side of the white matter, and end at the seventh and eighth layers. This tract is mainly involved in the control of the movement of the trunk and proximal limb muscles.

The tectospinal tract (顶盖脊髓束). This tract starts from the contralateral superior colliculus of the midbrain, and the fibers pass through the ventral side of the periaqueductal gray matter and the dorsal side of the tegmentum, cross and descend to the anterior funiculus of the spinal cord, and end at the layers Ⅵ and Ⅶ of the upper cervical spinal cord, participating in the completion of audio-visual reflex.

The medial longitudinal fasciculus (内侧纵束). It mainly starts from the bilateral vestibular nucleus, descends from the anterior funiculus to the cervical spinal cord, and ends at the seventh and eighth layers. It mainly coordinates the movement of the eyeball; the head and neck.

3. Function of the Spinal Cord

The spinal cord belongs to the lower center. Under the control of the brain's various levels of centers, the spinal cord can complete the transmission and relay of up and down information. Through the specific connection of neurons in the spinal cord, the intrinsic reflex activity of the spinal cord can be completed.

(1) **Stretch reflex** (牵张反射)

It is the most common skeletal muscle reflex. The reflex arc is composed of two neurons, afferent and efferent, and belongs to single-synaptic reflex. When skeletal muscle is stretched and lengthened, intramuscular receptors such as muscle spindles are stimulated to produce nerve impulses, which are transmitted to the spinal cord through the central process of pseudounipolar neurons in the posterior root ganglion, and its collateral branches can be directly excited by α- Motor neurons, reflexively causing the elongated muscles to contract. The commonly used deep reflex (tendon reflex) examinations in clinic include knee reflex, Achilles tendon reflex and biceps brachii reflex.

(2) **Flexion reflex** (屈曲反射)

It is a protective reflex activity, belonging to multi-synaptic reflex, and at least three neurons participate in the completion. That is, the skin receptor transmits information to the spinal cord through the central process of the dorsal root ganglion, and then via the intermediate neuron to α- Motor neurons that causes muscle contraction. This type of reflex occurs when the skin of a limb is subjected to harmful stimulation and it will be immediately retracted.

4. Common Manifestations of Spinal Cord Injury

(1) **Complete spinal cord transection**

All sensory and random movements below the injury plane of complete spinal cord transection (脊髓完全横断) are lost. At the early stage of spinal cord transection (several days to several weeks), various spinal cord reflexes disappear and are in a non-reflex state, which is called spinal cord shock. After that, various spinal cord reflexes can gradually recover, but the sensation and skeletal muscle movement below the injury plane cannot be recovered, which can be manifested by increased muscle tension, hyperreflexia of tendon, and inability to control defecation and urination reflexes at will.

(2) **Hemisection of the spinal cord** (脊髓半横断)

The position sense, vibration sense and fine touch sense (deep sense) below the ipsilateral plane of the spinal cord hemisection injury disappeared, and the ipsilateral limb paraplegia, and the contra-lateral pain and temperature sense (shallow sense) below the injury plane disappeared. These symptoms are called Brown-Square syndrome (布朗—色夸综合征)。

(3) **Syringomyelia** (脊髓空洞症)

The spinal cord central canal expansion in syringomyelia causes the central part of the spinal cord to be like a cavity. If the lesion damages the anterior commissure of white matter, the spinothalamic tract fibers that can conduct pain and temperature sensation are damaged here, resulting in the disappearance of bilateral segmental pain and temperature sensation below the injury plane. But the deep sense is normal. This phenomenon is called sensory separation.

(4) **Poliomyelitis** (脊髓灰质炎)

Poliomyelitis poliovirus infection causes lesions in the anterior horn of the gray matter of the spinal cord, which is characterized by flaccid paralysis of the skeletal muscle (such as one lower limb) in the area under its control, hypotonia, disappearance of tendon reflex, muscle atrophy, but normal sensation.

9.5   Brain

The brain (or encephalon) (脑) is located in the cranial cavity, and the average weight of adult brain is about 1, 400 g. Generally, the brain is divided into six parts: telencephalon, diencephalon, midbrain, pons, medulla oblongata and cerebellum (Figs.9-10 & 9-11). Traditionally, the midbrain, pons and medulla oblongata are collectively called brainstem. The medulla oblongata is connected to the spinal cord through the foramen magnum.

9.5.1   Brain Stem

The brain stem (脑干, Fig.9-12) is the distal part of the brain that is located between the spinal cord and the diencephalon. It is made up of the midbrain, pons, and medulla oblongata from the top to the bottom. Each of the three components has its own unique structure and function. Together, they help to regulate breathing, heart rate, blood pressure, and several other important functions. The back of the medulla oblongata and pons is connected to the cerebellum through the cerebellar peduncle. The ventricular cavity between them is the fourth ventricle, which connects with the central canal of the medulla oblongata and the spinal cord downward and connects with the midbrain aqueduct of the midbrain upward.

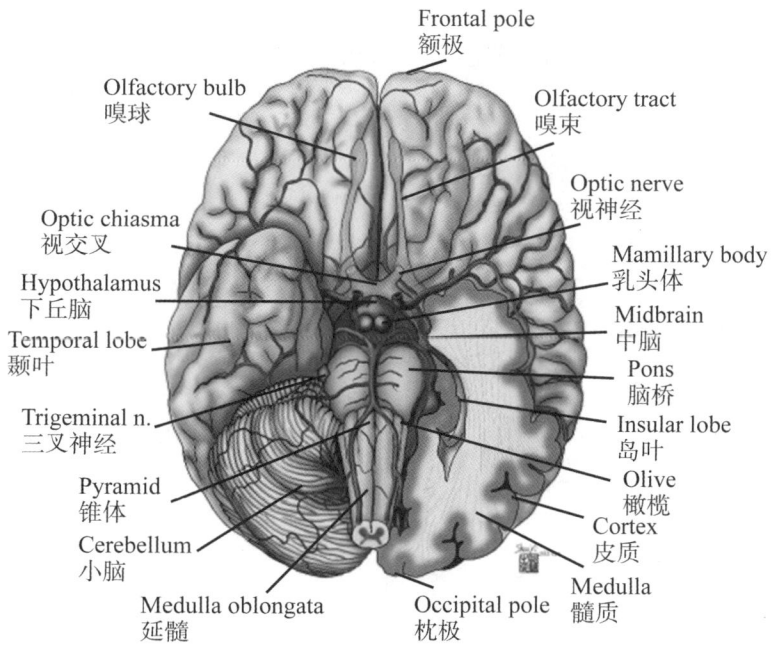

Frontal pole
额极

Olfactory bulb
嗅球

Olfactory tract
嗅束

Optic nerve
视神经

Optic chiasma
视交叉

Mamillary body
乳头体

Hypothalamus
下丘脑

Midbrain
中脑

Temporal lobe
颞叶

Pons
脑桥

Trigeminal n.
三叉神经

Insular lobe
岛叶

Olive
橄榄

Pyramid
锥体

Cortex
皮质

Cerebellum
小脑

Medulla
髓质

Medulla oblongata
延髓

Occipital pole
枕极

Fig.9-10   Bottom of the brain

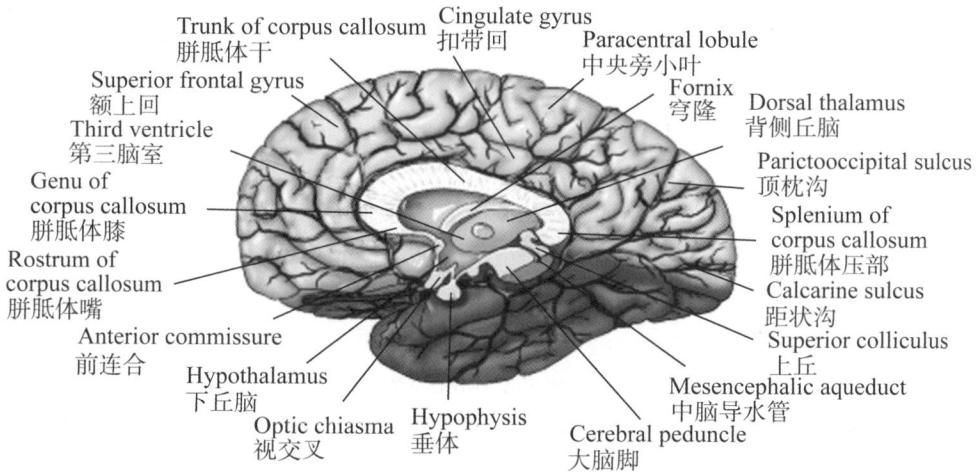

Trunk of corpus callosum
胼胝体干

Cingulate gyrus
扣带回

Paracentral lobule
中央旁小叶

Superior frontal gyrus
额上回

Fornix
穹隆

Dorsal thalamus
背侧丘脑

Third ventricle
第三脑室

Parietooccipital sulcus
顶枕沟

Genu of
corpus callosum
胼胝体膝

Splenium of
corpus callosum
胼胝体压部

Rostrum of
corpus callosum
胼胝体嘴

Calcarine sulcus
距状沟

Anterior commissure
前连合

Superior colliculus
上丘

Hypothalamus
下丘脑

Mesencephalic aqueduct
中脑导水管

Optic chiasma
视交叉

Hypophysis
垂体

Cerebral peduncle
大脑脚

Fig.9-11   Midsagittal section of the brain

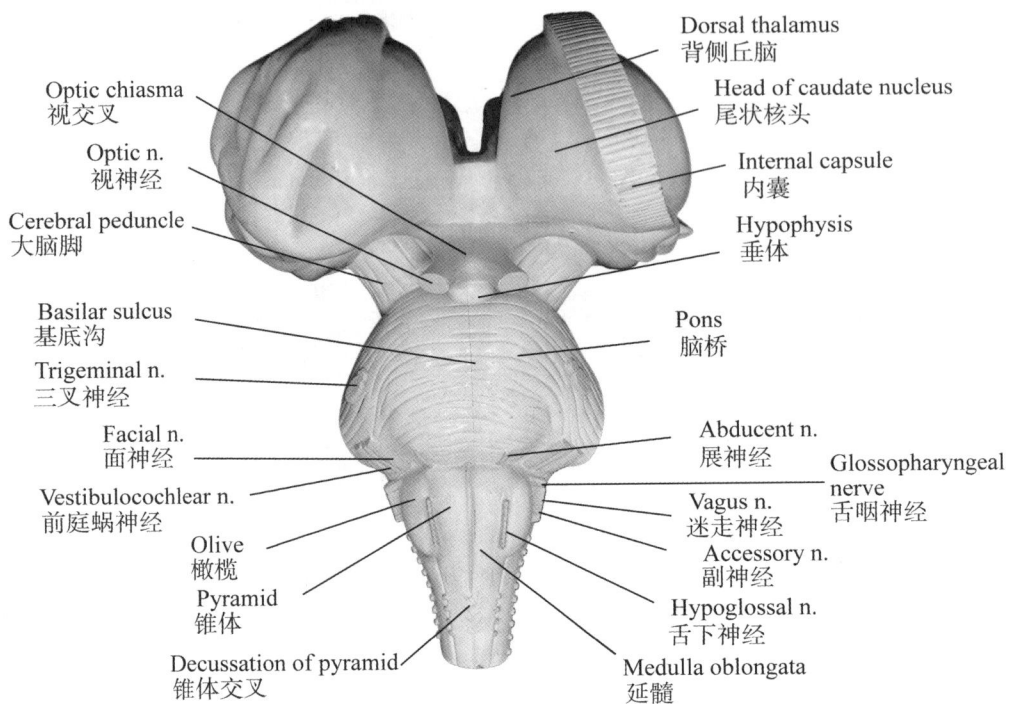

Fig.9-12　　The brain stem

1. Medulla Oblongata

The medulla oblongata (延髓) is like an inverted cone, which is located at the lower part of the brain stem. Its lower end is connected to the spinal cord at the foramen magnum of the occipital bone. The upper end of the medulla oblongata and the pons are bounded by the transverse bulbopontine sulcus (延髓脑桥沟) on the ventral side and the transverse medullary stria in the middle of the rhomboid fossa on the dorsal side.

The longitudinal projections on both sides of the anterior median fissure are called pyramids (锥体), which are mainly composed of corticospinal tract fibers. At the lower end of the medulla oblongata, most of the fibers in the pyramids cross the edge to the opposite side, forming a visible decussation of pyramid (锥体交叉) in shape. The oval raised olive (橄榄) can be seen at the each dorsolateral side of the pyramids, with the inferior olivary nucleus inside. In the anterolateral groove between the olive and the pyramid, the hypoglossal nerve (CN-Ⅻ) root filaments exit from the brain. On the dorsal side of the olive, the glossopharyngeal nerve (CN-Ⅸ), vagus nerve (CN-Ⅹ) and accessory nerve (CN-Ⅺ) root filaments are arranged from top to bottom. There are gracile tubercles (薄束结节) and cuneate tubercles (楔束结节) on both sides of the posterior median sulcus at the lower part of the dorsal side of the medulla oblongata, and there are gracile nuclei and cuneite nuclei on the deep side, which are the termination nuclei of the fasciculus gracilis and fasciculus cuneatus respectively. There is a raised inferior cerebellar peduncle (小脑下脚) at the latero-superior part of the cuneate tubercle. The central canal opens to form the fourth ventricle at the upper part of the dorsal medulla oblongata, forming the lower part of the rhomboid fossa.

2. Pons

The ventral side of pons (脑桥) has a broad swelling called the basilar part (基底部), and there is a longitudinal basilar sulcus (基底沟) in the middle to accommodate the basilar artery. The inferior margin of the pons is bounded by the bulbopontine sulcus with the medulla oblongata, and the superior end is the cerebral peduncle of the midbrain. In the bulbopontine sulcus, there are abducent nerve (CN - Ⅵ), facial nerve(CN - Ⅶ) and vestibulocochlear nerve (CN - Ⅷ) from middle to lateral. The basilar part gradually narrows posterolaterally, and moves to the middle cerebellar peduncle (小脑中脚), which is composed of fibers from the pons into the cerebellum. There is a trigeminal nerve (CN-Ⅴ) root between the middle cerebellar peduncle and the basilar part of the pons. At the lateral end of the bulbopontine sulcus, the area among the medulla oblongata, the pons and the cerebellum is clinically called the pontocere-bellar trigone (脑桥小脑三角), where the facial nerve root and the vestibulocochlear nerve root are located. Therefore, tumors at this site often cause various clinical symptoms involving facial nerve injury.

The back of the pons is the upper half of the bottom of the fourth ventricle. Its lateral wall is the left and right superior cerebellar peduncles (小脑上脚). The thin layer of white matter between the two superior cerebellar peduncles is called the superior medullary velum (上髓帆), which is involved in the formation of the top of the fourth ventricle. The trochlear nerve (CN-Ⅳ) root exits the brain from the superior medullary velum, which is the only cranial nerve that exits the brain from the back of the brain stem.

Rhomboid fossa (菱形窝) is the floor of the fourth ventricle (第四脑室底), and is located at the upper part of the medulla oblongata and the back of the pons. There is a longitudinal median sulcus (正中沟) in the middle of this fossa, and a longitudinal sulcus limitans (界沟) on the outside. The triangular area on the lateral side of the sulcus limitans is the vestibular area (前庭区) with the vestibular nucleus in deep. The small bulge at the lateral corner of the vestibular area is called the acoustic tubercle (听结节) with the dorsal nucleus of the cochlear nerve in deep. The area between the sulcus limitans and the median sulcus is called the medial eminence (内侧隆起). Two small triangular areas can be seen below the medullary stria: the hypoglossal triangle (舌下神经三角) with the hypoglossal nucleus in deep, and the vagal triangle (迷走神经三角) with the dorsal nucleus of the vagus nerve in deep. The narrow area between the vagal triangle and the inferolateral of the rhomboid fossa is called the area postrema (最后区), which contains abundant blood vessels and glia. On the medial eminence above the medullary stria, there is a round eminence called the facial colliculus (面神经丘) with abducent nucleus in deep. On fresh specimens, a small blue-black region called locus ceruleus (蓝斑) can be seen at the upper end of the sulcus limitans, containing pigmented noradrenergic neurons.

The fourth ventricle (第四脑室) (Fig.9-13) is the ventricular cavity located between the pons, medulla oblongata and cerebellum. Its top is towards the cerebellum, and the posterior part of the top is attached to the choroid tissue of the fourth ventricle, which is formed by the epithelial ependyma and its surface soft membrane and blood vessels. The blood vessels of part of the choroid tissue repeatedly wound into bundles and protruded into the ventricular cavity, forming the choroid plexus of the fourth ventricle, which can produce cerebrospinal fluid.

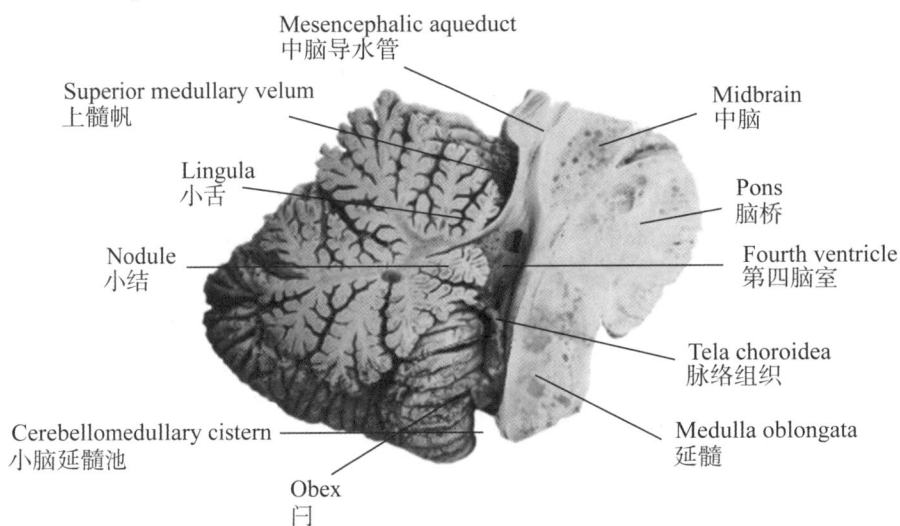

Fig.9-13   The choroid plexus of the fourth ventricle

There are three holes in the fourth ventricle that are connected with the subarachnoid space: The unmatched median aperture of the fourth ventricle (第四脑室正中孔) is located above the tip of the lower horn of the rhomboid fossa; the paired lateral apertures of the fourth ventricle (第四脑室外侧孔) are located at the tip of the lateral recess of the fourth ventricle.

3. Mesencephalon (or Midbrain) (中脑)

The upper boundary of the ventral side of the mesencephalon (or Midbrain) (中脑) is the optic tract of the diencephalon, and the lower boundary is the superior margin of the pons. A pair of large protuberances on the ventral side of the midbrain, called cerebral peduncle (大脑脚), are composed of a large number of descending fibers from the cerebral cortex. The depression between the two sides of the cruses cerebri is the interpeduncular fossa (脚间窝), in which the oculomotor nerve (CN-Ⅲ) root comes out of the brain. There are two pairs of round projections on the dorsal side of the midbrain, with a symmetric superior colliculus (上丘) that connects the lateral geniculate body with the brachium of superior colliculus (上丘臂) at the top and a symmetric inferior colliculus (下丘) that connects medial geniculate body with brachium of inferior colliculus (下丘臂) at the bottom. There is a mesencephalic aqueduct (中脑水管) in the midbrain, which leads down to the fourth ventricle and up to the third ventricle.

4.Internal Structure of the Brain Stem

The internal structure of the brain stem includes the gray matter, the white matter the and reticular formation. The gray matter divides into the nuclei of cranial nerve (脑神经核) and the noncranial nuclei (非脑神经核).

(1) Cranial nuclei properties and classification of cranial nuclei

The CN - Ⅲ to CN - Ⅻ pairs of cranial nerves all enter and exit the brain stem. Therefore, the cranial nuclei associated with these cranial nerves are located in the brain stem. The arrangement pattern of these cranial nuclei in the brain stem can be deduced from the arrangement pattern of the gray matter of the spinal cord. With the sulcus limitans at the bottom of the fourth ventricle as the boundary, the sensory nucleus is located on the lateral side of the sulcus limitans, and the motor nucleus is located between the sulcus limitans and the median sulcus. Cranial nuclei are divided into seven types according to their properties and are arranged into vertical functional columns in the brain stem.

Somatic motor nucleus (躯体运动柱/核) innervates the skeletal muscle derived from the sarcomere, namely the lingual muscle and extraocular muscle, which is equivalent to the motor nucleus of the anterior horn of the spinal cord (oculomotor nucleus, CN - Ⅲ; trochlear nucleus, CN - Ⅳ; abducens nucleus, CN - Ⅵ; and Hypoglossal nucleus, CN - Ⅻ). Special visceral motor nucleus (特殊内脏运动柱/核) innervates skeletal muscle derived from branchial arch, such as masticatory muscle, facial expression muscle, pharyngolaryngeal muscle that play a role in the digestive and respiratory activities (motor nucleus of trigeminal nerve, CN-Ⅴ; facial nucleus, CN-Ⅶ; nucleus ambiguus, CN-Ⅸ, Ⅹ, Ⅺ; accessory nucleus, CN-Ⅺ). General visceral motor nucleus (一般内脏运动柱/核), which dominates the smooth muscle, myocardium and glands of the head, neck, chest and abdominal organs, is equivalent to the sacral parasympathetic nucleus of the spinal cord (accessory oculomotor nucleus (CN - Ⅲ); Superior salivatory nucleus, CN - Ⅶ); Inferior salivatory nucleus, CN - Ⅸ; Dorsal nucleus of vagus nerve, CN - Ⅹ). General visceral sensory nucleus (一般内脏感觉柱/核), which receives primary sensory fibers from viscera and cardio-vascular system, is equivalent to the intermediomedial nucleus of spinal cord (accessory oculomotor nucleus, CN-Ⅲ; superior salivatory nucleus, CN-Ⅶ; inferior salivatory nucleus, CN - Ⅸ; dorsal nucleus of vagus nerve, CN - Ⅹ). Special visceral sensory nucleus (特殊内脏感觉柱/核) receives the primary afferent fibers of taste (nucleus of solitary tract, taste CN-Ⅶ & Ⅸ). General somatosensory nucleus(一般躯体感觉柱/核) receives the primary sensory afferent fibers from the skin of the head and face and the mucosa of the mouth and nose (mesencephalic nucleus of trigeminal nerve, CN-Ⅴ; pontine nucleus of trigeminal nerve, CN-V; spinal nucleus of trigeminal nerve, CN-Ⅴ,Ⅶ,Ⅸ,Ⅹ. Special somatosensory nucleus (特殊躯体感觉柱/核), which receives the primary afferent fibers of inner ear hearing and balance sense (cochlear nucleus & vestibular nucleus CN-Ⅷ)(Fig.9-14), shows the arrangement of cranial nuclei in the upper transverse section of the medulla oblongata.

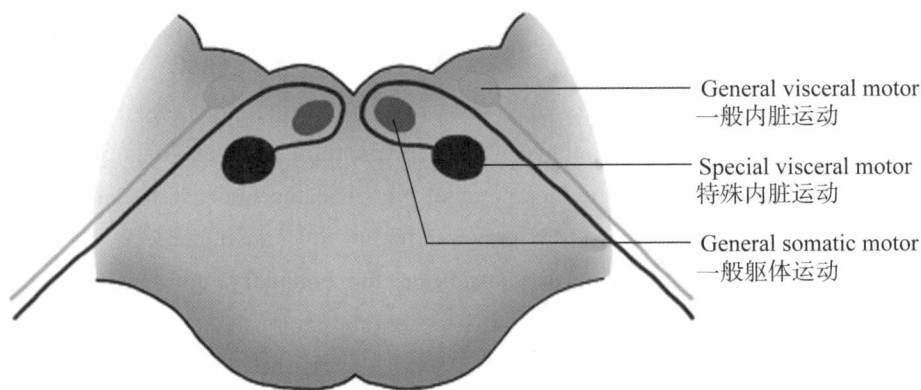

General visceral motor 一般内脏运动

Special visceral motor 特殊内脏运动

General somatic motor 一般躯体运动

Fig. 9-14   The cranial nuclei

1) Somatic motor column. This column is located on both sides of the median line and consists of four nuclei: i) Oculomotor nucleus (动眼神经核, CN-Ⅲ), located at the plane of the superior colliculus of the midbrain, is ventral to the midbrain aqueduct. The fibers from the nucleus run ventrally and go out of the brain through the interpedullary fossa, forming the general somatic motor fibers of the oculomotor nerve (CN-Ⅲ), and innervating the extraocular muscles and levator palpebrae superioris muscles except the rectus and superior oblique muscles. ii) The trochlear nucleus (滑车神经核, CN-Ⅳ), is located at the ventral side of the midbrain aqueduct at the plane of the inferior colliculus of the midbrain. The fibers from this nucleus run backward around the periaqueductal gray matter of the midbrain, completely cross the left and right fibers in the superior medullary velum, exit the brain at the dorsal side of the brainstem, and dominate the superior oblique muscle. iii) The abducens nucleus (展神经核, CN-Ⅵ): located in the deep surface of the facial nerve colliculus in the middle and lower part of the pons, the fibers from this nucleus run to the ventrolateral side, leaving the brain at the junction of the basilar part of the pons and the upper end of the pyramids, and innervating the lateral rectus muscle. iv) The hypoglossal nucleus (舌下神经核, CN-Ⅻ) is located in

the deep surface of the hypoglossal nerve triangle at the upper part of the medulla oblongata, the fibers from this nucleus form the root filaments of the hypoglossal nerve, which exits from the brain between the pyramids and the olive and innervates all the internal and external lingual muscles on the same side.

2) Special visceral motor column. This column is located at the ventrolateral side of the somatic motor column,innervates skeletal muscle derived from branchial arch, such as masticatory muscle, facial expression muscle, pharyngolaryngeal muscle that play a role in the digestive and respiratory activities, consists of four nuclei. i) The motor nucleus of trigeminal nerve (三叉神经运动核, CN-Ⅴ) is located in the middle of the pons, emitting fibers to the ventrolateral side, forming the trigeminal motor root and joining the mandibular nerve, innervating the masticatory muscle, mandibular hyoid muscle, front belly of digastric muscle, etc. ii) The facial nucleus (面神经核, CN-Ⅶ) is located in the middle and lower parts of the pons. The fibers from this nucleus first go to the dorsomedial side, bypass the abducent nucleus to form the genu of facial nerve, and then go to the ventrolateral side, exit the brain through the bulbopontine sulcus to form the facial nerve motor root, which innervates the facial muscle, the posterior belly of the digastric muscle, the styloid hyoid muscle, stapedius and platysma. iii) The nucleus ambiguus (疑核, CN-Ⅸ, Ⅹ, Ⅺ) is located in the reticular formation in the middle and upper part of the medulla oblongata, the fibers from this nucleus are respectively added to the glossopharyngeal nerve (CN-Ⅸ), vagus nerve (CN-Ⅹ) and accessory nerve (CN-Ⅺ) from top to bottom. The fibers of the glosso-pharyngeal nerve innervate the styloid pharyngeal muscle, the fibers of the vagus nerve innervate the skeletal muscle of the soft palate, pharynx and larynx and the upper esophagus, and the fibers of the accessory nerve innervates the palatal muscle and the internal laryngeal muscle. iv) The accessory nucleus (副神经核, CN-Ⅺ): located at the decussation of pyramid of the medulla oblongata to the dorsolateral area of the anterior horn of the upper fifth or sixth cervical cord. The fibers from this nucleus form the spinal root of the accessory nerve and innervate the sternocleidomastoid muscle and the trapezius muscle.

3) General visceral motor column is located at the lateral of the somatic motor column near the sulcus limitans. It is composed of four nuclei. i) Accessory oculomotor nucleus (动眼神经副核, CN-Ⅲ), also known as Edinger-Westphal nucleus, is located at the dorsomedial side of the oculomotor nucleus at the superior colliculus plane. This nucleus sends out parasympathetic preganglionic fibers to join the oculomotor nerve and leave the brain, forming synaptic contact with neurons in the ciliary ganglion. The parasympathetic postganglionic fibers from this ganglion innervate the pupil sphincter and ciliary muscle of the eye, make the pupil narrow and adjust the curvature of the lens, and participate in completing the pupil's light reflex and adjustment reflex. ii) The superior

salivatory nucleus (上泌涎核, CN-Ⅶ) is located in the reticular formation of the lower part of the pons, and its the boundary is unclear. The parasympathetic preganglionic fibers from the nucleus are added to the facial nerve (CN-Ⅶ), and the postganglionic fibers innervate the lacrimal gland after passing through the exchange neurons of the pterygopalatine ganglion; The exchange neurons through the submandibular ganglion control the secretion of sublingual gland and submandibular gland. iii) The inferior salivatory nucleus (下泌涎核, CN-Ⅸ) is located in the reticular formation of the upper part of the medulla oblongata olives, and its the boundary is also unclear. This nucleus sends out parasympathetic preganglionic fibers to join the glossopharyngeal nerve (CN-Ⅸ), and controls the secretion of parotid gland after exchanging neurons through the otic ganglion. iv) The dorsal nucleus of vagus nerve (迷走神经背核, CN-Ⅹ) is located in the deep surface of the vagus nerve triangle, inferolateral the hypoglossal nucleus. This nucleus sends out parasympathetic preganglionic fibers to join the vagus nerve, and exits the brain at the dorsal side of the olive. After exchanging neurons through the intramural ganglion of the target organ, it controls the activities of most organs in the neck, chest and abdominal cavity, and digestive canal until the left colic flexure.

4) General and special visceral sensory column is composed of a single nucleus of solitary tract (孤束核) that receives the input of general visceral sensation from the respiratory, cardiovascular, and gastrointestinal systems, and special visceral sensa-tion (taste). The nucleus is located at the lateral side of the sulcus limitans, with the upper end reaching the lower part of the pons and the lower end reaching the plane of the decussation of medial lemniscus (glossopharyngeal, CN-Ⅸ) nerve,facial nerve,CN-Ⅶ and vagus nerve, CN-Ⅹ).

5) General somatic sensory column is located at the ventrolateral side of the visceral sensory column, composed of three nuclei related to the trigeminal nerve. i) The mesencephalic nucleus of trigeminal nerve (三叉神经中脑核, CN-Ⅴ) is the most extreme end of the general somatosensory column. This nucleus is associated with proprioceptive conduction in the masticatory muscles, facial muscles, and teeth. ii) The pontine nucleus of trigeminal nerve (三叉神经脑桥核, CN-Ⅴ) is located in the middle of the pons. iii) The spinal nucleus of trigeminal nerve (三叉神经脊束核, CN-Ⅴ,Ⅶ,Ⅸ,Ⅹ) is formed by the downward continuation of the pontine nucleus of the trigeminal nerve. The spinal nucleus of trigeminal nerve continues downward into layers Ⅰ — Ⅳ of the posterior horn of the spinal cord. The pontine nucleus of the trigeminal nerve and the spinal nucleus of the trigeminal nerve mainly receive the general somatic sensory input from the teeth, the facial skin, the mouth and the nasal mucosa. These fibers enter the brain mainly through the trigeminal nerve (Ⅴ). The fibers ending in the spinal nucleus of trigeminal nerve descend from the lateral side of the nucleus in the brain stem to form the

spinal tract of trigeminal nerve (三叉神经脊束).

6)Special somatic sensory column is located at the lateral side of the visceral sensory column, the level of the lower pons and upper medulla oblongata, and the deep side of the vestibular area of the lateral rhomboid fossa, which is composed of two nuclei. i) The cochlear nucleus (蜗神经核) (Ⅷ) receives the primary auditory fibers from the spiral ganglion (cochlear ganglion); ii) The vestibular nucleus (前庭神经核) (Ⅷ) receives the primary balance sensory fibers transmitted through the vesti-bular ganglion and the fibers transmitted from the cerebellum (Fig.9-15).

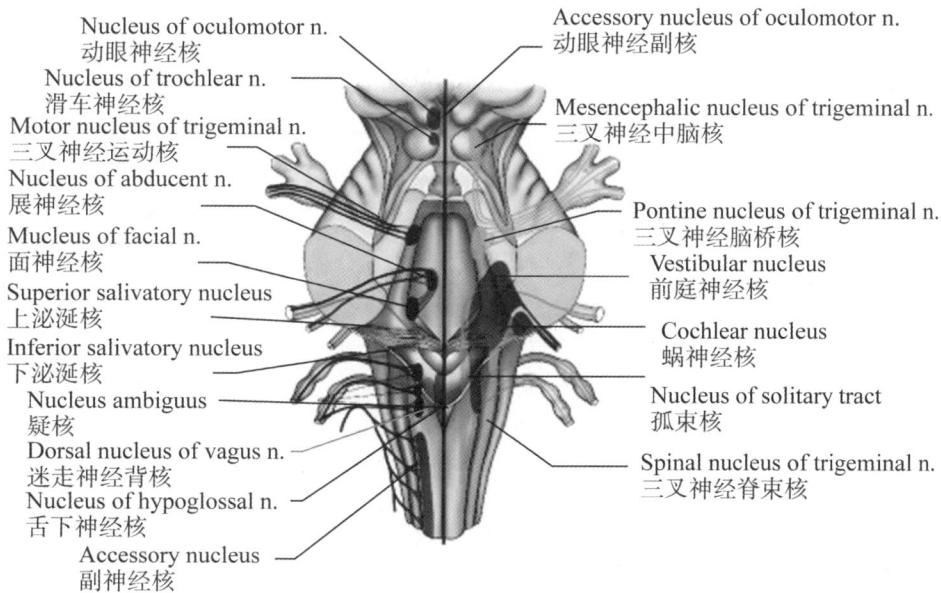

Fig.9-15   Nuclei of the cranial nerve

(2) Noncranial nuclei

They are generally not directly associated with the cranial nerves. As the relay nucleus of the ascending or descending conduction pathway in the brain stem, they have extensive afferent and efferent fiber connections, realizing the connection with the brain and spinal cord at all levels.

1) Noncranial nuclei of medulla oblongata

Gracile nucleus (薄束核) and *cuneate nucleus* (楔束核). They are located at the deep side of the gracile tubercle and cuneate tubercle in the middle and lower dorsal medulla oblongata, respectively, and the fibers of the fasciculus gracilis and fasciculus cuneatus end at these two nuclei. After relay, two nuclei send fibers arcuate around the center to the ventral side, crossing left and right on the midline, called the decussation of medial lemniscus (内侧丘系交叉). The crossed fibers ascended on both sides of the midline and became the medial lemniscus (内侧丘系). Therefore, the gracile nucleus and cuneate nucleus are the relay nuclei of conscious proprioception and fine touch of the trunk and limbs.

Inferior olivary nucleus (下橄榄核). It is located in the deep surface of the olive of the medulla oblongata, involved in the regulation of cerebellar control of movement, especially for motor learning and memory.

2) Noncranial nuclei of pons

Superior olivary nucleus (上橄榄核). It is located at the dorsomedial side of the lateral lemniscus in the middle and lower part of the pons, and mainly receives the ascending fibers from the bilateral cochlear nucleus, and sends the ascending fibers to join the bilateral lateral lemniscus. Its function is to locate the sound source in space according to the time difference and intensity difference of the sound transmitted by the two ears.

Pontine nucleus (脑桥核). It is composed of a number of neurons scattered between the longitudinal and transverse fibers at the basilar part of pons, and is the most important relay nucleus for transmitting motor information from the cerebral cortex to the cerebellum.

3) Noncranial nuclei of the midbrain

Inferior colliculus (下丘). It is located in the lower dorsal part of the midbrain, it is an important relay nucleus in the auditory conduction pathway. This nucleus mainly receives the lateral lemniscus fibers from the cochlear nerve nucleus, and sends out the fibers to form the brachium of inferior colliculus to the medial geniculate body of the diencephalon to transmit the auditory information. In addition, the inferior colliculus nucleus is the auditory reflex center, which sends fibers to the superior colliculus and participates in the audiovisual reflex activities caused by sound, that is, the head and eye turn to the direction of the sound source.

Superior colliculus (上丘). It is located in the upper dorsal part of the midbrain. The superior colliculus is the human visual reflex center. It mainly receives afferent fibers from the retina and the visual area of the cerebral cortex, as well as fibers from the inferior colliculus, the spinal cord and other brain. Most of the fibers from the superior colliculus encircle the central gray matter and intersect at the left and right sides of the ventral midbrain aqueduct, which is called the dorsal tegmental decussation (被盖背侧交叉), and then descends along both sides of the midline to form the tectospinal tract, ending at the intermediate zone and the medial part of the anterior horn of the cervical cord. Partially uncrossed fibers from the superior colliculus descend in the ipsilateral brain stem and stop at the motor nucleus related to eye movement in the brain stem, participate in and complete reflex activities caused by sound and light stimulation.

Pretectal area (顶盖前区). It refers to the cell group at the junction of the midbrain and diencephalon, adjacent to the head of the superior colliculus. This area receives the fibers from the retina through the superior colliculus arm, sends the fibers to the accessory nucleus of the bilateral oculomotor nerve, and participates in completing the pupillary light reflex. Pretectal region is the center of the pupillary light reflex.

Red nucleus (红核). It is located in the tegmental part at the level of the superior colliculus of the midbrain, the posteromedial side of the substantia nigra, and a round nucleus in the transverse section. The red nucleus includes the small cell part and the large cell part. The afferent fibers of the red nucleus mainly come from the cerebellum and cerebral cortex. The efferent fibers from the large cell part of the red nucleus cross the ventral tegmentum (ventral decussation of tegmentum) at the lower part of the superior colliculus to the opposite side, forming the rubrospinal tract, which mainly terminates in the intermediate zone of the cervical spinal cord and the lateral part of the anterior horn. In function, the red nucleus participates in the regulation of somatic movement.

Substantia nigra (黑质). It is located between the midbrain tegmentum and the soles of the crus cerebri. The dopaminergic neurons in the substantia nigra have round-trip fiber connections with the neostriatum of the telencephalon. Through the projection from substantia nigra to the neostriatum, the dopamine synthesized by substantia nigra is transported to the neostriatum. Parkinson's disease (or tremor paralysis)(帕金森病或震颤性麻痹) is caused by the degeneration of dopaminergic neurons in the substantia nigra due to some reasons, and the decrease of dopamine levels in the substantia nigra and neostriatum. The patient showed muscle rigidity, movement limitation, reduction and tremor. Under physiological conditions, substantia nigra is an important center for regulating voluntary movement.

Ventral tegmental area (腹侧被盖区). It is located between the substantia nigra and the red nucleus of the midbrain, and is rich in dopaminergic neurons and belongs to the limbic system. The efferent fibers in this area mainly terminate in the structures of the limbic system such as hypothalamus, hippocampal formation and amygdala, forming the midbrain limbic dopaminergic system (中脑边缘多巴胺能系统), and participating in the regulation of human learning, memory, emotion and mental activities.

(4) **Long ascending and descending fasciculus**

1) Long ascending fasciculus

Medial lemniscus (内侧丘系). The fibers from the gracile nucleus and the cuneate nucleus go up after crossing the ventral side of the central canal of the medulla oblongata, which is called the medial lemniscus. In the medulla oblongata, this system is located between the midline and the inferior olivary nucleus, on the dorsal side of the pyramis. After the pons, it is located on the ventral side of the tegmentum, adjacent to the basilar part. In the midbrain, it moves to the lateral side of the red nucleus and finally stops at the ventral posterolateral nucleus of the dorsal thalamus(背侧丘脑腹后外侧核). The medial lemniscus conducts the conscious proprioception and fine touch of the opposite half of the trunk and limbs.

Spinothalamic tract or spinothalamic lemniscus (脊髓丘脑束或称脊髓丘系). After entering the brain stem, the spinothalamic tract, parallel to some fibers projecting from the spinal cord to the superior colliculus, is called the spinothalamic lemniscus. This system runs in the lateral medulla oblongata, equivalent to the dorsolateral side of the inferior olivary nucleus, and in the dorsolateral side of the medial lemniscus in the pons and midbrain, and terminates in the ventral posterolateral nucleus of the dorsal thalamus. It conducts pain, temperature sensation and rough touch of the opposite trunk, upper and lower limbs.

Lateral lemniscus (外侧丘系). It is composed of the ascending auditory fibers from the bilateral superior olivary nucleus and the contralateral cochlear nucleus. The lemniscus runs at the ventrolateral margin of the tegmentum at the pons, stops at the inferior colliculus at the midbrain, and projects to the medial geniculate body of the diencephalon after relay, transmitting bilateral auditory information. Before forming the lateral lemniscus, part of the auditory fibers cross the ascending medial lemniscus on the ventral side of the pontine tegmentum, and these fibers form a trapezoid body.

Trigeminal lemniscus (三叉丘系). The fibers from the spinal nucleus of trigeminal nerve and the pontine nucleus of trigeminal nerve go up from the opposite side to form the trigeminal lemniscus. The fibers of the trigeminal lemniscus run along the lateral side of the medial lemniscus and accompany it, and end at the ventral posterior medial nucleus of the dorsal thalamus (背侧丘脑腹后内侧核), transmitting the information of pain, temperature and touch pressure from the skin and mucosa of the opposite head and face.

Medial longitudinal fasciculus (内侧纵束). It is mainly from the vestibular nucleus, part of the fibers cross the border to the opposite side, go up to both sides of the midline of the fourth ventricle, and stop at the various motor nuclei innervating the extraocular muscles. Some fibers descend to the cervical segment of the spinal cord and end at the intermediate zone and the medial part of anterior horn.

Anterior spinocerebellar tract (脊髓小脑前束) and *posterior spinocerebellar tract* (脊髓小脑后束). They line at the lateral periphery of the medulla oblongata, the dorsal spinocerebellar tract enters the cerebellum through the inferior cerebellar peduncle at the upper part of the medulla oblongata, and the ventral spinocerebellar tract ascends to the suprapontine part and enters the cerebellum through the superior cerebellar peduncle. These two tracts are involved in conducting unconscious proprioception.

2) Long descending fasciculus

Pyramidal tract (锥 体 系). It starts from the cerebral cortex and controls the voluntary movement of skeletal muscle. Some of the fibers go down to the spinal cord and end directly or indirectly at the motor cells of the anterior horn of the spinal cord, called the corticospinal tract (皮质脊髓束); The other part of the fibers stop at the somatic motor nucleus and the special visceral motor nucleus in the brain stem, which is called the corticonuclear tract (皮 质 核 束). The pyramidal tract descends to the brain stem through the internal capsule, first in the middle of the 3/5 of the sole of the cerebral peduncle of the midbrain, and then passes through the basilar part of pons and is separated into several small tracts by the transverse fibers of the pons, which are re-aggregated at the lower end of the pons to form the pyramis of the medulla oblongata. At the lower part of the medulla oblongata, most of the fibers of the corticospinal tract descend from the side to the opposite side to form the lateral corticospinal tract (皮 质 脊 髓 侧 束), and a few non-overlapping fibers descend on the same side to form the anterior corticospinal tract (皮质脊髓前束).

Descending fasciculus from the brain stem. The rubrospinal tract (红核脊髓束) and the tectospinal tract (顶 盖 脊 髓 束) originate from the red nucleus and the superior colliculus of the midbrain, respectively, and immediately cross to the opposite and descend after the two tracts are sent out, and end at the gray matter of the spinal cord. The vestibulospinal tract from the pontine vestibular nucleus, the reticular spinal tract from the brainstem reticular formation, and the two tracts also end in the gray matter of the spinal cord, participating in the regulation of voluntary movement.

(5) Brainstem reticular formation

In the brain stem, in addition to the cranial nucleus, the well-defined noncranial nucleus and the long distance fiber tracts, the nerve fibers are crisscrossed, and a large number of nerve cell groups of different sizes are scattered in the area, which is called the reticular formation (网状结构) .There are Nuclei projected to cerebellum (lateral reticular nucleus, paramedian reticular nucleus and pontine tegmental reticular nucleus) which transmit information from the spinal cord, sensory and motor areas of cerebral cortex and vestibular nucleus to cerebellum; Raphe nucleus (中缝核) is located on both sides of the raphe of the brain stem, forming a longitudinal column of cells, mainly composed of 5-hydroxytryptaminergic neurons. Central group nuclei is located on both sides of the midline of the medulla oblongata and pons. The central group nuclei receive information from the spinal cord, the sensory nucleus of the cranial nerves, the superior colliculus, the cerebellum, the motor and sensory cortex of the brain, and send out long axons, which are projected to the cerebral cortex through multi-synaptic connections or descend to the motor cells of the anterior horn of the spinal cord through the reticular spinal tract. Therefore, it can be considered that the central group nuclei are the "effect area" of the reticular formation. Lateral nucleus group receives the lateral branches of various sensory fibers and forms synaptic contact with the medial area. It can be considered that the lateral nucleus group is the "sensory area" of the brainstem reticular formation; Locus coeruleus (蓝斑) is the largest nucleus in the brain stem that produces nore-pinephrine. The axons of neurons in this nucleus project to all parts of the central nervous system, and the dendrites are widely distributed. They play an important role in the overall activity of the brain, and also have a regulatory role in blood vessel movement.

1) Functions of reticular formation

Ascending reticular excitatory system (上行网状激动系统). This system includs sensory afferent to reticular formation, projection from reticular formation to intralaminar nuclei of thalamus, reticular nucleus and hypothalamus of dien-cephalon, and extensive projection from diencephalon to cerebral cortex. It does not cause specific sensations, but it can put the cerebral cortex in a state of wakefulness and alertness, maintain the conscious function of the cortex, make the cortex have a good perception of various incoming information, and play an important role in the maintenance of human wakefulness and sleep cycles. Some anesthetic drugs and sleeping drugs play their role by blocking some link in the ascending reticular system. In addition, if the system is damaged, it will cause different levels of consciousness disorder, until deep coma. In addition, there is also an ascending reticular inhibition system (上行网状抑制系统) in the reticular formation of the brain stem, and the dynamic balance between it and the ascending reticular excitatory system determines the changes of the sleep-wake cycle and the level of consciousness.

Regulation of somatic movement. The reticulospinal tract comes from the pontine and medullary reticular formations, and ends at the intermediate zone and the medial part of the anterior horn of the spinal cord on the same side, participating in the regulation of somatic movement and muscle tension. The neurons that send out the reticulospinal tract also receive information from the higher centers related to the trunk and limb motor control, such as the cerebral motor cortex, cerebellum and basal nuclei.

Regulation of visceral activities. There are important centers in the lower part of the pons and medulla oblongata reticular formations that regulate visceral activities, such as the respiratory center, cardiovascular motor center, etc. If these structures are damaged, they will cause respiratory and circulatory disorders, and even endanger life.

Regulation of somatic sensation. For example, 5-HT neurons are located in the raphe nucleus of the midbrain and pons mainly receive fibers from the limbic system and hypothalamus, which can modify, strengthen or inhibit the sensory information of the afferent center.

(6) **Representative transverse sections of the brain stem**

1) Transverse section of the middle part of the olive. The main changes in this plane include the follows. The inferior olivary nucleus appears on the deep side of the olives of the dorsal and the lateral side of the pyramid. The central canal opens to become the fourth ventricle, and the part between the floor of the ventricle and the pyramid is called the tegmental part. The gray matter of the ventricular floor is bounded by the sulcus terminalis. The medial side of the sulcus terminalis is the motor cranial nucleus, and the lateral side is sensory. From both sides of the median sulcus to the outside, there is sublingual nucleus, dorsal nucleus of vagus nerve, solitary nucleus and its surrounding solitary tract and vestibular nucleus. There is ambiguous nucleus in the reticular formation of the ventral gray matter of the ventricular floor. On both sides of the midline, there is the pyramidal tract, medial lemniscus, tectospinal tract and medial longitudinal tract from ventral to dorsal side. The spinocerebellar posterior tract has joined the inferior cerebellar peduncle. The spinal tract of trigeminal nerve and its medial spinal nucleus of trigeminal nerve can be seen in the ventromedial side of the inferior cerebellar peduncle. On the dorsal side of the inferior olivary nucleus, the glossopharyngeal nerve, vagus nerve and accessory nerve root exit the brain, and the hypoglossal nerve exits the brain between the pyramid and the olive.

2) Transverse section of the lower part of the pons (via the facial nerve colliculus). The pons can be divided into the ventral basal part and the dorsal tegmental part. The two parts are bounded by a transverse corpus trapezoideum. The longitudinal medial lemniscus passes through the middle of the corpus trapezoideum, and the fibers of the corpus trapezoideum turn upward at the lateral edge of the superior olivary nucleus to become the lateral lemniscus. The basal part of the pons contains longitudinal and transverse interlaced fibers, and the pontine nucleus is scattered in it. They emit transverse fibers that cross to the opposite side, and gather outward to form the middle cerebellar peduncle, and then enter the cerebellum backward. The longitudinal fibers include the pyramidal tract, etc. The former is divided into several small bundles by the transverse pontocerebellar fibers. The tegmental parts of the pons and medulla oblongata are continuous, and the inferior cerebellar peduncle enters the cerebellum on the lateral side. There are raised facial colliculus between the two sides of the midline of the ventricular floor and the sulcus terminalis, and there are genu of facial nerve and abducent nucleus on the deep side. The vestibular nucleus can be seen on the lateral side of the sulcus terminalis. The facial nucleus is located at the dorsomedial side of the lateral lemniscus. It sends out fibers around the abducent nucleus and then turns to the ventrolateral side to exit the brain. The spinal nucleus of trigeminal nerve and spinal tract of trigeminal nerve

are located at the dorsomedial side of the facial nucleus. The reticular formation is located in the center of the tegmentum, and the position of other fiber tracts is roughly the same as that of the upper section of the medulla oblongata.

3) Transverse section of the inferior colliculus. The transverse section of the midbrain from the dorsal to the ventral side includes the tectum, periaqueductal gray matter of the midbrain and the cerebral peduncle. The tectum consists of the anterior region of the tectum, the superior colliculus and the inferior colliculus; The crus cerebri is composed of longitudinal fiber tracts, which from the inside to the outside are the frontopontine tract, pyramidal tract and parietal, occipital and temporal pontine tracts; The dorsal side of the crus cerebri is substantia nigra, and the part between the dorsal side of substantia nigra and the ventrolateral side of the gray matter around the midbrain aqueduct is the midbrain tegmentum. The tectum of this plane is the inferior colliculus, and the fibers of the lateral lemniscus scatter into it. The medial longitudinal tract is located on both sides of the midline on the ventral side of the central gray matter of the aqueduct. The trochlear nucleus is located on the dorsal side of the tract. The ventral side of the tract has the decussation of the upper cerebellar peduncle, and the ventral side of the cross fiber is the rubrospinal tract. The medial lemniscus is located at the dorsal side of substantia nigra, while the spinal lemniscus is located at the dorsolateral side of the medial lemniscus, and the trigeminal lemniscus is located at its dorsomedial side. The reticular formation is located at the dorsolateral part of the tegmentum.

(7) Common manifestations of brain stem injury

1) Medial medullary syndrome (延髓内侧综合征). It is caused by the occlusion of the branch of the vertebral artery supplying the medulla oblongata on one side. If it is a unilateral injury, it is called hypoglossal nerve cross paralysis. The structures involved include the pyramid, medial lemniscus and root of the hypoglossal nerve. The clinical manifestations include the spastic paralysis of the upper and lower limbs on the opposite side, disappearance of the position, motion and fine touch of the trunk and limbs on the opposite side, and deviation of the tip of the tongue to the affected side when the tongue is extended.

2) Lateral medullary syndrome (or Wallenberg's syndrome) (延髓外侧综合征). It is caused by the occlusion of the posterior inferior cerebellar artery, a branch of the vertebral artery supplying the lateral medullary region. The damaged structures include the spinal tract of the trigeminal nerve and the spinal nucleus of the trigeminal nerve, the spinothalamic tract and the nucleus ambiguus. The symptoms of the patients are the pain and temperature sense of the injured head and face on the same side and the opposite trunk and limbs decrease or disappear. Paralysis of the ipsilateral soft palate and pharyngolaryngeal muscles causes dysphagia and hoarseness. If the sympathetic

descending pathway projected from the hypothalamus to the lateral nucleus of the intermedial zone of the thoracic cord is injured, Horner's syndrome can be caused, which is characterized by narrowing of the pupil on the injured side, ptosis of the upper eyelid, facial skin flushing and sweat gland secretion disorder. If the lesion extends dorsolateral, it can damage the inferior cerebellar peduncle or vestibular nucleus, and the patient will have cerebellar ataxia and vertigo.

3) Pontine basal syndrome (脑桥基底部综合征). An injury to the middle and lower part of one side of the pons can damage the pyramidal tract and abducent root. The manifestations are the opposite upper and lower limb paraplegia. The ipsilateral eyeball cannot be extended.

4) Weber syndrome (韦伯综合征或大脑脚综合征). It is caused by the injury of the crus cerebri of the midbrain. The structures involved include the pyramidal tract and the root of the oculomotor nerve. The patient's performance is that the opposite upper and lower limbs are paralyzed, the ipsilateral extraocular muscles are paralyzed except the rectus and superior oblique muscles, and the pupil is dilated.

9.5.2   Cerebellum

The cerebellum (小脑)(Fig. 9-16) is located in the posterior cranial fossa and is separated from the tentorium cerebelli on the underside of the occipital lobe of the telencephalon. The upper part of the cerebellum is flat, and the middle part is narrow, which is called the cerebellar vermis (小脑蚓). The two lateral sides are enlarged, which is called the cerebellar hemispheres (小脑半球). The middle part of the lower part is concave and hemispherical protrusions on both sides. Near the upper part of the foramen magnum, the hemispheres on both sides of the cerebellar vermis are more prominent, called the tonsil of cerebellum (小脑扁桃体). When intracranial hypertension is caused by craniocerebral injury or intracranial tumor, the cerebellar tonsil can be embedded into the foramen magnum, forming a tonsil of cerebellum hernia (or occipital foramen hernia), compressing the medulla oblongata and endangering life. The front of the cerebellum is connected to the back of the brain stem by three pairs of cerebellar peduncles. The inferior cerebellar peduncle is mainly composed of fibers originating from the spinal cord and the inferior olivary nucleus, which enter the cerebellum from the internal inferior part of the middle cerebellar peduncle. The fibers of the middle cerebellar peduncle originate from the contralateral pontine nucleus; The superior cerebellar peduncle is mainly composed of the efferent fibers of the cerebellum, and there is a thin superior medullary velum between the two superior peduncles.

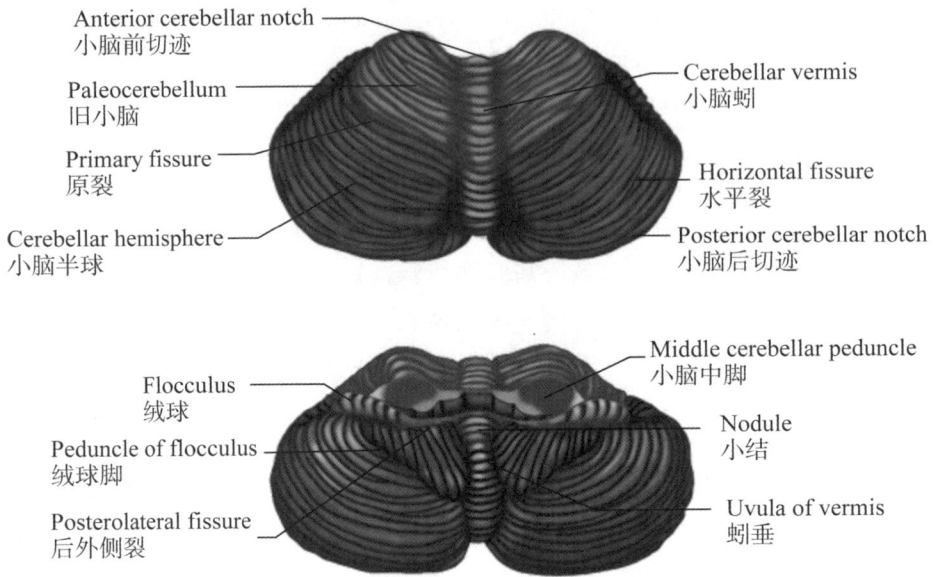

Anterior cerebellar notch
小脑前切迹

Paleocerebellum
旧小脑

Primary fissure
原裂

Cerebellar hemisphere
小脑半球

Cerebellar vermis
小脑蚓

Horizontal fissure
水平裂

Posterior cerebellar notch
小脑后切迹

Flocculus
绒球

Peduncle of flocculus
绒球脚

Posterolateral fissure
后外侧裂

Middle cerebellar peduncle
小脑中脚

Nodule
小结

Uvula of vermis
蚓垂

Fig.9-16　The cerebellum

The gray matter on the surface of cerebellum is called cerebellar cortex (小脑皮质). The white matter on the deep side of the cerebellum is called the cerebellar medulla (小脑髓质), and the gray matter mass in the medulla is called the cerebellar nuclei (小脑核). There are four pairs of cerebellar nuclei: the dentate nucleus (齿状核), the largest one with the emboliform nucleus (栓状核) and the globose nucleus (球状核) on the medial side, and the fastigial nucleus (顶核) on both sides of the midline above the top of the fourth ventricle. These nuclei mainly receive fibers from the cerebellar cortex and emit efferent fibers to the cerebellum (Fig.9-17).

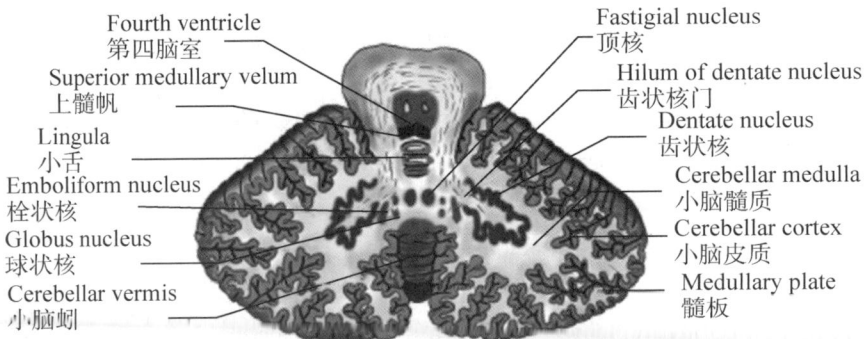

Fourth ventricle
第四脑室

Superior medullary velum
上髓帆

Lingula
小舌

Emboliform nucleus
栓状核

Globus nucleus
球状核

Cerebellar vermis
小脑蚓

Fastigial nucleus
顶核

Hilum of dentate nucleus
齿状核门

Dentate nucleus
齿状核

Cerebellar medulla
小脑髓质

Cerebellar cortex
小脑皮质

Medullary plate
髓板

Fig.9-17　The cerebellar nuclei

1. Lobation and Division of the Cerebellum

(1) **Lobation of the cerebellum**

There are two deep grooves on the surface of the cerebellum, which divide the cerebellum into three lobes: the deep groove at the junction of the anterior 1/3 and the posterior 2/3 of the upper cerebellum is called the primary fissure (原裂). The cerebellar hemisphere and cerebellar vermis before the primary fissure are the anterior lobe (前叶), and most of the cerebellar hemisphere after the primary fissure and below the cerebellum are the posterior lobe (后叶). Below the cerebellum, the posterolateral fissure (后外侧裂) is the boundary between the posterior cerebellar lobe and the flocculonodular lobe (绒球小结叶).

(2) **Functional division of the cerebellum**

The flocculonodular lobe is mainly associated with the vestibular nucleus and the vestibular nerve. It is called vestibulocerebellum (前庭小脑), which appears the earliest in evolution, so it is also called archecerebellum (原小脑). The cerebellar vermis and the middle part of the cerebellar hemisphere form the paleocerebellum (旧小脑), which mainly receives information from the spinal cord, also known as the spinocerebellum (脊髓小脑). The lateral part of the cerebellar hemisphere receives the information relayed by the cerebral cortex via the pontine nucleus, which is called the cerebrocerebellum (大脑小脑). It appears the latest in evolution and is related to the development of the cerebral cortex, so it is also called neocerebellum (新小脑).

2. Fiber Connection and Functions of the Cerebellum

(1) **Vestibulocerebellum (archicerebellum)**

It mainly receives fibers from the ipsilateral vestibular ganglion and vestibular nucleus, then enters the cerebellum through the inferior cerebellar peduncle. The efferent fibers are directly emitted from the cortex of the flocculonodular lobe, mainly to the ipsilateral vestibular nucleus, then through the vestibular spinal tract and the medial longitudinal tract, regulate the function of the motor neurons of the trunk muscle and extraocular muscle, and participate in the regulation of muscle tension, body balance, etc.

(2) **Spinocerebellum (paleocerebellum)**

Afferent fibers mainly come from the fibers of the spinocerebellar tract to obtain various information about changes inside and outside the body during movement. Its efferent fibers leave the cerebellum after being replaced by the fastigial nucleus and the intermediate nuclei (globular nucleus and emboliform nucleus). Among them, the vermis of the cerebellum sends out fibers to the fastigial nucleus, which are projected to the vestibular nucleus and the reticular formation after replacement. Through the vestibulospinal tract and the reticulospinal tract, it innervates the motor neurons in the medial part of the anterior horn, and regulates the muscle tension and motor coordination of the trunk muscle and the limb muscle.

(3) Cerebrocerebellum (neocerebellum)

The afferent fibers of the cerebellum come from the contralateral pontine nucleus, pass through the middle cerebellar peduncle to the cerebellar neocortex, and receive information from the contralateral cerebral cortex (especially the frontal and parietal lobes). After being replaced by the cerebellar dentate nucleus, the efferent fibers cross to the contralateral side through the superior cerebellar peduncle, terminate in the contralateral dorsal ventrolateral nucleus of the thalamus, and then project to the motor area of the cerebral cortex. Through cerebellum-brain feedback, it affects the brain's initiation, planning and coordination of fine movements of limbs, including determining the strength, direction and range of movements.

3. Common Manifestations of Cerebellar Injury

(1) Archicerebellar syndrome (原小脑综合征)

The vestibulocerebellar injury caused by archicerebellar syndrome is characterized by imbalance of balance, unstable standing, wide distance between legs when walking, and faltering gait.

(2) Neocerebellar syndrome (新小脑综合征)

It is caused by cerebellar hemisphere injury and often involves the paleocerebellum. The patient's symptoms include: the ataxia of the affected side of the limb, incongruity between the joints and muscles during movement, inability to accurately point the nose with fingers (positive finger-nose test). and inability to make rapid alternating movement (unable to rotate movement). When the limbs are moving, they show a non-voluntary rhythmic swing. When they are close to the target, the swing is intensified (intentional tremor).

9.5.3   Diencephalon

The diencephalon (间脑, Fig.9-18) is located between midbrain and telence-phalon. In addition to the ventral chiasma, optic tract, tuber cinereum, infundibulum, pituitary and papillary body exposed at the bottom of the brain, other parts of the diencephalon are covered by the cerebral hemisphere. The diencephalon can be divided into five parts: dorsal thalamus, epithalamus, subthalamus, metathalamus and hypothalamus. Its volume is less than 2% of that of the central nervous system, but its structure and function are quite complex, and it is the central advanced part only next to the telencephalon. The sagittal narrow space in the middle of the diencephalon is the third ventricle (第三脑室), which is connected to the fourth ventricle through the midbrain aqueduct, and the dorsal thalamus and hypothalamus are on both sides.

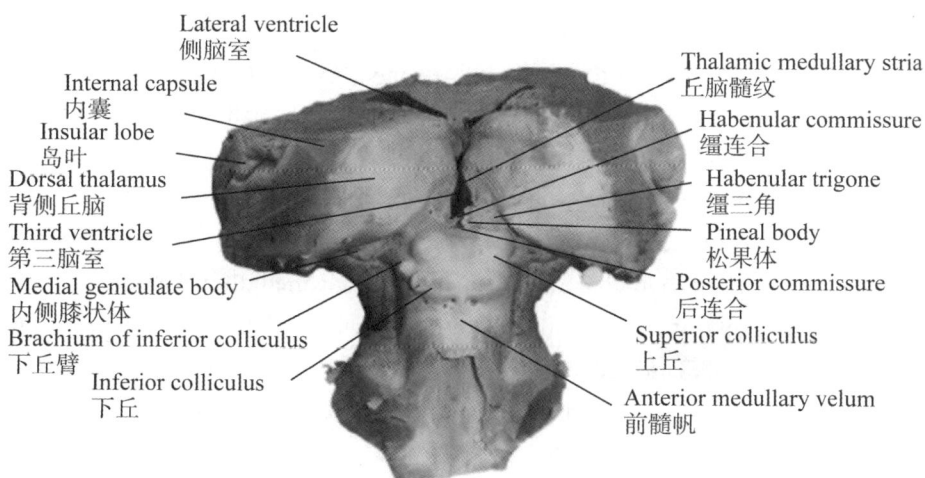

Fig.9-18   Dorsal view of diencephalon

1. Dorsal Thalamus

Dorsal thalamus (背侧丘脑), also known as thalamus (Fig.9-19), is composed of two oval gray matter masses connected by adhesion between the thalamus. Between the two dorsal thalamus is the third ventricle. The lateral wall of the third ventricle has a shallow groove from the interventricular foramen to the midbrain aqueduct, called the hypothalamic sulcus (下丘脑沟), which is the boundary between the dorsal thalamus and the hypothalamus.

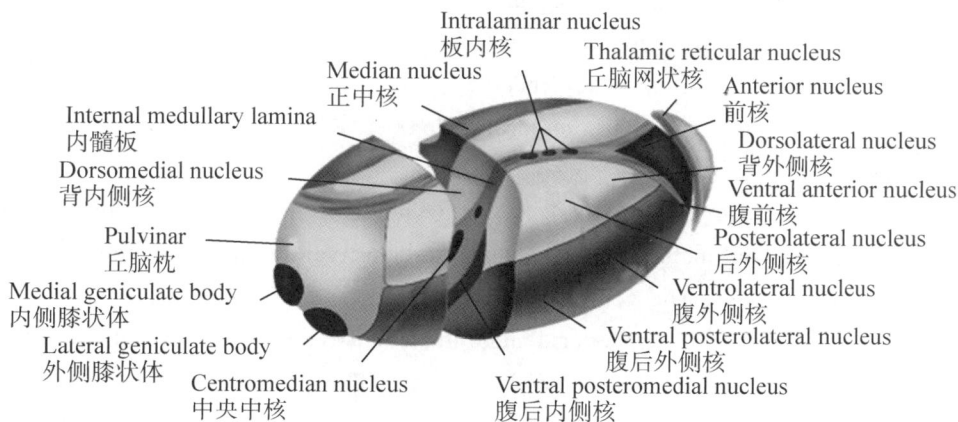

Fig.9-19   Stereoscopic view of dorsal thalamic nucleus

In the dorsal thalamus, there is a "Y" shaped white matter plate from the outside up to the inside down, called the internal medullary lamina (内髓板), which divides the dorsal thalamus into three parts: the anterior nucleus group in front of the fork of the anterior part of the internal medullary lamina, the medial nucleus group and lateral nucleus group are located at the medial and lateral sides of the inner medullary lamina respectively. The lateral nuclear group is divided into two layers: dorsal and ventral. The ventral nucleus group is divided from front to back into ventral anterior nucleus (腹前核), ventral intermediate nucleus (腹中间核) (also called ventral lateral nucleus) and ventral posterior nucleus (腹后核). The ventral posterior nucleus is also divided into ventral posterolateral nucleus (腹后外侧核) and ventral posteromedial nucleus (腹后内侧核). In addition, there are several lamellar nuclei in the internal medullary lamina, and the thin gray matter in the lateral wall of the third ventricle is called the median nucleus; There is also a thin layer of the thalamic reticular nucleus outside the dorsal thalamus.

The above numerous dorsal thalamic nuclei can be classified into the following three categories.

(1)Non-specific projection nuclei

Non-specific projection nuclei (非特异性投射核团) are relatively old in evolution, including the median nucleus and the lamellar nucleus. They mainly receive the afferent fibers of the brainstem reticular formation, and the efferent fibers reach the structures such as the hypothalamus and striatum, and form a round-trip fiber connection with these structures. The fibers of the ascending excitatory system of the brainstem reticular formation, after being relayed by these nuclei, project to a wide area of the cerebral cortex to maintain the awake state of the body.

(2)Connective nuclei

Connective nuclei (联络性核团) are the latest dorsal thalamic nucleus group in evolution. They include the medial nucleus, the dorsal layer of the lateral nucleus group and the anterior nucleus group. They receive a wide range of afferent fibers and have round-trip fiber connections with the cerebral cortex.

(3)Specific relay nuclei

Specific relay nuclei (特异性中继核团) are relatively new dorsal thalamic nucleus groups in evolution, and include ventral anterior nucleus, ventral intermediate nucleus and ventral posterior nucleus. The ventral anterior nucleus and ventral intermediate nucleus mainly receive the fibers of cerebellar dentate nucleus, striatum and substantia nigra, and send the fibers to the motor area of cerebral cortex. The ventral posteromedial nucleus receives the trigeminal lemniscus and taste fibers from the solitary nucleus, the ventral posterolateral nucleus receives fibers from the medial and spinal lemniscuses. The fibers from the ventral posterior nucleus project to the somatosensory center of the central posterior gyrus of the cerebral cortex with the sensory information of the head and face project to the medial ventral nucleus and the sensory information of the upper limb. The trunk and lower limb project to the ventral posterolateral nucleus from inside to outside. These relay information to the primary somatosensory cortex by way of the posterior limb of the internal capsule then through the corona radiate (projection fibers).

When the dorsal thalamus is damaged, it can cause sensory dysfunction, hyperalgesia, spontaneous pain, etc. In addition, the ventral intermediate nucleus and ventral anterior nucleus connect the cerebral cortex with the cerebellum, striatum and substantia nigra to realize the regulation of body movements.

2. Metathalamus

The metathalamus (后丘脑) is located at the lower posterior occipital part of the thalamus, including the medial geniculate body (内侧膝状体) and the lateral geniculate body (外侧膝状体), which is a specific relay nucleus. The medial geniculate body receives the auditory fibers from the inferior colliculus through the brachium of inferior colliculus, and then sends out the fibers to form the auditory radiation, which projects to the auditory center of the temporal lobe. The lateral geniculate body receives the afferent fibers of the optic tract, and after relaying, sends out fibers to form optic radiation, which projects to the visual center of the occipital lobe.

3. Epithalamus

The epithalamus (上丘脑) is located around the top of the third ventricle, inclu-ding the pineal body (松果体), the habenular triangle and the medullary stria of the thalamus. The pineal body is an endocrine gland that produces melatonin, which has the function of inhibiting gonads and regulating biological clock. The calcification of pineal body after 16 years old can be used as a localization marker for X-ray diagnosis of intracranial space-occupying lesions.

4. Subthalmus

The subthalmus (底丘脑) is a transitional area between the diencephalon and the midbrain, which contains the subthalmus nucleus and has close fiber connections with the striatum, substantia nigra and red nucleus. It is an important structure of the extrapyramidal system.

5. Hypothalamus

The hypothalamus (下丘脑) is located below the dorsal thalamus and forms the lower half and bottom wall of the lateral wall of the third ventricle. The upper part is bounded by the hypothalamic sulcus and the dorsal thalamus. At the bottom of the brain, the optic chiasma (视交叉) and the lamina terminalis are located at the forefront of the hypothalamus and extend backward to the optic tract. There is a tuber cinereum (灰结节) behind the optic chiasma. The tuber cinereum moves forward and downward to the infundibulum (漏斗) and hypophysis (垂体). There is a mamillary body (乳头体) behind the tuber cinereum (Fig.9-20).

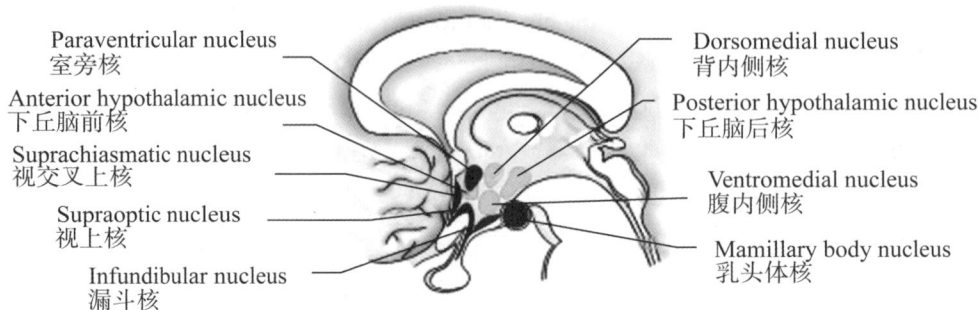

Fig.9-20   Main nuclei of the hypothalamus

(1) The hypothalamic nuclei

It mainly includes the supraoptic nucleus (视上核) at the dorsolateral side of the chiasma, the paraventricular nucleus (室旁核) at the upper part of the lateral wall of the third ventricle, the infundibular nucleus (漏斗核) at the deep side of the infundi-bulum, the suprachiasmatic nucleus (视交叉上核) above the chiasma on both sides of the midline, and the papillary body nucleus (乳头体核) at the deep side of the papillary body.

(2)The fiber connection of the hypothalamus

The fiber connection of the hypothalamus (Fig.9-21) is complex, and its afferent fibers are of two types: the medial forebrain bundle (前脑内侧束), which starts from the septal nuclei and olfactory brain of the telencephalic limbic system, passes through the lateral hypothalamic area to the mesencephalic tegmentum, and has a round-trip fiber connection with the hypothalamus. The fornix (穹隆), the largest afferent tract of the hypothalamus, starts from the hippocampus and ends at the nucleus of the papillary body. The somatic and visceral information transmitted through the brain stem and the spinal cord is mainly relayed to the hypothalamus via the reticular formation. The efferent fibers of the hypothalamus mainly include: i) The mamillothalamic tract (乳头丘脑束) and the mamillo-tegmental tract(乳头被盖束), which project from the nucleus of the papillary body to the anterior nucleus group of dorsal thalamus and the mesencephalic tegmentum, respectively, and the former has a round-trip fiber connection with the cerebral cortex cingulum; ii) hypothalamic-brain stem and spinal cord fibers (Fig.9-22) from paraventricular nucleus to dorsal nucleus of vagus nerve and lateral horn of spinal cord; iii) dorsal longitudinal fasciculus (背侧纵束), from periventricular gray matter to midbrain central gray matter and tegmental, iv) hypothalamohypophyseal tract (下丘脑垂体束): The supraoptic and supraopticohypophyseal tracts (视上垂体束和室旁垂体束) originate from the supraoptic and paraventricular nuclei respectively, and transport vasopressin and oxytocin produced by hypothalamic neuroendocrine neurons to the median eminence or the posterior pituitary (neurohypophysis), and then spread to the whole body through the blood vessels of the posterior pituitary. v) Tuberohypophysial tract or tuberoinfundibular tract (结节垂体束或结节漏斗束): Some neurons from the infundibulum nucleus and the basal medial part of the hypothalamus stop at the capillaries of the median eminence, transport ACTH, hormone release or inhibin and other neuroendocrine substances to the anterior pituitary through the hypophyseal portal system(垂体门脉系统), and control the endocrine function of the anterior pituitary.

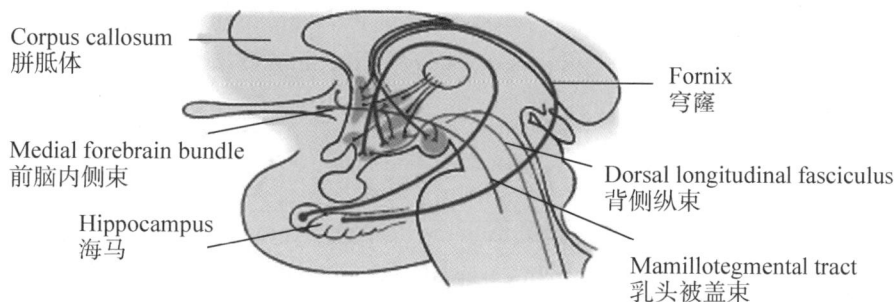

Fig.9-21   Fiber connection of hypothalamus

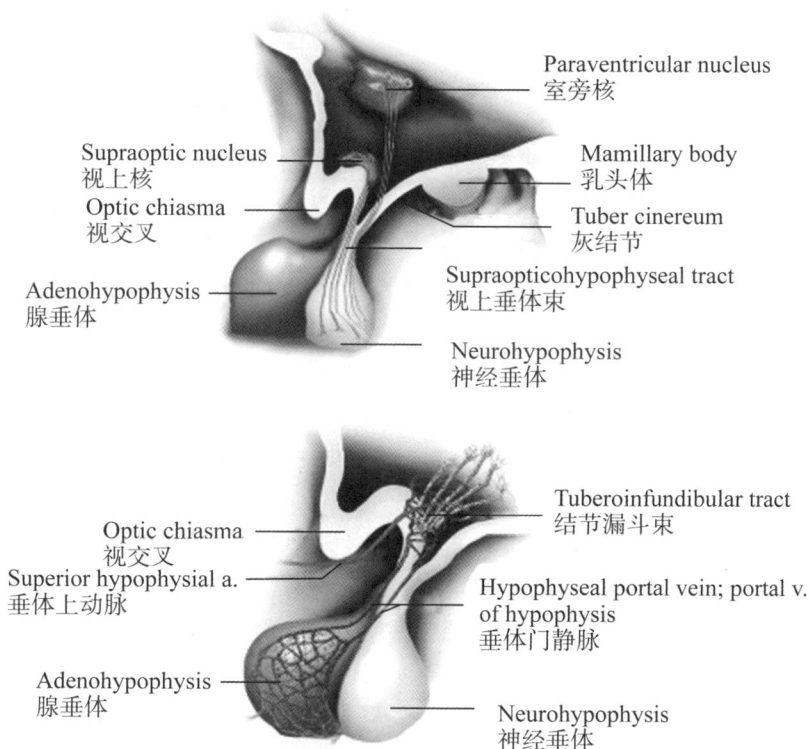

Fig.9-22   The connection between hypothalamus and hypophysis

(3) Function of the hypothalamus

The hypothalamus is the neuroendocrine center, which integrates the neuroregulation and humoral regulation through the connection between the hypothalamus and the pituitary body. The hypothalamus is the high-level center of the subcortical visceral regulation, which participates in the regulation of body temperature, food intake, reproduction, water and salt balance and endocrine activities. Through the connections between the hypothalamus and the limbic system, it participates in the regulation of emotional activities. In addition, the suprachiasmatic nucleus is related to the human circadian rhythm and regulates the human circadian rhythm.

9.5.4　Telencephalon

The telencephalon (端脑), including the left and right hemispheres, is the most advanced part of the brain. The human cerebral hemisphere is highly developed, covering the diencephalon and the midbrain, and the left and right cerebral hemispheres are connected by the corpus callosum. The structures of the cerebral hemisphere include the cerebral cortex, medulla, basal nuclei and lateral ventricle.

1. Shape and Lobulation of Telencephalon

There are many protruding gyri and deep sulci on the surface of the cerebral hemisphere (Fig.9-23). The cerebral longitudinal fissure (大脑纵裂) separates the left and right cerebral hemispheres, and the bottom of the longitudinal fissure is the corpus callosum. The cerebral transverse fissure (大脑横裂) separates the brain from the cerebellum. Each hemisphere has three surfaces, namely the superolateral surface, the medial surface and the basal surface. There are three constant sulcuses on the surface of the hemisphere, which divide the hemisphere into five lobes. The lateral sulcus (外侧沟) is the deepest groove in the hemisphere, which starts from the bottom of the hemisphere, turns to the superolateral surface, and goes up and back. The central sulcus (中央沟) starts from slightly behind the midpoint of the upper edge of the hemisphere, oblique forward and downward. The lower end is separated from the lateral sulcus by a gyrus, and the upper end extends to the medial surface of the hemisphere. The parietooccipital sulcus (顶枕沟) is located at the rear of the medial surface of the hemisphere, which is inclined from the inferoanterior to the postero-superior and extends to the superolateral surface. The part before the central sulcus and above the lateral sulcus is the frontal lobe (额叶); the part after the central sulcus and before the parietooccipital sulcus is the parietal lobe (顶叶); the part below the lateral sulcus is the temporal lobe (颞叶); the part behind the parietooccipital sulcus is the occipital lobe (枕叶); the anterior boundary of the occipital lobe on the supero-lateral surface is the line from the parietooccipital sulcus to the anterior occipital notch (about 4 cm in front of the occipital pole). In the deep side of the lateral sulcus, the insular cortex covered by the frontal, parietal and temporal lobes is called the insular lobe (岛叶).

(1) Superolateral surface

In front of the central sulcus of the frontal lobe, there is a parallel precentral sulcus (中央前沟), between which is the precentral gyrus (中央前回). Behind the central sulcus of the parietal lobe, there is also a parallel sulcus called the postcentral sulcus (中央后沟), and the gyrus between the two sulcus is called the postcentral gyrus (中央后回). In front of the precentral sulcus, there are two grooves roughly parallel to the upper edge of the hemisphere, which are called the superior frontal sulcus (额上沟) and the inferior frontal sulcus (额下沟). The two grooves divide the rest of the superolateral frontal lobe into the superior frontal gyrus (额上回), the middle frontal gyrus (额中回) and the inferior frontal gyrus (额下回). There is a groove parallel to the upper edge of the hemisphere behind the postcentral gyrus, which is called the intraparietal sulcus (顶内沟). The rest of the parietal

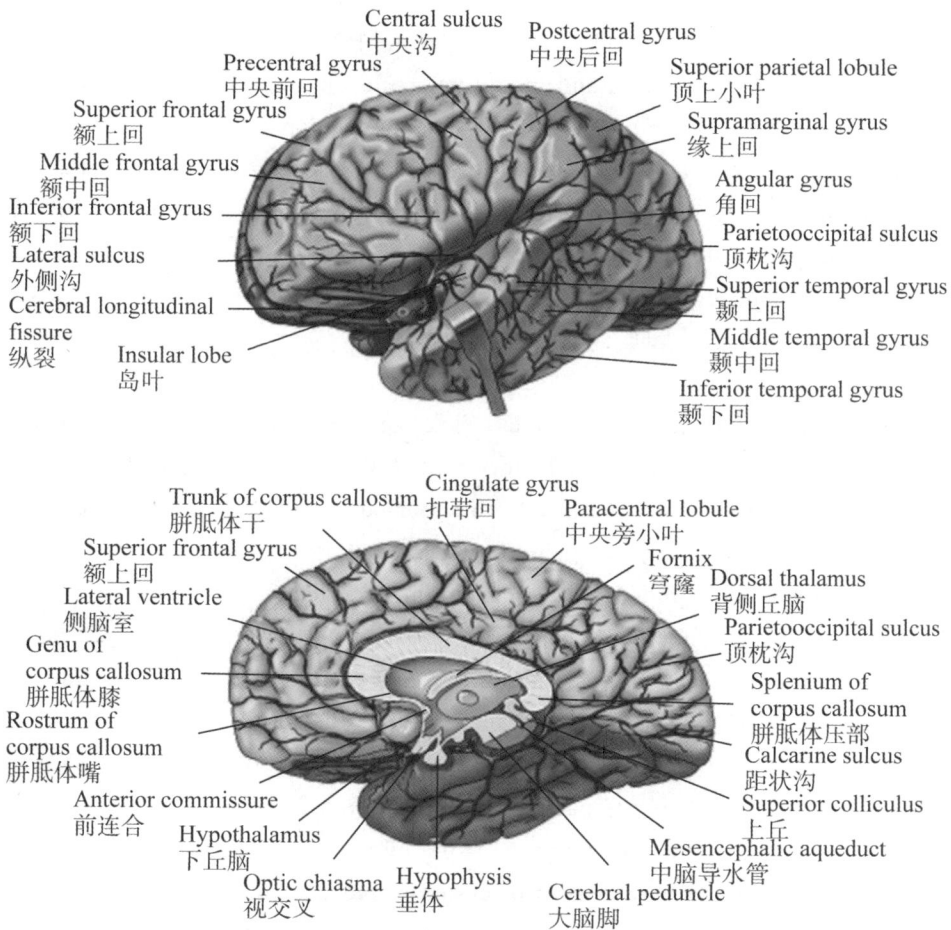

Fig.9-23   The cerebral hemisphere

lobe is divided into the upper superior parietal lobule (顶上小叶) and the lower inferior parietal lobule (顶下小叶). The part of the inferior parietal lobule around the end of the lateral sulcus is called the supramarginal gyrus (缘上回), and the part around the end of the superior temporal sulcus is called the angular gyrus (角回). In the temporal lobe, there are two superior temporal sulcus (颞上沟) and inferior temporal sulcus (颞下沟) which are roughly parallel to the lateral sulcus. The two sulcus divide the temporal lobe into superior temporal gyrus (颞上回), middle temporal gyrus (颞中回) and inferior temporal gyrus (颞下回). There are 2－3 transverse temporal gyrus (颞横回) from the top to the bottom of the lateral sulcus.

(2) Medial surface

The part extending from the dorsolateral surface of the precentral and post-central gyrus to the medial surface is the paracentral lobule (中央旁小叶). In the middle, there is a large fiber tract section with an arch in the anterior-posterior direction, called the corpus callosum (胼胝体). On the back of the corpus callosum, there is a callosal sulcus (胼胝体沟), above which there is a parallel cingulate sulcus (扣带沟). The gyrus between the two is the cingulate gyrus (扣带回), and the corpus callosum sulcus bypasses the posterior part of the corpus callosum, moving forward is the hippocampal sulcus (海马沟). There is an arc-shaped calcarine sulcus (距状沟) below the posterior part of the corpus callosum, which runs backward to the posterior part of the occipital lobe. The middle part of this sulcus is connected with the parietooccipital sulcus (顶枕沟). Between the calcarine sulcus and the parietoocci-pital sulcus is called the cuneus (楔叶), and below the calcarine sulcus is the lingual gyrus (舌回).

(3) The basal surface

There is a longitudinal olfactory tract (嗅束) on the medial side of the frontal lobe. Its front end is expanded into the olfactory bulb (嗅球), connected with the olfactory nerve, and its rear end is expanded into the olfactory trigone (嗅三角). The area between the olfactory triangle and the optic tract is called the anterior perforated substance (前穿质). There are many small blood vessels penetrating into the cerebral parenchyma (Fig.9-24). Under the temporal lobe, there is an occipitotemporal sulcus (枕颞沟) parallel to the lower edge of the hemisphere. The shallow groove parallel to the medial side of this sulcus is the collateral sulcus (侧副沟). The medial side of the collateral sulcus is the parahippocampal gyrus (海马旁回) (also known as the hippocampal gyrus), and the anterior curved hook end of the parahippocampal gyrus is called the uncus (钩). The medial side of the parahippo-campal gyrus is the hippocampal sulcus, and the upper part of the sulcus is a serrated narrow strip of cortex called dentate gyrus (齿状回). On the lateral side of the dentate gyrus, there is an arched hippocampus (海马) on the bottom wall of the inferior horn of the lateral ventricle. The hippocampus and dentate gyrus form the hippocampal formation (海马结构, Fig.9-25).

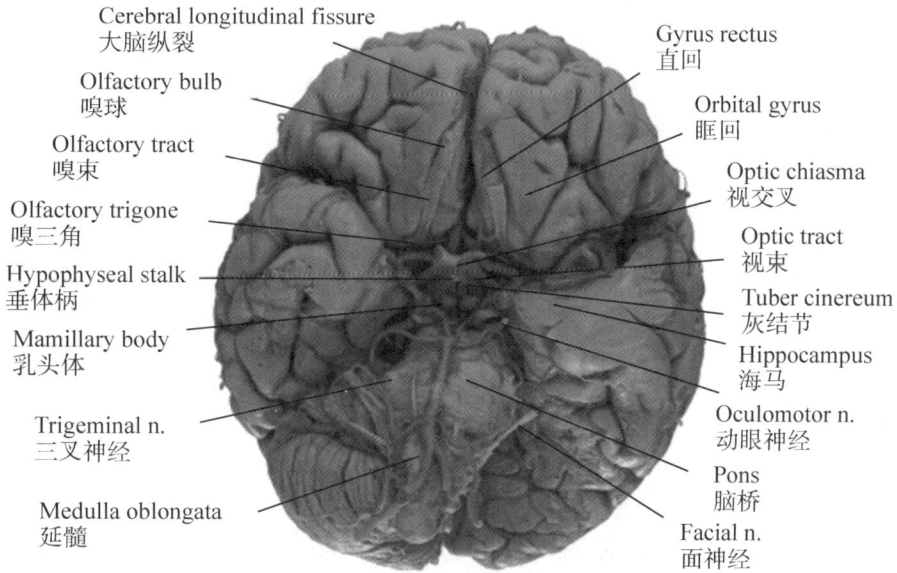

Cerebral longitudinal fissure
大脑纵裂

Olfactory bulb
嗅球

Olfactory tract
嗅束

Olfactory trigone
嗅三角

Hypophyseal stalk
垂体柄

Mamillary body
乳头体

Trigeminal n.
三叉神经

Medulla oblongata
延髓

Gyrus rectus
直回

Orbital gyrus
眶回

Optic chiasma
视交叉

Optic tract
视束

Tuber cinereum
灰结节

Hippocampus
海马

Oculomotor n.
动眼神经

Pons
脑桥

Facial n.
面神经

Fig.9-24　Basal surface of the brain

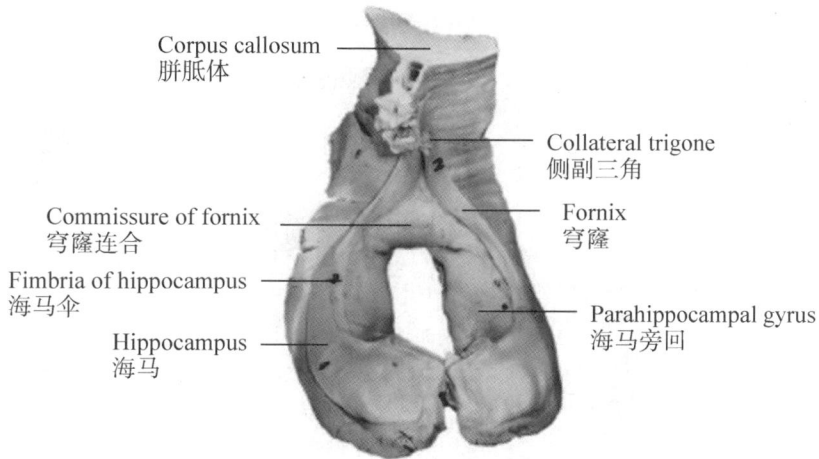

Corpus callosum
胼胝体

Collateral trigone
侧副三角

Commissure of fornix
穹窿连合

Fornix
穹窿

Fimbria of hippocampus
海马伞

Hippocampus
海马

Parahippocampal gyrus
海马旁回

Fig.9-25　Hippocampal formation

On the medial surface of the hemisphere, a circle of arc-shaped structures can be seen around the corpus callosum and the bottom wall of the lower horn of the lateral ventricle, including the septal area (the inferior area of the corpus callosum and the paralamina terminalis gyrus), the cingulate gyrus, the parahippocampal gyrus, the hippocampus and the dentate gyrus, etc., which belong to the original and old cortex in evolution. The above structures, together with the anterior part of the insula and the temporal pole, are collectively called the limbic lobe (边缘叶).

In terms of function, frontal lobe is related to somatic movement, language and advanced thinking activities. The parietal lobe is related to somatic feeling, taste and language. Occipital lobe is related to visual information integration. The temporal lobe is related to hearing, language, learning and memory. The insula is related to visceral sensation. The limbic lobe is related to emotion, behavior and visceral activity.

2. Internal Structure of Telencephalon

The gray matter on the surface of the cerebral hemisphere is called the cerebral cortex, while the white matter on the deep side is called the medulla, and several gray matter masses in the white matter are the basal nuclei. The ventricular cavity in the hemisphere is the lateral ventricle.

(1) Lateral ventricles

There are two lateral ventricles (侧脑室) on the left and the right respectively, containing cerebrospinal fluid, and extend to each lobe of the hemisphere in a "C" shape. The lateral ventricles (Fig.9-26) span the cerebrum, including the occipital, frontal and parietal lobes. It has a body or central part and three extensions, namely the anterior, posterior and inferior horns. The lateral ventricle (Fig.9-27) is connected with the third ventricle through the interventricular foramen (室间孔). There is choroid plexus of lateral ventricle in the central part and inferior horn, producing cerebrospinal fluid.

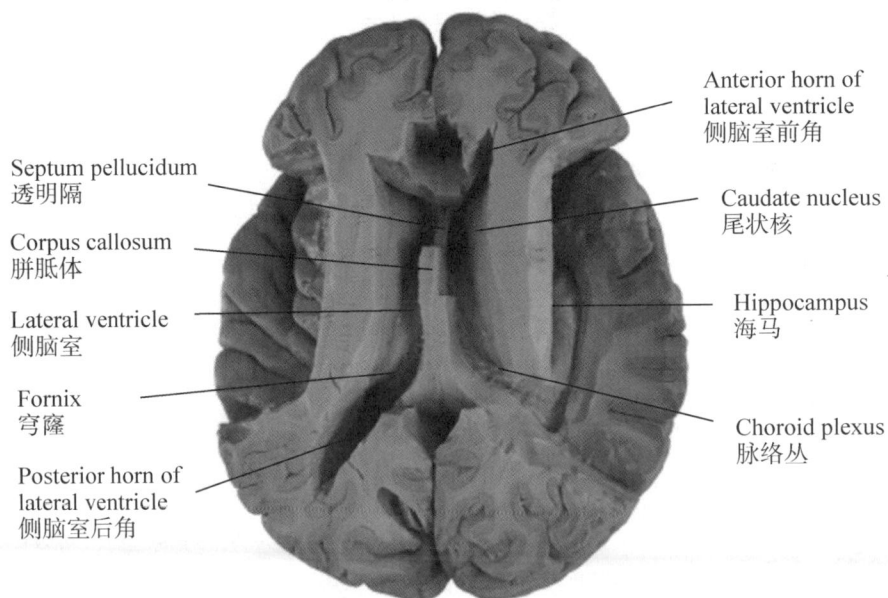

Fig.9-26   Lateral ventricles

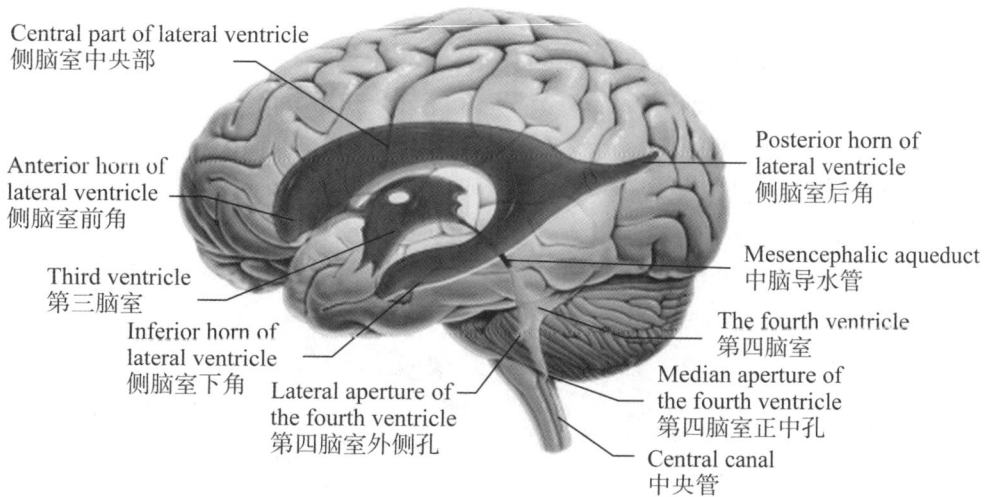

Central part of lateral ventricle
侧脑室中央部

Posterior horn of
lateral ventricle
侧脑室后角

Anterior horn of
lateral ventricle
侧脑室前角

Mesencephalic aqueduct
中脑导水管

Third ventricle
第三脑室

The fourth ventricle
第四脑室

Inferior horn of
lateral ventricle
侧脑室下角

Median aperture of
the fourth ventricle
第四脑室正中孔

Lateral aperture of
the fourth ventricle
第四脑室外侧孔

Central canal
中央管

Fig.9-27   Projection of lateral ventricle

(2) Basal nuclei

The basal nuclei include the corpus striatum, claustrum and amygdaloid body.

1) The corpus striatum (纹状体) includes caudate nucleus and lentiform nucleus. The two nuclei at the front end are connected with each other by gray matter bands, and this appearance is striatum, so it is called corpus striatum. The caudate nucleus (尾状核) is located on the lateral side of the dorsal thalamus, and is "C" shaped around the lentiform nucleus and the dorsal thalamus. The lentiform nucleus (豆状核) is located in the lateral part of the dorsal thalamus and the deep part of the insula. In the horizontal section, the nucleus is a wedge-shaped shape from the tip to the medial side, and is divided into three parts by two white matter plates: the outer part is called putamen (壳), and the inner two parts are collectively referred to as the globus pallidus (苍白球). In phylogeny, the caudate nucleus and putamen belong to the neostriatum (新纹状体), and the globus pallidus is a relatively old part, called the paleostriatum (旧纹状体). The striatum is an important part of the extrapyramidal system and a major regulatory center of somatic movement.

2) The claustrum (屏状核) is the thin layer of gray matter between the insula and lentiform nucleus, the thin layer of white matter between the claustrum and the putamen is the external capsule (外囊), and the white matter between the claustrum and the insula is the extreme capsule (最外囊). The function of the claustrum is unknown.

3) The amygdaloid body (杏仁体), located in the deep side of the parahippocampal gyrus uncus and connected with the caudate nucleus, is a component of the limbic system, and is related to the regulation of emotion, endocrine and visceral activities.

3. Cerebral Cortex

The cerebral cortex (大脑皮质) is the most advanced center of the nervous system. According to phylogeny, the cerebral cortex can be divided into the protocortex (hippocampus and dentate gyrus), old cortex (olfactory cortex) and most of the rest of the neocortex. Scholars divide the whole cerebral cortex into several areas according to the cellular architecture of the cortex and the distribution of nerve fibers. The more commonly used method is the Brodmann partition method (布罗德曼分区法), which divides the cerebral cortex into 52 regions (Fig.9-28).

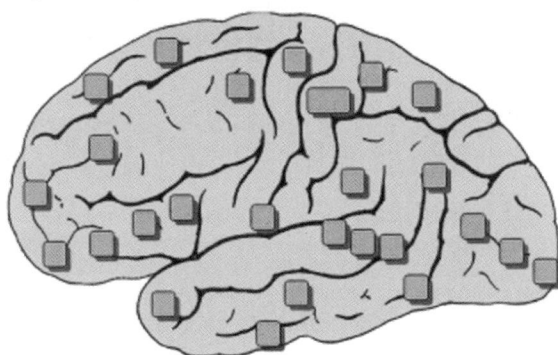

Fig.9-28　The cerebral cortex (lateral surface)

(1) Functional orientation of the cerebral cortex

Different areas of the cerebral cortex have different main functions. These cerebral areas with certain functions are called "centers". However, these centers are only the core parts that perform certain functions, and their adjacent cortex may also have similar functions. For example, the precentral gyrus is mainly responsible for the voluntary movement of the skeletal muscles of the whole body, but also receives some sensory information. The postcentral gyrus is somatosensory, but stimulation of it can also trigger a small amount of movement. Therefore, the functional orientation of the cerebral cortex is relative. When a certain center is damaged, other relevant cerebral regions can produce certain compensation. In addition, most areas of the cerebral cortex are not limited to certain functions, but process and integrate all kinds of information to complete higher-level neuropsychiatric activities, called the contact area (联络区).

1) The first somatic movement area (第一躯体运动区). This area is located in the precentral gyrus and the anterior paracentral lobule (areas 4 and 6)(Fig.9-29). This area manages the contraction of skeletal muscles in all parts of the body as follows. i) Upside down: feet up, head down, but head and face upright, that is, the uppermost part of the precentral gyrus and the anterior paracentral lobule are related to the lower limb movement; The middle part is related to the movement of the trunk and the upper limbs.

The lower part is related to the movement of face, tongue, pharynx and larynx. ii) Left and right crossing: One side of the motor area controls the movement of the opposite limb, but some muscles related to joint movement are controlled by the bilateral motor area, such as the upper facial muscles, masticatory muscles, respiratory muscles, trunk and perineum muscles. iii) Projection area just with functional complexity but without its size of the body: This area receives fibers from the postcentral gyrus, ventral anterior nucleus of the dorsal thalamus, ventrolateral nucleus and ventral posterior nucleus. It sends out fibers to form pyramidal tracts to the brainstem somatic motor nucleus and the anterior horn of the spinal cord to control the voluntary movement of skeletal muscles.

2) The first somatosensory area (第一躯体感觉区). This area is located in the postcentral gyrus and the posterior part of the paracentral lobule (areas 3, 1 and 2)(Fig.9-30), receiving the opposite half of the somatic pain, temperature, touch, pressure, position and motion information from the ventroposterior nucleus of the dorsal thalamus. The projection of body parts in this area is similar to that of the first somatic movement area. i) Upside down: The head is upright; ii) left and right crossing; iii) projection area just with sensitivity of the sense but without its size of the body.

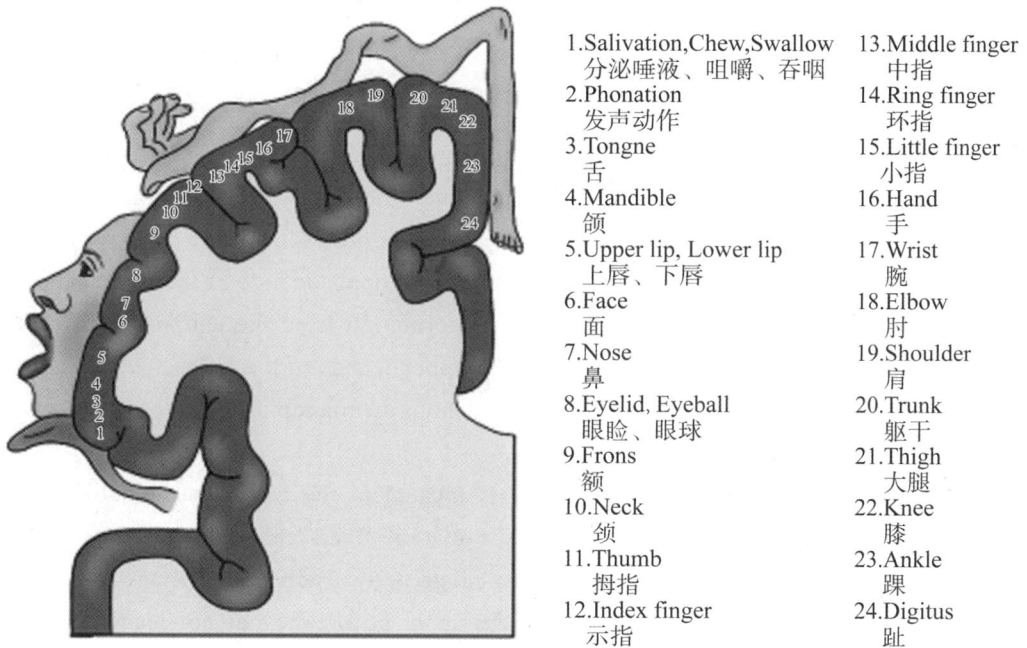

1.Salivation,Chew,Swallow	13.Middle finger
分泌唾液、咀嚼、吞咽	中指
2.Phonation	14.Ring finger
发声动作	环指
3.Tongne	15.Little finger
舌	小指
4.Mandible	16.Hand
颌	手
5.Upper lip, Lower lip	17.Wrist
上唇、下唇	腕
6.Face	18.Elbow
面	肘
7.Nose	19.Shoulder
鼻	肩
8.Eyelid, Eyeball	20.Trunk
眼睑、眼球	躯干
9.Frons	21.Thigh
额	大腿
10.Neck	22.Knee
颈	膝
11.Thumb	23.Ankle
拇指	踝
12.Index finger	24.Digitus
示指	趾

Fig.9-29　Positioning of human parts in the first somatic movement area

1.Abdominal organs 腹内器官	15.Hand 手
2.Pharynx 咽	16.Wrist 腕
3.Tongue 舌	17.Forearm 前臂
4.Gingiva, Mandible 牙龈、颌	18.Elbow 肘
5.Lower lip 下唇	19.Upper arm 上臂
6.Upper lip 上唇	20.Shoulder 肩
7.Face 面	21.Neck 颈
8.Nose 鼻	22.Head 头
9.Eye 眼	23.Trunk 躯干
10.Thumb 拇指	24.Thigh 大腿
11.Index finger 示指	25.Leg 小腿
12.Middle finger 中指	26.Foot 足
13.Ring finger 环指	27.Digitus 趾
14.Little finger 小指	28.Genital organ 生殖器

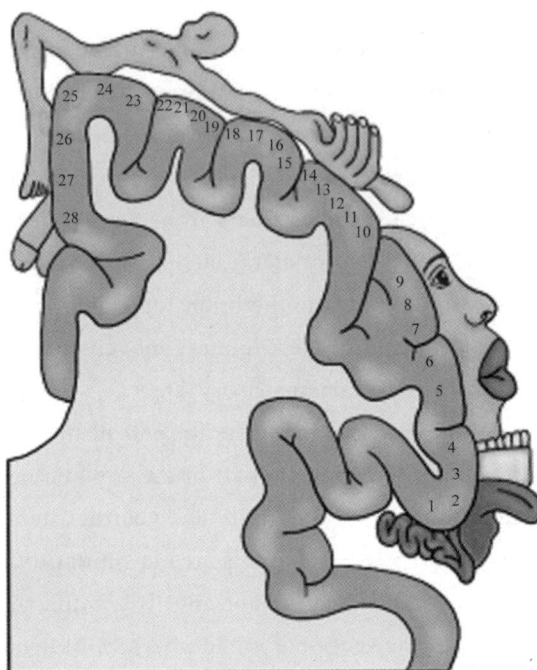

Fig.9-30　Location of human parts in the first somatosensory area

3) Visual area (视觉区). This area is located in the cortex on both sides of the calcarine sulcus on the medial surface of the occipital lobe (area 17), receiving the optical radiation fiber from the lateral geniculate body. Because the axons of the optic nerve from the nasal half of the retinal ganglion cells cross to the opposite side at the optic chiasma, one side of the visual area receives the visual information from the temporal half on the same side of the retina and the nasal half on the opposite side of the retina. The damage of one side of the visual area can lead to homonymous hemianopia of the opposite visual field of both eyes.

4) Auditory area (听觉区). This area is located in the transverse temporal gyrus (areas 41 and 42). It receives the auditory radiation fibers that transmit the auditory information of both ears from the medial geniculate body. Therefore, damage to one side of the hearing area can cause hearing decreasing in both ears, but not leading to total deafness.

5) Balance perception area (平衡觉区). This area is located near the head and face representative area at the lower part of the postcentral gyrus.

6) Taste area (味觉区). This area may be located nearby the insula below the postcentral gyrus.

7) Olfactory area (嗅觉区). This area is located near the parahippocampal gyrus hook.

8) Language center (语言中枢). Higher neural functional activities such as thinking, consciousness and language conducted by this area are unique to human cerebral cortcx. Therefore, there is the language center in human cerebral cortex (Fig.9-31). The language center usually develops in one hemisphere. For most people, the language center is located in the left hemisphere. Only a few people who are good at using the left hand (left-handed) have their language center in the right hemisphere. The language center includes four areas: speaking, listening, writing and reading.

Motor language center (*speech center*) (运动性语言中枢、说话中枢) is located in the posterior part of the inferior frontal gyrus (areas 44 and 45), also known as Broca area. If this area is damaged, although the patients' vocal organs are not paralyzed, they can also make sounds, but cannot speak continuous words and sentences, which is called motor aphasia (运动性失语症).

Writing center (书写中枢) is located at the posterior part of the middle frontal gyrus (area 8), the upper limb near the precentral gyrus, especially the representative area of the hand. If the area is damaged, although there is no obstacle to the movement of the hand, the patients are unable to write the correct words, which is called agraphia (失写症).

Auditory language center (*auditory speech area*) (听觉性语言中枢, 听话中枢) is located in the posterior part of the superior temporal gyrus (area 22), which can adjust its own language, listen to and understand others' language. If this area is damaged, although the patients' hearing is normal and can hear others' speech, they couldn't understand the

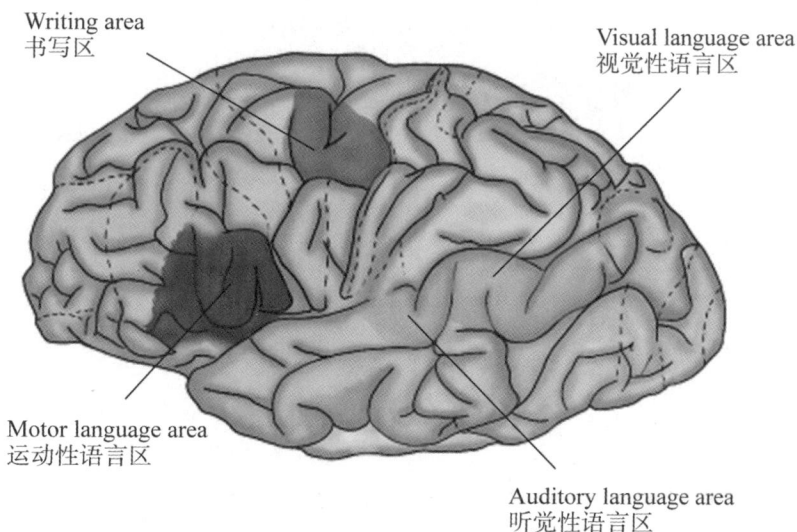

Fig.9-31　Language center

meaning of others' speech, and their speech would be often confused without self-knowledge, so they can't answer questions correctly and speak normally, which is called sensory aphasia (感觉性失语症).

Visual language center (*reading center*) (视觉性语言中枢, 阅读中枢) is located in angular gyrus (area 39), close to the visual center. If the area is damaged, the patients would have no visual impairment, they cannot understand the meaning of the text symbols, which is called dyslexia (失读症).

In addition, the language centers do not exist in isolation from each other. They are closely related. Language ability can only be achieved through the coordination of relevant regions of the cerebral cortex.

The functions of human's left and right hemispheres are basically the same, but because of long-term evolution and development, the functions of the left and right hemispheres are asymmetric. The left hemisphere is closely related to language, consciousness and mathematical analysis. The right hemisphere mainly perceives nonverbal information, music, graphics and space-time concepts. Therefore, the left and right hemispheres have their own advantages, and the coordination and cooperation between the two hemispheres can complete various high-level neuropsychiatric activities.

(4)**Medulla of the cerebral hemisphere.** It is composed of a large number of nerve fibers, which can be divided into the following three categories: the fibers connecting in the same hemisphere, between the left and right hemisphere, between the cerebral cortex and subcortical centers (Fig.9-32).

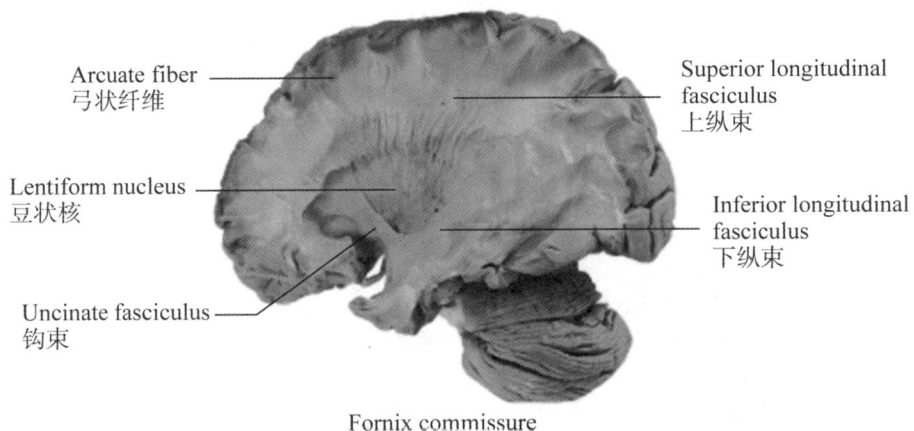

Arcuate fiber 弓状纤维

Superior longitudinal fasciculus 上纵束

Lentiform nucleus 豆状核

Inferior longitudinal fasciculus 下纵束

Uncinate fasciculus 钩束

Fornix commissure

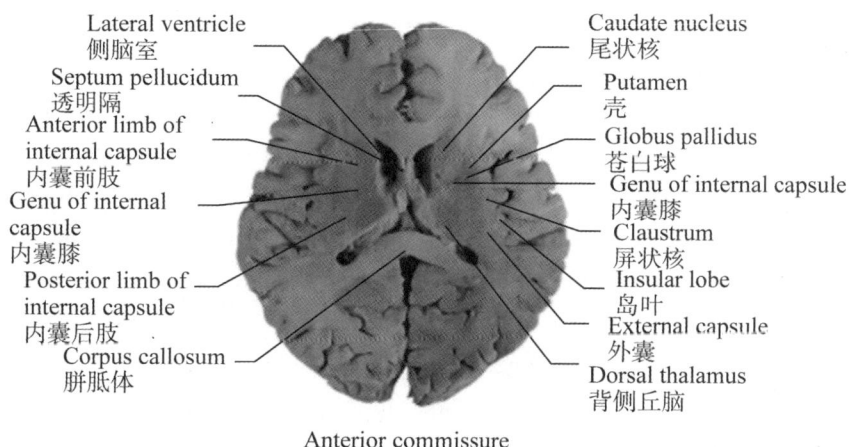

Lateral ventricle
侧脑室
Septum pellucidum
透明隔
Anterior limb of
internal capsule
内囊前肢
Genu of internal
capsule
内囊膝
Posterior limb of
internal capsule
内囊后肢
Corpus callosum
胼胝体

Caudate nucleus
尾状核
Putamen
壳
Globus pallidus
苍白球
Genu of internal capsule
内囊膝
Claustrum
屏状核
Insular lobe
岛叶
External capsule
外囊
Dorsal thalamus
背侧丘脑

Anterior commissure

Fig.9-32　The corpus callosum, anterior commissure and fornix commissure

1) Association fibers (联络纤维). Association fibers refer to the fibers connecting the different gyrus in the same hemisphere, and the short fiber connecting the adjacent gyrus is called arcuate fiber. Long fibers connect the lobes of the ipsilateral cerebral hemisphere, and the main areas as follows: i) the hook tract connecting the front of the frontal and temporal lobes; ii)the superior longitudinal tract, connecting frontal, parietal, occipital and temporal lobes; iii)the inferior longitudinal tract, connecting occipital and temporal lobes; iv)the cingulate, located in the deep part of the cingulate gyrus and the parahippocampal gyrus, connecting the various parts of the limbic lobe.

2) Commissural fibers (连合纤维). Commissural fibers refer to the fibers connecting the left and right hemispheric cortex, including the corpus callosum, the anterior commissure and the fornix commissure.

Corpus callosum (胼胝体). Located at the bottom of the longitudinal cerebral fissure, it is the largest connective fiber, connecting the corresponding parts of the cortex of the two hemispheres of the brain. It is arcuate on the midsagittal plane of the brain. The corpus callosum is divided into four parts: rostrum, genu, body/trunk, and splenium.

Anterior commissure (前连合). It is close to the rear of the lamina terminalis and the front of the column of fornix, connecting the left and right olfactory bulbs and temporal lobes.

Fornix and fornical commissure (穹隆和穹隆连合). The fornix is an arc-shaped fiber tract from the hippocampus to the hypothalamic papillary body, which is close to the lower part of the corpus callosum. A part of the fibers reach the contralateral side and connect the contralateral hippocampus, which is called fornix commissure, and connect each part of the limbic lobe.

3) Projection fibers(投 射 纤 维). They are upstream and downstream fibers that

connect the cerebral cortex and subcortical centers. Most of these fibers pass through the internal capsule.

Internal capsule (内囊). It is a broad and thick white matter located between the caudate nucleus, dorsal thalamus and lenticular nucleus(Fig. 9-33). On the horizontal section of the telencephalon, the internal capsule is in the shape of " > < " from the tip to the inside, and can divides into three parts: i) Anterior limb of internal capsule (内囊前肢) is located between the lentiform nucleus and the caudate nucleus, with the frontopontine tract and anterior thalamic radiation passing through; ii) The posterior limb of internal capsule (内囊后肢) is located between the lenticular nucleus and the dorsal thalamus, with the corticospinal tract, the corticorube tract, the thalamic central radiation, the parietooccipitopontine and temporopontine tract, the visual radiation and the auditory radiation passing through; iii) genu of the internal capsule (内囊膝) is located at the junction of the anterior and posterior limbs of the internal capsule, and there is corticonuclear tract passing through.

When the internal capsule is injured, the patient may suffer from superficial and deep sensory loss of the contralateral half of the body (damage to the thalamic central radiation), spastic paralysis of the contralateral half of the body (damage to the corticospinal tract and the corticonuclear tract), nasal hemianopia of the injured side of the field of vision and temporal hemianopia of the healthy side of the field of vision (damage to the visual radiation), which is the so-called "trisection syndrome"(三偏征).

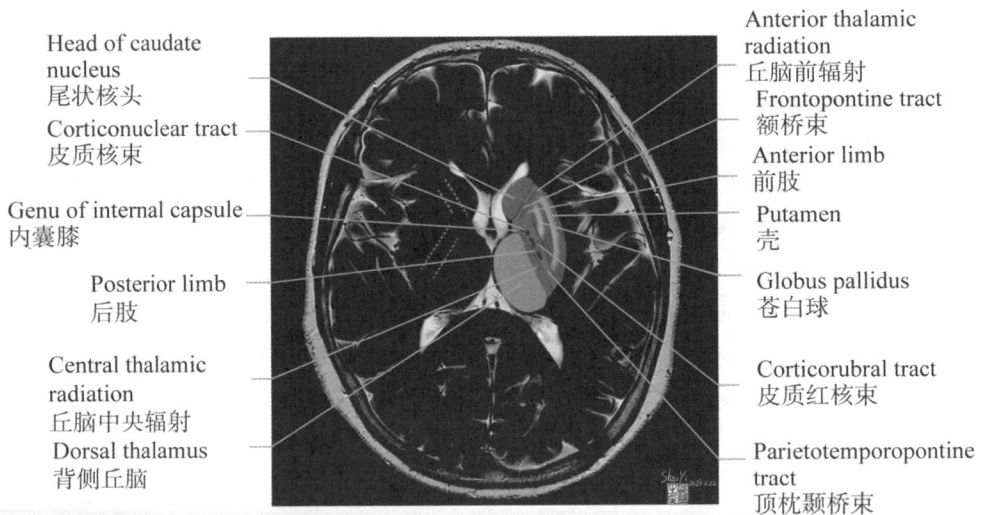

Fig.9-33   Pattern of the inner capsule

4. Limbic System

The limbic system (边缘系统) is composed of the limbic lobe and other related cortical and subcortical structures, such as amygdala, hypothalamus, suprathalamus, anterior nucleus of the dorsal thalamic and mesencephalic tegmentum (Fig. 9-34). The system is an ancient part of the brain in evolution, closely related to the regulation of olfactory and visceral activities, emotional response and sexual activities, and also related to individual survival functions (such as foraging, defense, attack, etc.) and lineage continuation. The hippocampus is also related to learning and memory functions.

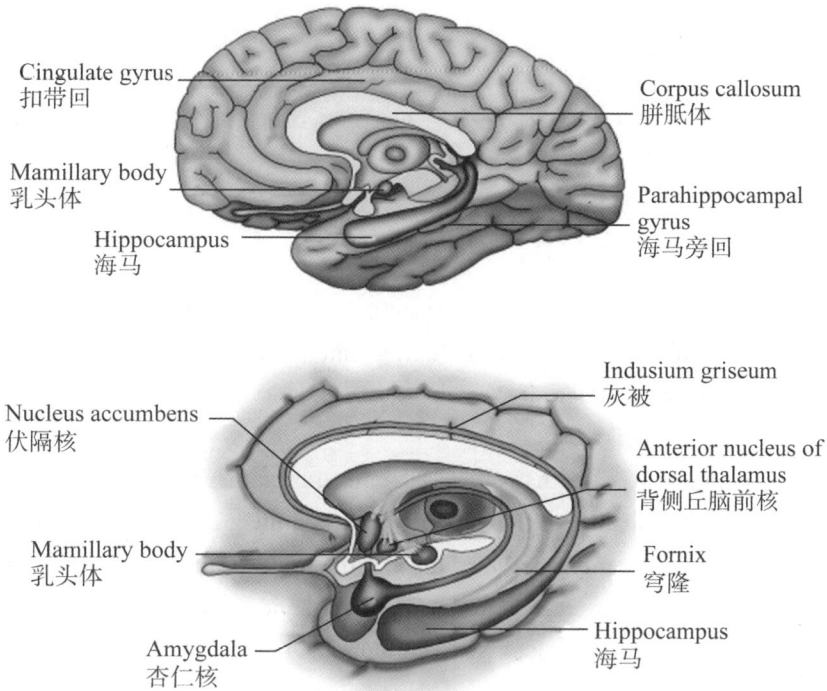

Fig.9-34   Illustration of the rhinencephalon and limbic system

Exercise

1. A 77-year-old man had been lying in bed for half a year due to a fracture. He is now doing rehabilitation exercises; however, he presented an unsteady gait, slow and slurred speech, and inaccurate sight. Neurologic examination revealed hypotonia and intention tremor. It suggested that this patient's injury is in the brain. Which of the following structure does this damage?

(A) Medulla oblongata.

(B) Pons.

(C) Cerebellum.

(D) Midbrain.

(E) Diencephalon.

2. Two chefs were fighting in the kitchen. One of them was stabbed with an ice pick which passed through the superior orbital fissure. Which of the following was most likely to be severed as the ice pick passed through this fissure?

(A) The abducens nerve.

(B) The facial nerve.

(C) The mandibular nerve.

(D) The maxillary nerve.

(E) The optic nerve.

Answer

1. The correct answer is C.

It is obviously that the patient has a cerebellar lesion. Cerebellar dysfunction can lead to a variety of motor dysfunction, including intention tremor, dysdiado-chokinesia, dysmetria, hypotonia and nystagmus.

2. The correct answer is A.

The abducent nerve (Choice A) is the sixth pair of brain nerves, belonging to the motor nerve. It exits brain on both sides of the midline of the pontine groove, enters the orbit through the superior orbital fissure, and innervates the external rectus muscle of the eye. When this nerve is damaged, the affected eye cannot turn outward and the esotropia occurs.

The facial nerve (Choice B) passes through the internal auditory meatus, and the mandibular nerve (Choice C) passes through the foreman rotundum, while the maxillary nerve (Choice D) passes through the foreman spinosum, and the optic nerve (Choice E) passes through the optic canal.

（温州医科大学　崔怀瑞）

Chapter 10   Peripheral Nervous System

The peripheral nervous system refers to all the nervous structures and tissues distributed throughout the body that are structurally connected to the spinal cord and the brain of the central nervous system, including the ganglia, nerve plexuses, and nerve terminal devices. It is generally divided into spinal nerves and cranial nerves according to the characteristics of its connection with the spinal cord and the brain. The former refers to the 31 pairs of nerves connected to the spinal cord; the latter refers to the 12 pairs of nerves connected to the brain.

Different fiber components in peripheral nerves are distributed in different parts of the body. Some nerve fibers are distributed in the skeletal muscles, and skin of the whole body, while some fibers are distributed in the smooth muscles, cardiac muscles and glandular tissues. Therefore, it can be divided into two parts: somatic nerves and visceral nerves. Both spinal nerves and cranial nerves contain somatic nerve fibers and visceral nerve fibers.

Functionally, peripheral nerves are composed of two parts: sensory nerves conducting sensory signals and motor nerves conducting motorial signals. Sensory nerves conduct nerve impulses from the peripheral receptors to the central nervous system, also known as afferent nerves; motor nerves transmit nerve impulses from the central nervous system to the peripheral effectors, also known as efferent nerves. Furthermore, the visceral motor nerve can be divided into two parts: the sympathetic nerve and the parasympathetic nerve.

10.1   Spinal Nerve

10.1.1   Introduction

The spinal nerves are the peripheral nerves connected to the spinal cord, and there are 31 pairs in total. Each pair of spinal nerves connects to a segment of the spinal cord, consisting of an anterior root and a posterior root. The anterior root is composed of motor nerve root filaments. The posterior root is composed of sensory nerve root filaments. The anterior and posterior roots meet at the intervertebral foramen to form the spinal nerve, so the spinal nerve is a mixed nerve that contains both sensory and motor fibers.

According to the connection between the spinal nerve and the spinal cord, it is divided into five parts: Eight pairs of cervical nerves, 12 pairs of thoracic nerves, five pairs of lumbar nerves, five pairs of sacral nerves and one pair of coccygeal nerves. Thus, there are 31 pairs of spinal nerves in total.

Spinal nerves are mixed nerves, composed of somatic nerve fibers and visceral nerve fibers, and both somatic nerves and visceral nerves contain motor fibers and sensory fibers. Therefore, spinal nerves contain four fiber components (Fig.10-1).

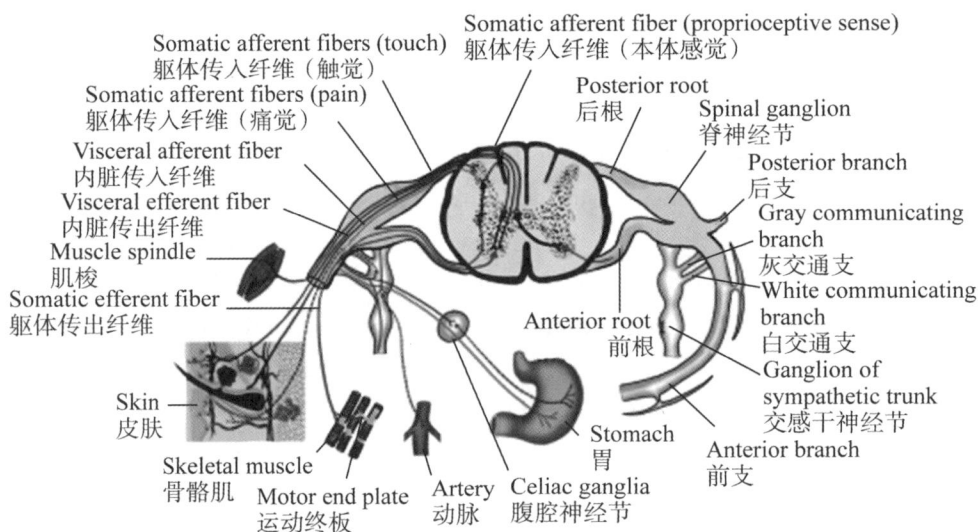

Fig.10-1　Diagram showing the constitution and distribution of the spinal nerves

1. Somatic Sensory (Afferent) Fibers

Somatic sensory (afferent) fibers［SS/SA, 躯体感觉(传入)纤维］come from the pseudounipolar neurons in the spinal ganglion. The central processes of these neurons form the posterior root of the spinal nerve and enter the spinal cord; and the peripheral processes of these neurons form the spinal nerves that distribute in the skin, skeletal muscles, tendons, joints and other body parts. They transmit exteroceptive (pain, temperature and touch) and proprioceptive (kinesis and position) sensory nervous impulses from the body to the spinal cord.

2. Somatic Motor (Efferent) Fibers

Somatic motor (efferent) fibers［SM/SE, 躯体运动(传出)纤维］are composed of the axons of motor neurons located in the anterior horn of the gray matter of the spinal cord, distributed in the skeletal muscles of the trunk and limbs, and control their voluntary movements. They transmit motor nervous impulses from the spinal cord to the skeletal muscles of trunk and limbs.

3. Visceral Sensory (Afferent) Fibers

Visceral sensory (afferent) fibers [VS/VA, 内脏感觉(传入)纤维] also come from the pseudounipolar neurons of the spinal ganglion. The central processes of these neurons form the posterior root and enter the spinal cord, and the peripheral processes of these neurons distribute in the viscera, cardiovascular and glands. They transmit interoceptive sensory nervous impulses from the viscera, cardiovascular and glands to the spinal cord.

4. Visceral Motor (Efferent) Fibers

Visceral motor (efferent) fibers [VM/ VE, 内脏运动(传出)纤维] originate from the intermediolateral nucleus (lower sympathetic nerve center) of T1—L3 segments of the spinal cord; and the sacral parasympathetic nucleus (lower parasympathetic nerve center) of the S2—S4 segments of the spinal cord. The axons of these neurons are distributed in the viscera, cardiovascular and glands, control the movement of the smooth muscle and the cardiac muscle, and the glands.

10.1.2   Branches of the Spinal Nerves

After the anterior root and posterior root of the spinal nerve merge into the spinal nerve trunk at the intervertebral foramen, they immediately divides into four branches: the anterior branch, posterior branch, communicating branch and meningeal branch.

1. Anterior Branch

The anterior branch, the thickest and largest branch of the spinal nerve trunk, is a mixed nerve branch and the widest distribution range, mainly distributed in the muscles and skin of the front and outside of the trunk, and limbs. In addition to the 12 pairs of thoracic nerves, the anterior branches of the remaining spinal nerves form a total of four nerve plexuses: cervical plexus, brachial plexus, lumbar plexus and sacral plexus. Nerve branches are sent from these plexuses to the body's effectors and receptors.

2. Posterior Branch

The posterior branch is a series of branches from the spinal nerves that travel to the back of the trunk and distribute in the nape, back and lumbosacral region, and are also mixed nerve branches. The posterior branch of the first cervical nerve, also known as the suboccipital nerve, passes between the upper part of the posterior arch of the atlas and the lower part of the vertebral artery, innervating the vertebral occipital muscles. The cutaneous branch of the posterior branch of the second cervical nerve is called the greater occipital nerve, which passes through the trapezius tendon to reach the subcutaneous, and distributes in the occipital and nuchal skin. The medial branch of the posterior branch of the third cervical nerve is called the third occipital nerve, which also passes through the trapezius muscle to subcutaneous, and distributes in the skin below the occipital. The lateral branches of the posterior branches of the first to the third lumbar nerves are thick and distributed in the skin of the upper buttocks, called the superior clunial cutaneous nerves. The cutaneous branches of the posterior branches of the first to the third sacral nerves are distributed in the middle gluteal region and are called the middle clunial nerves.

3. Communicating Branch

The communicating branch belongs to the structure of the sympathetic nervous system, and is a thin branch connected between the spinal nerve and the sympathetic trunk. It can be divided into two categories: The white communicating branch enters the sympathetic trunk from the spinal nerve, and its fiber components belong to visceral motor fibers, which are preganglionic nerve fibers originating from the lateral horn of the gray matter of the spinal cord; the gray communicating branches are unmyelinated nerve fibers originating from the sympathetic trunk, composed of postganglionic fibers originating from the ganglia of sympathetic trunk.

4. Meningeal Branch

The meningeal branch is a thin branch that returns to the spinal canal after the spinal nerve exits the intervertebral foramen. After the branch returns to the spinal canal, it distributes in the spinal dura mater, blood vessel wall, periosteum, ligaments and intervertebral discs.

10.1.3   Spinal Nerve Plexus

The nerve fibers supplying the neck and limbs are from the anterior rami, which have been redistributed within a network of nerves, called the nerve plexus. The anterior rami of the upper cervical spinal nerves (C1—C4) form the cervical plexus (supplies the anterior neck). The lower cervical and first thoracic anterior rami (C5—C8 & T1) form the brachial plexus (supplies upper limb). The lower lumbar and upper sacral anterior rami form the lumbar plexus (L1—L4) and sacral plexus (L4—L5 & S1—S4, supplies lower limb). The thoracic anterior rami remain segmental becoming the intercostal nerves in the intercostal spaces (Fig.10-2).

1. Cervical Plexus

(1) Formation and position of the cervical plexus

It is formed by interweaving anterior branches of the first to fourth cervical nerves. This plexus is located deep to the upper part of the sternocleidomastoid.

(2) Branches and distribution of the cervical plexus

The branches of the cervical plexus are divided into three categories: the cutaneous branches distributed in the skin; the muscular branches to deep muscles; the communicating branches descending from the superior cervical ganglion (which is the largest of the three cervical ganglia) (Figs.10-3 & 10-4).

The cutaneous branches of the cervical plexus emerge superficially near the midpoint of the posterior edge of the sternocleidomastoid, the important block point for infiltration anesthesia of the superficial structure of the neck, so it is also called the nerve point in clinical practice. The main branches of the cervical plexus are as follows. It mainly consists of the four cutaneous branches and one muscular branch. i) The lesser occipital nerve (C2)(枕小神经) ascends along the posterior edge of the sternocleidomastoid, and distributes in the skin of occipital and upper back of the auricle. ii) The great auricular nerve (C2－C3)(耳大神经) goes upward along the surface of the sternocleidomastoid toward the earlobe, and distributes in the auricle and nearby skin. iii)The transverse nerve of neck (C2－C3)(颈横神经) is sent out and traverses across the surface of sternocleidomastoid and runs forward, distributes in the skin of the front of neck. iv) The supraclavicular nerves (C3－C4) (锁 骨 上 神 经) have 2－4

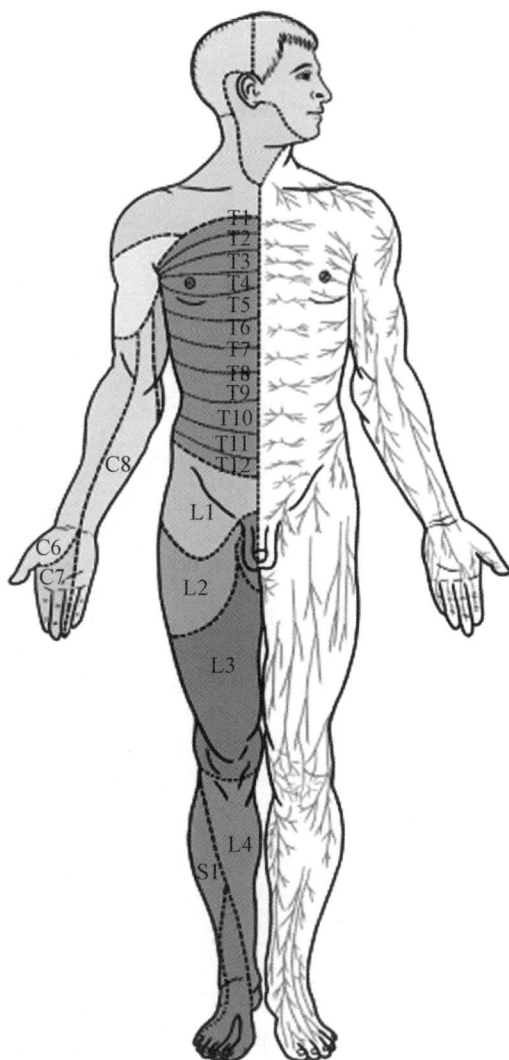

Fig.10-2 Segmental distribution of the spinal nerve

branches in total, which radiate downward and laterally, cross the clavicle and reach the upper part of the anterior chest wall and the shoulder. v) The phrenic nerve (C3－C5)(膈神经) first descends on the outer side of the upper end of the anterior scalene muscle, then enters the thoracic cavity between the subclavian artery and vein through the superior aperture of thorax. After entering the chest, it is accompanied by pericardiophrenic blood vessels, passes through the front of the lung root, and finally penetrates into the muscle fibers of the diaphragm near the central tendon. The motor fibers of phrenic nerve distribute in the diaphragm and control its movement. Hiccups occur when the phrenic nerve is stimulated. The sensory fibers of phrenic nerve distribute in the pleurae, pericardium and diaphragmatic peritoneum; usually the right one may be distributed in the liver, the gallbladder and the biliary system. Therefore, the diseases of the liver, the gallbladder and the biliary system may cause pain in the right shoulder. This situation is called referred pain.

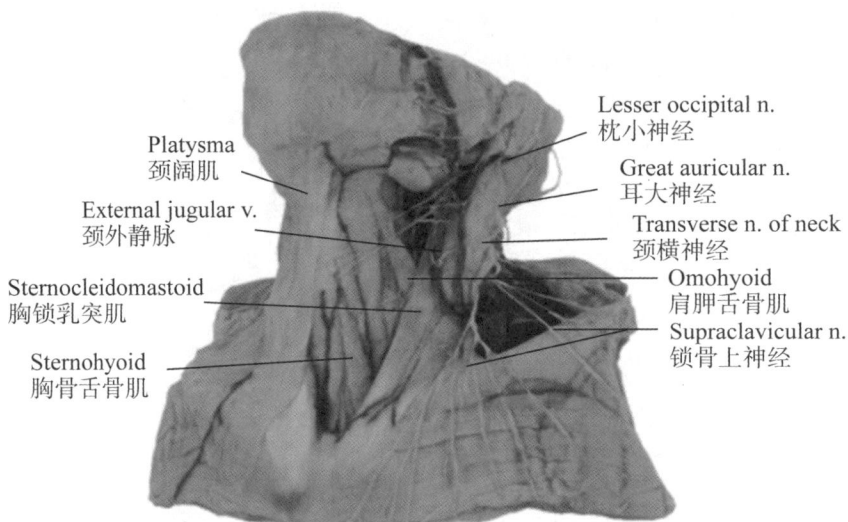

Fig.10-3　Distribution of the cutaneous branch of the cervical plexus

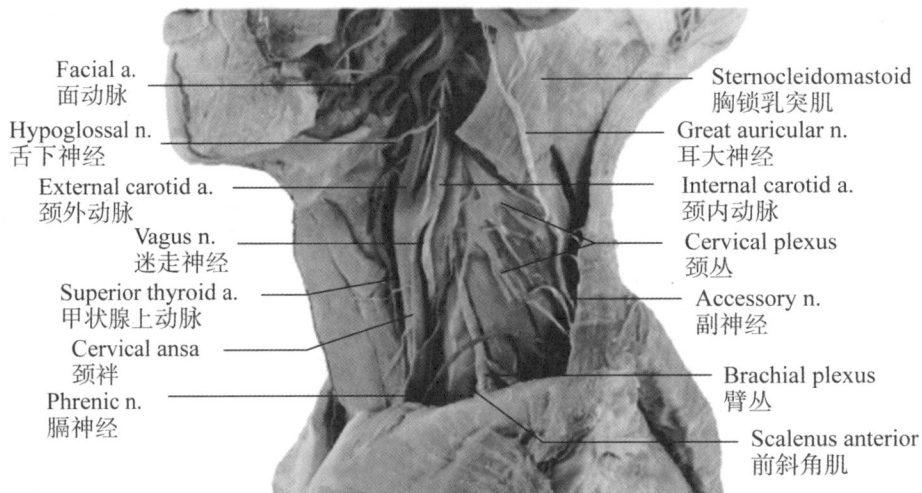

Fig.10-4　The nerves, muscles, and blood vessels of the neck

2. Brachial Plexus

(1) Formation and position of the brachial plexus

The brachial plexus is formed by the anterior branches of the fifth to the eighth cervical nerves and the great part of anterior branch of the first thoracic nerve. The main structures of this plexus first pass laterally through the scalene fissure, and then travel laterally and inferiorly behind the clavicle into the axillary cavity. The five roots (C5－C8 and T1) of brachial plexus merge into three trunks, namely, superior trunk, middle trunk and inferior trunk with anterior and posterior divisions. So there are six divisions in all. Finally, the divisions merge into cords of the brachial plexus (the posterior cord which is behind the axillary artery, the lateral cord which is lateral to the axillary artery, the medial cord) that give off the terminal branches of the brachial plexus. The branches of the brachial plexus are divided into supraclavicular branches and infraclavicular branches according to the origin of each branch above the clavicle or below the clavicle (Fig.10-5).

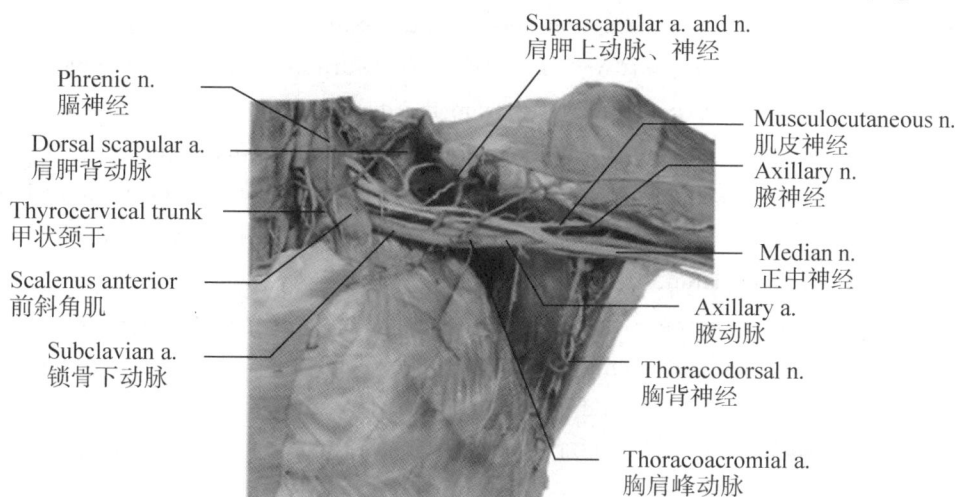

Fig.10-5   Brachial plexus

(2) The branches above the clavicle

The supraclavicular branches mostly belong to short stroke muscle branch, distributed in the deep neck muscles, superficial back muscles (except trapezius), some upper chest muscles and upper limb girdle muscles. Their main branches are as follows.

1) The long thoracic nerve (C5－C7) (胸长神经) descends along the lateral surface of the serratus anterior with the lateral thoracic artery / vein, distributed in the serratus anterior and the outer part of the breast. An injury to this nerve can lead to paralysis of the serratus anterior, with the sign of "winged shoulder" characterized by a raised medial border of the scapula.

2) The suprascapular nerve (C5－C6) (肩胛上神经) travels backward through the suprascapular notch into the supraspinous fossa, then turns around the lateral edge of the scapular spine together with the suprascapular artery / vein into the infra-spinous fossa, distributed in the supraspinatus, infraspinatus and shoulder joint.

3) The dorsal scapular nerve (C4—C5) (肩胛背神经) passes through the middle scalene muscle and crosses the levator scapulae posteriorly, descends between the scapula and the spine with the dorsal scapular artery/vein, and distributes to the rhomboid muscle and levator scapulae.

(3) The branches below the clavicle

The infraclavicular branches are widely distributed, including the muscles, joints and skin of the shoulder, thoracolumbar region, arm, forearm and hand. They can be divided into five short branches and six long branches according to their length.

1) Five short branches include the medial pectoral nerve, the lateral pectoral nerve, the thoracodorsal nerve, the subscapular nerve and the axillary nerve.

The medial pectoral nerve (C8—T1) (胸内侧神经) originates from the medial cord of the brachial plexus, enters and innervates from the deep surface in the pectoralis minor, some fibers pass through the muscle, and distributed to the pectoralis major.

The lateral pectoral nerve (C5—C7) (胸外侧神经) originates from the lateral cord of the brachial plexus, passes through the clavipectoral fascia, travels deep to the pectoralis major and distributes to it.

The thoracodorsal nerve (C6—C8) (胸背神经) originates from the posterior cord of the brachial plexus, descends along the lateral edge of the scapula with the subscapular and thoracodorsal blood vessels, and distributes to the latissimus dorsi.

The subscapular nerve (C5—C7) (肩胛下神经) originates from the posterior cord of the brachial plexus and is often divided into upper and lower branches, which control the movement of subscapularis and teres major respectively.

The axillary nerve (C5—C6) (腋神经)originates from the posterior cord of the brachial plexus, and is accompanied by the posterior humeral circumflex blood vessels in a posterior outward direction. After passing through the quadrangular foramen on the posterior wall of the axillary fossa, it goes around the surgical neck of the humerus to innervate the deltoid and teres minor. Fracture of the surgical neck of humerus may damage the axillary nerve and lead to paralysis of the deltoid muscle and the patient's shoulder also loses its rounded shape, which will be shown as "square shoulder" and with loss of sensation over the deltoid region.

2) Six long branches include the musculocutaneous nerve, median nerve, ulnar nerve, radial nerve, medial cutaneous nerve of the arm, and medial cutaneous nerve of the forearm (Fig.10-6).

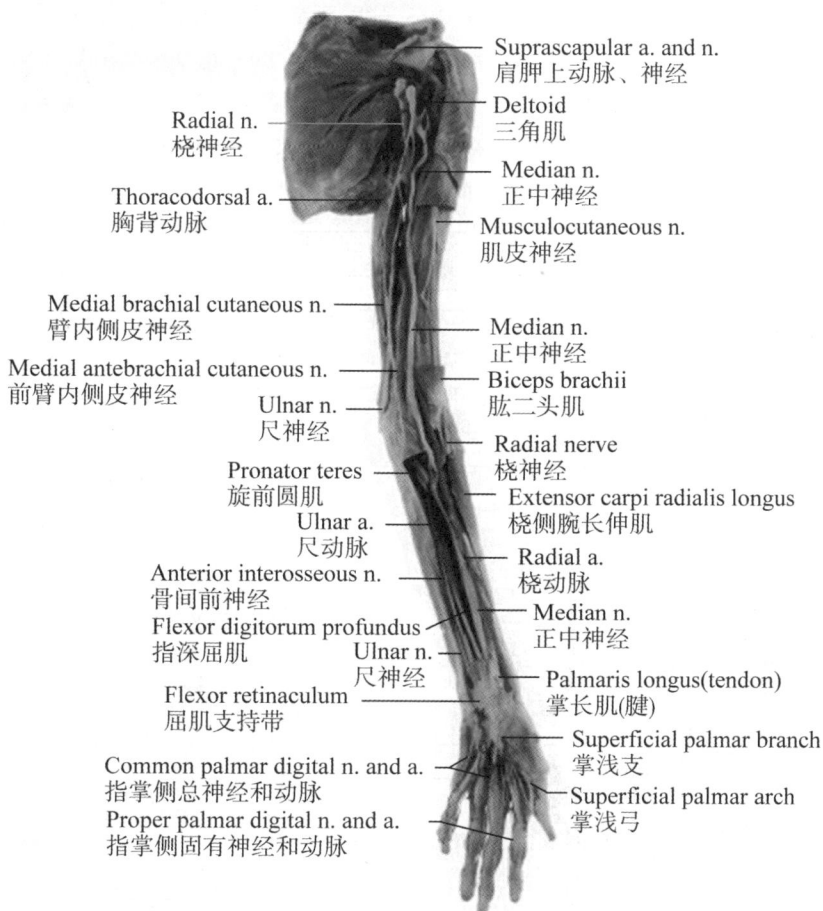

Suprascapular a. and n.
肩胛上动脉、神经

Deltoid
三角肌

Median n.
正中神经

Musculocutaneous n.
肌皮神经

Median n.
正中神经

Biceps brachii
肱二头肌

Radial nerve
桡神经

Extensor carpi radialis longus
桡侧腕长伸肌

Radial a.
桡动脉

Median n.
正中神经

Palmaris longus(tendon)
掌长肌(腱)

Superficial palmar branch
掌浅支

Superficial palmar arch
掌浅弓

Radial n.
桡神经

Thoracodorsal a.
胸背动脉

Medial brachial cutaneous n.
臂内侧皮神经

Medial antebrachial cutaneous n.
前臂内侧皮神经

Ulnar n.
尺神经

Pronator teres
旋前圆肌

Ulnar a.
尺动脉

Anterior interosseous n.
骨间前神经

Flexor digitorum profundus
指深屈肌

Ulnar n.
尺神经

Flexor retinaculum
屈肌支持带

Common palmar digital n. and a.
指掌侧总神经和动脉

Proper palmar digital n. and a.
指掌侧固有神经和动脉

Fig.10-6   Muscles, blood vessels and nerves of the anterior aspect of the upper limb

The musculocutaneous nerve (C5－C7) (肌皮神经). It originates from the lateral cord of the brachial plexus, and leaves the axilla by obliquely piercing through the coracobrachialis which it supplies, then descends between the biceps brachii and brachialis. gives off branches to supply the above three muscles (anterior group muscles of arm), pierces the deep fascia between the tendons of the biceps brachii and brachioradialis as lateral cutaneous nerve of the forearm, which distributes to the skin of the lateral side of the forearm.

The median nerve (C6－C8 & T1) (正中神经, Fig. 10-7). It originates from the medial and lateral cords of the brachial plexus, then goes down along the medial groove of the biceps brachii in the arm, and descends to the cubital fossa with the brachial artery/vein. From the cubital fossa, it goes down through the pronator teres, and continues downward between the flexor digitorum superficialis and flexor digitorum profundus in the middle of the forearm. At the wrist,the median nerve emerges from the lateral border of the flexor digitorum superficialis, and lies between the tendons of the flexor carpi radialis and palmaris longus. It finally enters the palm by passing through the carpal canal and deep to the palmar aponeurosis. The median nerve innervates all the anterior group muscles of forearm except the brachioradialis, flexor carpi ulnaris, and the ulnar half of the flexor digitorum profundus. In the palm the median nerve gives off a thick and short recurrent branch, and enters the thenar, innervating the thenar muscles except the adductor pollicis and the first and the second lumbrical muscles. The sensory fibers are distributed in the skin of the two-thirds of the radial side of palm, and three and a half fingers of the radial side of palmar aspect including middle and distal fingers on dorsum, but the distribution of the thumb is only the skin of the distal fingers on dorsum.

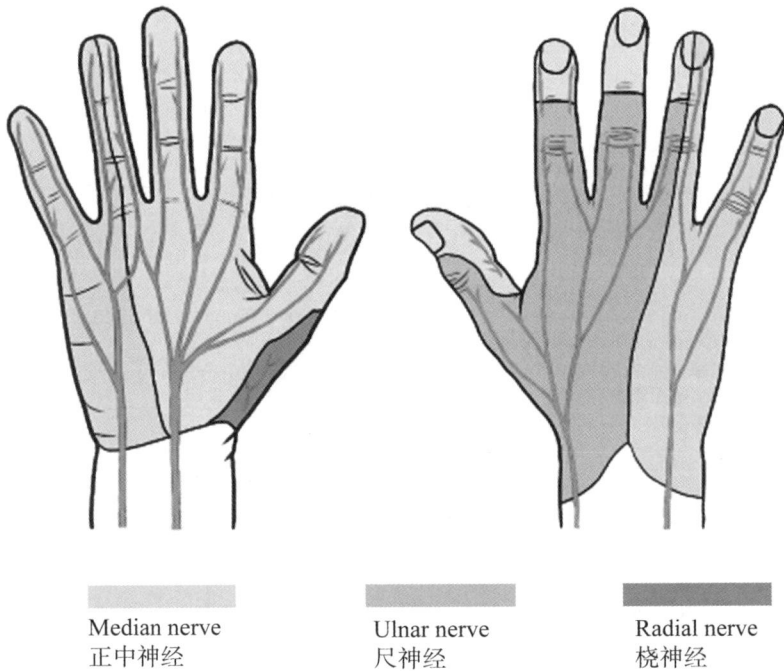

Median nerve
正中神经

Ulnar nerve
尺神经

Radial nerve
桡神经

Fig.10-7　Cutaneous innervation of hands

In the forearm the median nerve damage can result in a loss of pronation of the forearm; flexion of the second, the third fingers and the distal phalanx of the thumb and opposition of the thumb. Wrist flexion is severely affected (carpal tunnel syndrome). The thenar muscles are paralyzed, manifested as the thenar muscles atrophy, and the palm becomes flattened into an "ape-like" hand. At the same time, there is also a loss or weakness of sensation from the skin of the lateral part of the palm (2/3) and palmar surface of the thumb, index, middle and the radial half of the ring finger (3.5), especially at the tip of the thumb and index fingers.

The ulnar nerve (C8—T1) (尺神经, Fig.10-7). It originates from the medial cord of the brachial plexus, and travels along the medial side of the brachial artery to the middle of the arm in the medial groove of the biceps brachii. Then it descends into the groove of the ulnar nerve behind the medial epicondyle of the humerus. After reaching the forearm, the ulnar nerve accompanies the ulnar artery/vein and descends on its medial side between the flexor carpi ulnaris and the flexor digitorum profundus. The ulnar nerve does not give off any branches in the arm, but gives out muscular branches in the upper forearm to innervate the flexor carpi ulnaris and the ulnar half of the flexor digitorum profundus; the deep branch is distributed in the adductor pollicis, hypothenar muscles, palmar interossei and dorsal interossei, and the 3rd and the 4th lumbrical muscles. The superficial branch is distributed in the skin of the hypothenar (one-third of the ulnar side of palm), the little finger and the ulnar half of the ring finger of the palmar aspect; the dorsal branch is distributedin the skin of the ulnar half of dorsum of hand, posterior aspect of ulnar two and one-half fingers except supplied by the median nerve.

When the ulnar nerve is injured in the upper two parts, the movement disorder mainly manifests as weakened wrist flexion force, inability to flex the distal knuckles of the ring finger and little finger, atrophy of the hypothenar muscle and interosseous muscles, inability to adduct the thumb, and inability to interact with each other. At the same time, the metacarpophalangeal joints are hyperextended, and a "claw-shaped hand" appears. At the same time, the senation from the skin of the hypothenar and the little finger is also lost

The radial nerve (C5－T1) (桡神经, Fig.10-7). It is from the posterior cord of the brachial plexus and turns around the back of the middle part of the humerus along the sulcus of radial nerve and descends outside the humerus accompanying the deep brachial vessels. Above the lateral epicondyle of humerus, it passes through the lateral fascial septum and runs between the brachioradialis and brachialis, and then continues downward between the brachialis and the extensor carpi radialis longus. Above the elbow, the radial nerve is usually divided into the superficial branch and the deep branch.

The superficial branch of the radial nerve turns to the dorsal side at the junction of the middle and lower 1/3 of the forearm, continues down to the back of the hand, and is divided into 4－5 dorsal digital nerves, distributed in the skin on the radial half of the back of the hand and the skin on the back of the proximal two and a half fingers on the radial side. The deep branch of the radial nerve, also known as the posterior interosseous nerve, passes through the supinator muscle on the outside of the radial neck to the back of the forearm, along the back of the interosseous membrane of the forearm, between the superficial and deep extensor groups of the forearm, descending to the back of the wrist joint, and along the way, branches are distributed to the all posterior group muscles of forearm (extensor group), distal radioulnar joint, wrist joint and intermetacarpal joint.

The radial nerve also sends out many branches in the arm, among which the muscular branches are mainly distributed in the triceps brachii (posterior group muscles of arm), anconeus, brachioradialis and extensor carpi radialis longus; the articular branch is distributed in the elbow joint. The cutaneous branches have three nerves: The posterior brachial cutaneous nerve is distributed in the skin of the posterior region of the arm after it emanates from the armpit; the inferior lateral brachial cutaneous nerve emerges superficially far from the insertion point of the deltoid muscle, and is distributed in the skin of the lower lateral part of the arm; the posterior antebrachial cutaneous nerve is superficial from the middle lateral part of the arm. It goes out and goes down to the back of the forearm, then reaches the wrist, and branches along the way to the skin of the back of the forearm.

Radial nerve injury is the most common large nerve injury in the whole body, and the signs of different parts of the injury are different. The radial nerve is most vulnerable to injury during fractures of the midshaft of the humerus and radial neck. At the back of the middle part of the arm, the radial nerve runs close to the radial nerve groove of the humerus. Therefore, the fracture of the middle part of the humerus or the junction of the middle and lower 1/3 is likely to be combined with the injury of the radial nerve, resulting in paralysis of the extensor muscles of the forearm, manifested as raising the forearm it is in the shape of "hanging wrist" or "wrist-drop", and at the same time, there is also a loss of sensation in the areas of skin supplied by the radial nerve, the skin sensory disturbance on the back between the first and second metacarpal bones is obvious. Radial head dislocation, radial neck fracture, or supinator muscle disease can damage the deep branch of the radial nerve, causing symptoms such as weakness in wrist extension and inability to extend fingers.

The medial brachial cutaneous nerve (C8—T1) (臂内侧皮神经). It originates from the medial cord of the brachial plexus, descends on the medial side of the axillary vein, then descends along the medial side of the brachial artery and the basilic vein to emerge superficially near the middle of the arm, and distributes in the skin on the inside of the arm and the front of the arm. This nerve branch often communicates with the intercostobrachial nerve in the axilla.

The medial antebrachial cutaneous nerve (C8—T1) (前臂内侧皮神经). It originates from the medial cord of the brachial plexus, first travels between the axillary artery and the vein, then descends along the medial side of the brachial artery until the middle part of the arm emerges superficially, and accompanied by the basilic vein, the terminal can be as far as the wrist. The nerve is divided into front and rear branches in the forearm, distributed in the front and back of the skin of the inner forearm.

3. Anterior Branch of Thoracic Nerve

There are 12 pairs of anterior branches of thoracic nerves (Fig.10-8). The first to the eleventh pairs of thoracic nerves are located in the corresponding intercostal spaces and are called intercostal nerves. The twelvth pair of thoracic nerves is located below the twelvth rib, named subcostal nerves. The intercostal nerve runs between the internal and external muscles of the intercostals, under the intercostal blood vessels, and runs forward in the costal groove at the lower edge of the ribs until it leaves the costal groove near the anterior axillary line, and continues in the middle of the intercostal space.

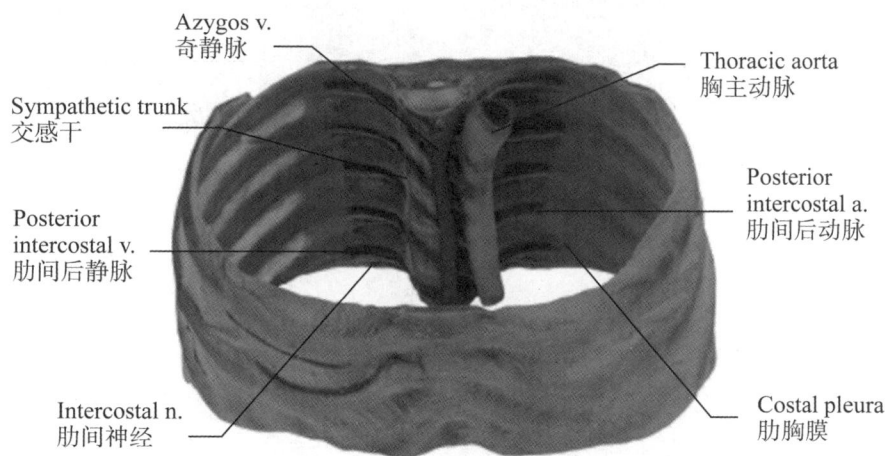

Azygos v.
奇静脉

Sympathetic trunk
交感干

Posterior
intercostal v.
肋间后静脉

Intercostal n.
肋间神经

Thoracic aorta
胸主动脉

Posterior
intercostal a.
肋间后动脉

Costal pleura
肋胸膜

Fig.10-8   Thoracic nerves

The distribution of the anterior branch of the thoracic nerve in the skin of the thoracic and abdominal walls has very obvious segmental distribution characteristics. For example, the distribution area of T2 corresponds to the plane of the sternal angle, T4 corresponds to the plane of the nipple, T6 corresponds to the plane of the xiphoid process, and T8 corresponds to the plane of the costal arches on both sides (midpoint between the xiphoid process and umbilicus), T10 is equivalent to the umbilical plane, and the distribution area of T12 is equivalent to the plane of the midpoint between the umbilicus and symphysis pubis (about at the level of the anterior superior iliac spine). In clinical practice, specific damaged thoracic nerves can be analyzed and inferred based on the plane of somatocutaneous sensory disorders. At the same time, the plane of the skin sensory disturbance can also be deduced after the specific injured thoracic nerve is identified.

4. Lumbar Plexus

(1) **Formation and position of the lumbar plexus**. The lumber plexus is composed of a part of the anterior branch of the twelvth thoracic nerve (small), the anterior branches of the first to the third lumbar nerves, and a part of the anterior branch of the fourth

lumbar nerve (most). The lumbar plexus is located deep to the psoas major and anterior to the transverse process of the lumbar spine (Fig.10-9).

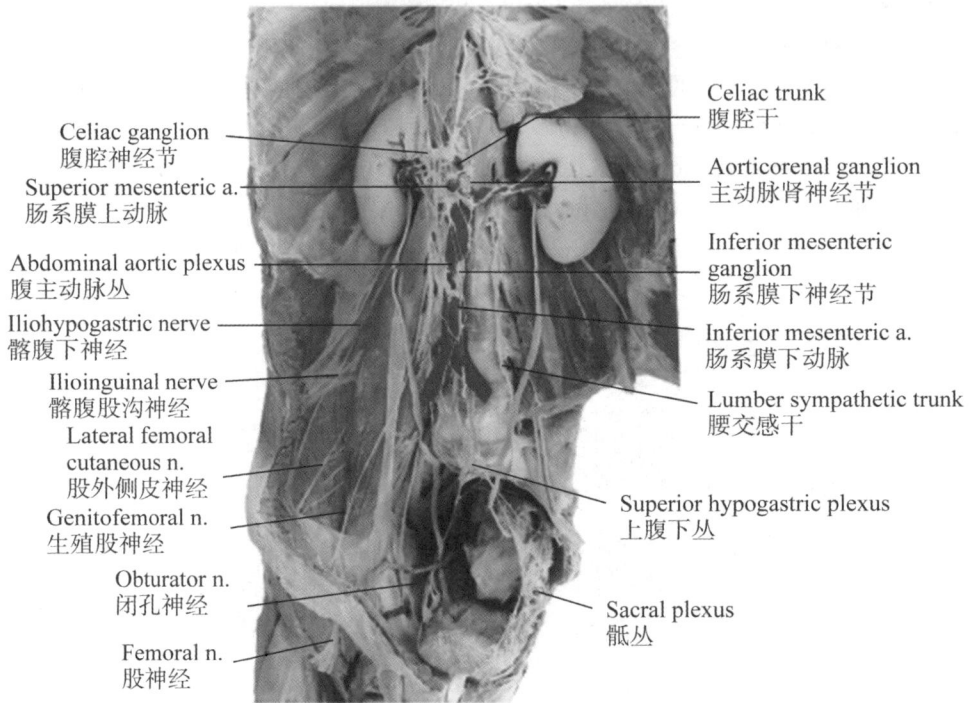

Celiac ganglion 腹腔神经节
Superior mesenteric a. 肠系膜上动脉
Abdominal aortic plexus 腹主动脉丛
Iliohypogastric nerve 髂腹下神经
Ilioinguinal nerve 髂腹股沟神经
Lateral femoral cutaneous n. 股外侧皮神经
Genitofemoral n. 生殖股神经
Obturator n. 闭孔神经
Femoral n. 股神经

Celiac trunk 腹腔干
Aorticorenal ganglion 主动脉肾神经节
Inferior mesenteric ganglion 肠系膜下神经节
Inferior mesenteric a. 肠系膜下动脉
Lumber sympathetic trunk 腰交感干
Superior hypogastric plexus 上腹下丛
Sacral plexus 骶丛

Fig.10-9　Lumbar plexus

(2) Branches and distribution of the lumbar plexus

The lumbar plexus gives off many branches that distribute in the inguinal region, the front and the medial part of the thigh.

1) The iliohypogastric nerve (T12—L1)(髂腹下神经). It passes through the lateral border of the psoas major, the back of the kidney and the front of the quadratus lumborum, and goes outward and downward, enters between the transversus abdominis and the obliquus internus abdominis above the posterior part of the iliac crest, and finally penetrates the aponeurosis of obliquus externus abdominis about 3 cm above the superficial ring of inguinal canal to the skin.

2)The ilioinguinal nerve (L1)(髂腹股沟神经). It exits the lateral border of the psoas major under the iliohypogastric nerve, crosses the quadratus lumborum and the upper part of the iliacus obliquely, passes through the transversus abdominis near the front of the iliac crest, and goes forward into the inguinal canal, accompanies the spermatic cord (uterine round ligament). Its cutaneous branch distributes to the skin of the inguinal region, scrotum or greater lip of pudendum.

3) The lateral femoral cutaneous nerve (L2—L3)(股外侧皮神经). It passes through the lateral border of the psoas major, runs anterolaterally, crossesthe surface of the iliacus to the medial side of the anterior superior iliac spine, and then passes out of the deep fascia and distributes to the skin of the anterolateral thigh.

4) The femoral nerve (L2—L4)(股神经). As the largest branch from the lumbar plexus, it originates from the lateral border of the psoas major, descends between the psoas major and the iliacus to reach the inguinal region, passes through the ligament from the deep side slightly lateral to the midpoint of the inguinal ligament, and enters the femoral triangle of the thigh on the lateral side of the femoral artery. The muscular branches of the femoral nerve are mainly distributed in the iliacus, the pectineus, the quadriceps femoris and the sartorius (the anterior group muscles of thigh). The cutaneous branches are medial femoral cutaneous nerve and middle femoral cutaneous nerve, which are distributed in the skin of the front of the thigh and the knee joint. The longest cutaneous branch is the saphenous nerve, descending on the medial side of the knee joint, going out superficially behind the lower end of the sartorius to subcutaneous. Then, along with the great saphenous vein, it descends along the medial surface of the calf to the medial border of the foot, and along the way, it sends out branches, distributed in the skin of the infrapatella, the medial surface of calf and the medial border of foot. The main manifestations of the femoral nerve injury include hip flexion weakness, inability to extend the knee while sitting, an difficulty in walking, disapperance of knee jerk reflex, and skin sensory disturbance in front of the thigh and inner side of the calf.

5) The obturator nerve (L2—L4)(闭孔神经). It originates from the lumbar plexus and passes out from the lateral border of the psoas major, runs close to the inner surface of the pelvic wall, and passes through the obturator canal along with the obturator blood vessels. Then, the obturator nerve is divided into the anterior and posterior branches, superficially in front and behind the adductor brevis respectively to the medial region of the thigh. The muscular branches from the obturator nerve mainly innervate the obturator externus, adductor longus, adductor brevis, adductor magnus and gracilis, and occasionally to the pectineus; its cutaneous branches are mainly distributed in the skin of the medial region of thigh.

6) The genitofemoral nerve (L1—L2) (生殖股神经). It pierces the anterior surface of psoas major and goes down in front of the psoas major, and soon obliquely crosses the back of the ureter to the inguinal region, and divides into the genital branch and femoral branch above the inguinal ligament. The genital branch enters the inguinal canal at the deep ring of the inguinal canal and distributes to the cremaster and scrotum along with the structures inside the inguinal canal; in the female, it distributes to the greater lip of

pudendum along with the round ligament of uterus. The femoral branch passes through the femoral sheath and fascia lata to the skin of the femoral triangle. Care should be taken not to damage this nerve during inguinal hernia repair and appendix surgery.

5. Sacral Plexus

(1) Formation and position of the sacral plexus

The sacral plexus is composed of the lumbosacral trunk formed by a part of the anterior branch of the fourth lumbar nerve (small) and the anterior branch of the fifth lumbar nerve, and all the anterior branches of the sacral and coccygeal nerves. From the perspective of the number of spinal nerves participating in the composition, the sacral plexus is the largest spinal plexus in the whole body. The sacral plexus is located in the pelvic cavity, just in front of the sacrum and piriformis, behind the iliac vessels, with the sigmoid colon in front of the left sacral plexus, and the ileal loop in front of the right sacral plexus (Fig.9-44).

(2) Branches and distribution of the sacral plexus

The branches of the sacral plexus are divided into two categories: One is the short distance running branches, which are directly distributed to the adjacent pelvic wall muscles, such as piriformis, obturator internus, and quadratus femoris; the other is the long distance running branches, which are distributed in the muscles and skin of the buttocks, perineum, posterior femoral region, calf and feet.

1) The superior gluteal nerve (L4－S1)(臀上神经)originates from the sacral plexus, along with the superior gluteal blood vessels, exits the pelvic cavity through the superior piriformis foramen to the buttocks, and runs between the gluteus medius and gluteus minimus, distributed in the gluteus medius, gluteus minimus and tensor fascia lata.

2) The inferior gluteal nerve (L5－S2)(臀下神经) goes out of the pelvic cavity to the buttocks along with the inferior gluteal blood vessel through the subpiriformis foramen, runs deep to the gluteus maximus, and innervates this muscle.

3) The posterior femoral cutaneous nerve (S1－S3)(股后皮神经) originates from the sacral plexus, passes through the subpiriformis foramen along with the inferior gluteal nerve, exits the pelvic cavity to the buttocks, descends deep to the gluteus maximus, and gives branches to the skin of the gluteal region, retrofemoral region, and popliteal fossa.

4) The pudendal nerve (S2－S4) (阴部神经) originates from the sacral plexus and passes through the subpiriformis foramen along with the pudendal blood vessels to the buttocks, then goes around the ischial spine through the lesser sciatic foramen and enters the ischioanal fossa of the perineum, and branches along the way to distribute in the muscles and skin of the perineum, and the skin of the external genitals. The main branches: the anal nerve (inferior rectal nerve), the perineal nerve, and the dorsal nerve of

penis (clitoris). The nerve is distributed in the external anal sphincter and the skin of the anus; the perineal nerve accompanying with pudendal blood vessels are distributed in the perineal muscles and the skin of the scrotum or greater lip of pudendum; the dorsal nerve of penis (clitoris) walks in the dorsal side of the penis or clitoris, and is distributed in the cavernous body and skin of the penis or clitoris.

5) The sciatic nerve (L4—S3) (坐骨神经) is the nerve with the largest diameter and the longest course in the whole body. It exits the pelvic cavity through the infrapiriformis foramen to the deep surface of the gluteus maximus, descends deep to the midpoint between the sciatic tubercle and the greater trochanter, reaches the posterior femoral region, and then travels through the deep surface of the long head of biceps femoris and is generally divided into two terminal branches of the tibial nerve and the common peroneal nerve above the popliteal fossa. The sciatic nerve supplies the biceps femoris, semitendinosus and semimembranosus (posterior group muscles of the thigh) in the posterior thigh region, and also has branches to the hip joint.

6) The tibial nerve (L4—S3) (胫神经). It is the continuation of the main trunk of the sciatic nerve. It goes down along the midline at the lower part of the posterior femoral region and enters the popliteal fossa accompanied by the popliteal blood vessels located in their deep surface. It descends to the posterior region of the calf in the deep surface of the soleus muscle, Then, it continues to descend to the posterior of the medial malleolus accompanied by the posterior tibial blood vessels, and finally is divided into the two terminal branches of the medial and lateral plantar nerves in the ankle canal to the plantar region. After the tibial nerve injury, due to the weak contraction of the posterior calf muscles, the main manifestations are that the foot cannot plantar flex, cannot stand on the toes, and the varus force is weakened. Thus, the so-called "hook-like foot" deformity occurs.

7) The common peroneal nerve (L4—S2) (腓总神经). After the proximal end of the popliteal fossa is sent out by the sciatic nerve, it wraps around the neck of fibula and passes through the peroneus longus forward and is divided into two terminal branches of the superficial peroneal nerve and the deep peroneal nerve. The superfi-cial peroneal nerve descends deep to the peroneus longus, then continues to run between the peroneus longus and the peroneus brevis, and distributes to the peroneus longus and peroneus brevis along the way. The terminal branch emerges superficially at the junction of the middle and lower 1/3 of the calf as the cutaneous branch, and is distributed in the skin of the lateral surface of the calf, the dorsum of the foot, and the dorsum of the second to the fifth toes. The deep peroneal nerve runs obliquely forward between the fibula and peroneus longus, along with the anterior tibial blood vessels between the tibialis anterior and extensor digitorum longus, then descends between the tibialis anterior and extensor

hallucis longus, and finally through the front of the ankle joint to the dorsum of the foot. Along the way, the branches of the deep peroneal nerve are distributed in the anterior group muscles of the calf, the dorsal muscles of the foot, and the skin of the opposite edges of the first and second toes.

The common peroneal nerve is superficial at the fibular neck and easily injured. After the common peroneal nerve injury, due to the weak contraction of the anterior and lateral calf muscles, the main manifestations are that the foot cannot dorsiflex, the toes cannot extend, the foot droops and turns inward, showing the deformity of "talipes equinovarus" or "foot-drop". At the same time, obvious sensory disturbances appeared in the anterior and lateral sides of the calf, and the dorsum of the foot.

（徐州医科大学　刘志安）

10.2　Cranial Nerve

The cranial nerve (脑神经) is connected with the brain, so it is called cranial nerve. There are 12 pairs of cranial nerves (Table 10-1 & Fig. 10-10), which are numbered sequentially using Roman number (I — XII). Their numerical order (I — XII, using Roman numerals to show) is determined by their skull exit location (rostral to caudal). All cranial nerves originate from the nuclei in the brain. Two of them originate from the forebrain (olfactory and optic nerves.). One has its nucleus in the spinal cord (the accessory nerve) while the remainder originate from the brainstem.

Table 10-1 Name, nature and location of the cranial nerve

Name	Type	Location in the brain	Location in or out of the cranial cavity
I Olfactory nerve	Sensory	Telencephalon	Foramina in cribriform plate
II Optic nerve	Sensory	Diencephalon	Optic canals
III Oculomotor nerve	Motor	Midbrain	Superior orbital fissure
IV Trochlear nerve	Motor	Midbrain	Superior orbital fissure
V Trigeminal nerve	Mixed nerve	Pons	The ophthalmic nerve through the superior orbital fissure The maxillary nerve through the foramen rotundum The mandibular nerve through the foramen ovale

Name	Type	Location in the brain	Location in or out of the cranial cavity
Ⅵ Abducens nerve	Motor cranial nerve	Pons	Superior orbital fissure
Ⅶ Facial nerve	Mixed nerve	Pons	Internal acoustic pore → stylomastoid foramen
Ⅷ Vestibulocochlear nerve	Sensory cranial nerve	Pons	Internal acoustic pore
Ⅸ Glossopharyngeal nerve	Mixed nerve	Medulla oblongata	Jugular foramen
Ⅹ Vagus nerve	Mixed nerve	Medulla oblongata	Jugular foramen
Ⅺ Accessory nerve	Motor cranial nerve	Medulla oblongata	Jugular foramen
Ⅻ Hypoglossal nerve	Motor cranial nerve	Medulla oblongata	Hypoglossal canal

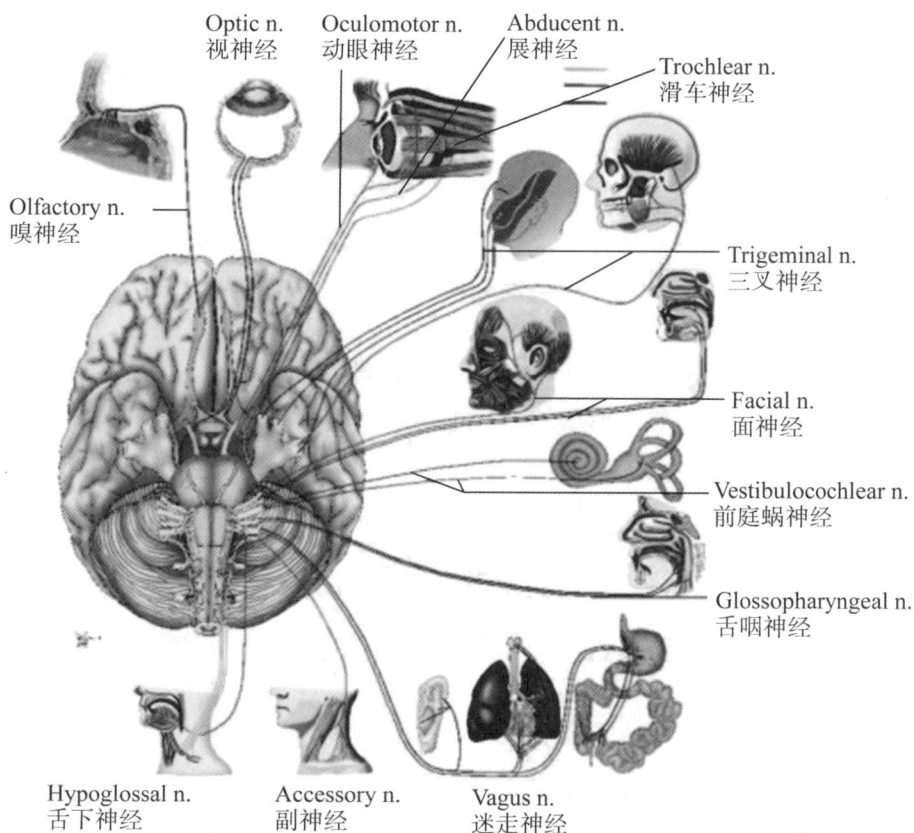

Fig.10-10　Cranial nerve profile

The fiber components of the cranial nerve are classified based on their functions and the type of information they carry. Special fibers are associated with special somatic senses (vision, hearing and balance) and special visceral senses(smell and taste), while general refers to sensory or motor information orginating from or directed to all other areas of the body. The information carried by a nerve is called somatic if it involves the skin and skeletal muscles, or visceral if it pertains to the our internal organs. So the cranial nerves can be divided into the following seven fiber components according to the characteristics of embryogenesis, nerve fiber inner-vation and function.

General somatic afferent fibers (GSA, 一般躯体感觉纤维) transmit exteroceptive and proprioceptive impulses from the head and the face to the somatic sensory nuclei.

Special somatic afferent fibers (SSA, 特殊躯体感觉纤维) transmit sensory impulses from special sense organs of vision, equilibrium and hearing to the brain.

General visceral afferent fibers (GVA, 一般内脏感觉纤维) transmit interoceptive impulses from the viscera to the visceral sensory nuclei.

Special visceral afferent fibers (SVA, 特殊内脏感觉纤维) transmit sensory impulses from special sense organs of smell and taste to the brain.

General somatic efferent fibers (GSE, 一般躯体运动纤维) innervate skeletal muscles of the eye and the tongue.

Special visceral efferent fibers (SVE, 特殊内脏运动纤维) transmit motor impulses from the brain to skeletal muscles derived from brachial (gill) arches of embryo. These include the muscles of mastication, facial expression and swallowing.

General visceral efferent fibers (GVE, 一般内脏运动纤维) transmit motor impulses from the general visceral motor nuclei, relayed in parasympathetic ganglions. The postganglionic fibers supply cardiac muscles, smooth muscles and glands.

Although there are seven types of fiber components in general, each pair of cranial nerve contains somewhat different types of fiber components. Cranial nerves can be devided into sensory, motor and mixed nerves. Some cranial nerves only contain only motor fibers called motor nerve (the oculomotor nerve, trochlear nerve, abducens nerve, accessory nerve and hypoglossal nerve); contain soly sensory fibers called sensory nerve (the olfactory nerve, optic nerve and vestibulocochlear nerve); contain both types of fibers called mixed nerve (the trigeminal nerve, facial nerve, glossopharyngeal nerve and vagus nerve).

1. Olfactory Nerve

The olfactory nerve (嗅神经) is composed of special visceral sensory fibers (特殊内脏感觉纤维) and is classified as a sensory cranial nerve. It carries information related to smell to the brain. Olfactory nerves are the central process derived from olfactory receptor neurons located in the superior conchae and its opposite nasal septum olfactory mucosa.

The bundles converge into as many as 20 branches that cross the cribriform plate, and enter the overlying olfactory bulb. In severe injuries involving the anterior cranial fossa, the olfactory bulb may be separated from the olfactory nerves or the nerves may be torn, leading to anosmia. Fractures may involve the meninges, causing cerebrospinal fluid may leak into the nasal cavity, resulting in cerebrospinal rhinorrhoea. Additionally, inflammation of the upper nasal mucosa, as seen in rhinitis, can cause temporary reduction in the sense of smell.

2. Optic Nerve

The optic nerve (视神经) is composed of special somatic sensory fibers (特殊躯体感觉纤维) that transmit visual information to the brain. The optic nerve contains the axons of retinal ganglion cells and gathers in the optic disk, pierces the sclera at the lamina cribrosa, continues to run to the optic nerve. The introorbital portion of the optic nerve is approximately $2.5-3.0$ cm in length and runs backward, through the optic canal into the middle cranial fossa, and then two optic nerves converge to form the optic chiasma, which is usually positioned over the diaphragma sellae and pituitary gland. The nerve fibers representing the temporal visual fields uncrossed, representing the nasal half visual fields decussate within the chiasma. The nerve fibers then continue to run as the two optic tracts to the lateral geniculate body of the thalamus.

3. Oculomotor Nerve

The oculomotor nerve (动眼神经) is a motor nerve, which contains general visceral motor fibers (一般躯体运动纤维) and general somatic motor fibers (一般内脏运动纤维). The general somatic motor fibers come from the oculomotor nucleus (动眼神经核) located in the superior colliculus plane of the midbrain. The general visceral motor fibers come from the accessory nucleus of the oculomotor nerve (动眼神经副核) (also called Edinger-Westphal nucleus) in the midbrain. As the name suggests, the oculomotor nerve is the primary motor nerve responsible for eye movement. It exits the interpeduncular fossa at the midbrain, passes the upper part of lateral wall of the cavernous sinus, and enters the orbit through the superior orbital fissure. Upon entering the orbit, it divides into superior and inferior divisions. The superior division of the oculomotor nerve enter the inferior (ocular) surface of superior rectus. It supplies this muscle and gives off a branch that runs to innervate levator palpebrae superioris. The inferior division of the oculomotor nerve is divided into the medial, central and lateral branches, innerrating inferior, medial rectus and inferior oblique muscle. The lateral branch enters the inferior oblique and also communicates with the ciliary ganglion (睫状神经节) for relay, and then postganglionic parasympathetic fibers will pass anteriorly to supply two intrinsic muscles of the eye as sphincter pupillae and the ciliary muscle, involved in constricting the pupil and accommodation of the lens of the eye respectively (Fig.10-11).

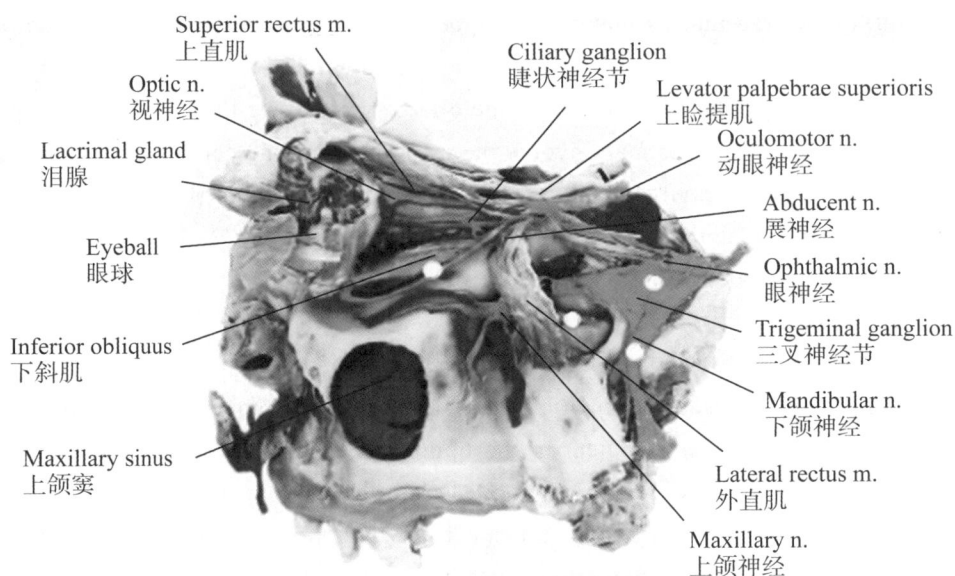

Fig.10-11　Nerves in the orbit

The ciliary ganglion (睫状神经节) is a small, flat, reddish-grey swelling parasynpathetic ganglion, approximately 1－2 mm in diameter. It is located between the optic nerve and the lateral rectus. The parasympathetic ganglion of the cranial nerve generally has some small nerve branches connected with it, and customary to call these nerve branches the root of the ganglion. The ciliary ganglion receives input via three roots (parasympathetic, sympathetic and sensory roots). i) The parasympathetic root(副交感根) is termed the short ciliary nerves. The general visceral motor fibers from the oculomotor nerve pass through this root into the ciliary ganglion, where they exchange neurons. ii) The sympathetic root (交感根) contains fibres from the plexus around the internal carotid artery within the cavernous sinus. The fibres traverse the ganglion without synapsing to emerge into the short ciliary nerves innervate dilator pupillae and are distributed to the blood vessels of the eyeball. iii) The sensory root(感觉根) that passes through the ciliary ganglion is derived from the nasociliary nerve. It enters the short ciliary nerves and carries sensation from the cornea, the ciliary body and the iris. Eight to ten delicate filaments, referred to as the short ciliary nerves, emerge anteriorly from the ciliary ganglion.

In ophthalmology, ganglion anesthesia (retrobulbar anesthesia, 球后麻醉) is often performed to induce vasoconstriction in the eye shrink and reduces the intraocular pressure.

The oculomotor nerve injury will result in paralysis of the levator palpebrae superioris muscle, superior rectus muscle, internal rectus muscle, inferior rectus muscle and inferior oblique muscle. This leads to ptosis, exotropia (outward and downward displacement of the pupil), and pupil dilation, the loss of the light reflex.

4. Trochlear Nerve

The trochlear nerve (滑车神经) is a motor cranial nerve, containing only general somatic motor fibers (一般躯体运动纤维). Interestingly, the trochlear nerve has the longest intracranial course despite being the smallest one of all the cranial nerves (by number of axons) and is the only cranial nerve that from the dorsal surface of the brain. The trochlear nerve originates from the trochlear nucleus (滑车神经核) of the inferior colliculus plane and crosses backward to the contralateral side, emerge from the dorsal surface of the brainstem, lateral to the lower edge of the inferior colliculus. After leaving the brainstem, the trochlear nerve runs laterally around the cerebral peduncle, passes through the lateral wall of the cavernous sinus, and enters the orbit through the superior orbital fissure to reach and innervate superior oblique (Fig.10-12).

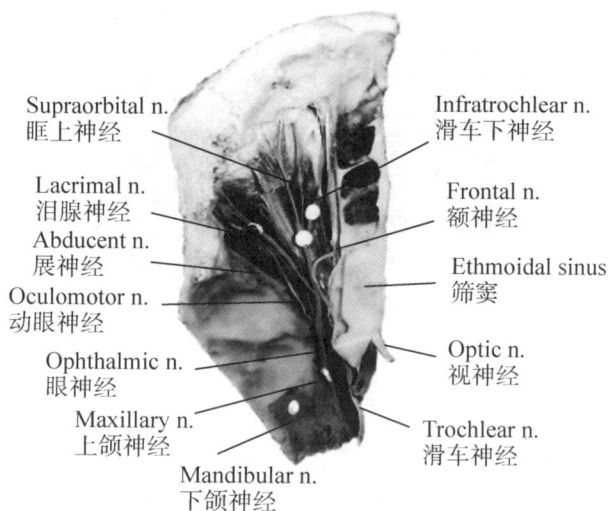

Supraorbital n.
眶上神经

Infratrochlear n.
滑车下神经

Lacrimal n.
泪腺神经

Frontal n.
额神经

Abducent n.
展神经

Ethmoidal sinus
筛窦

Oculomotor n.
动眼神经

Optic n.
视神经

Ophthalmic n.
眼神经

Maxillary n.
上颌神经

Trochlear n.
滑车神经

Mandibular n.
下颌神经

Fig.10-12   Nnerve in the orbit (superior aspect)

5. Trigeminal Nerve

The trigeminal nerve (三叉神经) is the largest mixed cranial nerve, containing both general somatic sensory fibers (一般躯体感觉纤维) and special visceral motor fibers (特殊内脏运动纤维). It has four nuclei that send fibers to form its tracts and is associated with three separate branches. The special visceral motor fibers originate from the motor nucleus of the trigeminal nerve (三叉神经运动核) in the middle part of the pons. The fibers form the motor root of the trigeminal nerve together with sensory fibers They exit and enter the brain from the basal part of the pontine. The fibers that conduct pain and temperature sensation form the pinal nucleus of the trigeminal nerve (三叉神经脊束核),

which terminates in the trigeminal spinal tract nucleus. The fibers that conduct touch terminate in the pontine nucleus of the trigeminal nerve (三叉神经脑桥核). The peripheral processes of neurons of the trigeminal ganglion formed three branches: the ophthalmic division (CN V1, 眼神经), the maxillary nerve (CN V2, 上颌神经), and the mandibular nerve (CN V3, 下颌神经). The three sensory branches of the trigeminal nerve unite within a shallow depression on the posteromedial side of the middle cranial fossa to unite and form the trigeminal ganglion (Fig.10-13).

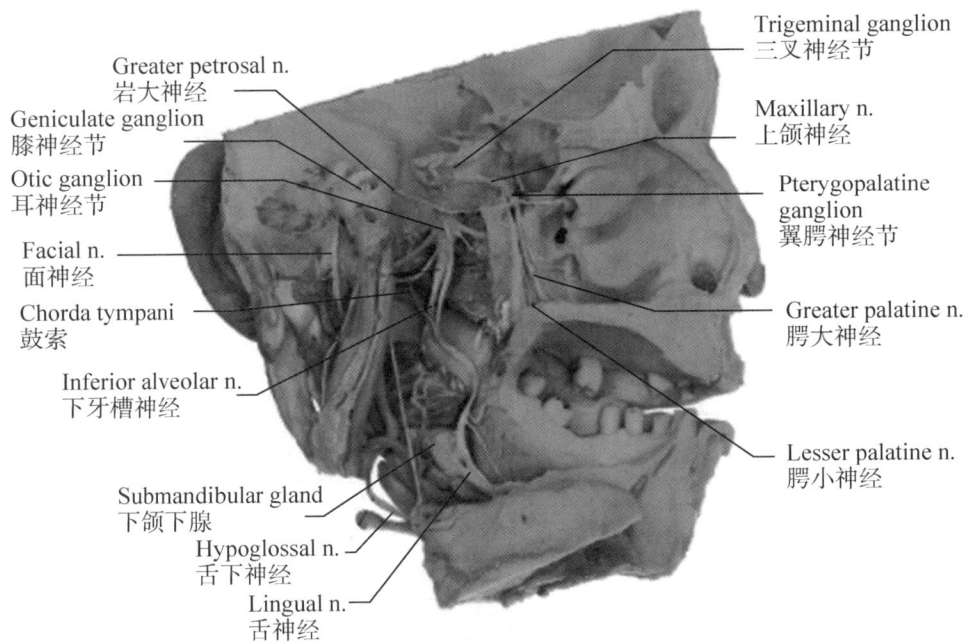

Fig.10-13　Nerves in the pterygopalatine fossa

(1) The ophthalmic nerve

It is the first division of the trigeminal nerve and is purely sensory nerve containing general somatic sensory fibers (一般躯体感觉纤维). It arises from the trigeminal ganglion located in the middle cranial fossa, passes forwards along the lateral dural wall of the cavernous sinus, and enters the orbit through the superior orbital fissure. The branch carries afferent stimuli of pain, light touch, and tempera-ture from the upper eyelids, cornea, conjunctiva of the eye and supraorbital region of the face, extending up to the vertex of the head. Furthermore, the ophthalmic branch also carries fibers arising from the dura mater of the anterior cranial fossa, the frontal sinus, and the superior aspect of the nasal cavity. The three main nerves that come together to form CN V1 are the nasociliary, frontal, and lacrimal nerves.

(2) **The maxillary nerve** (CN V2)

It is also a purely sensory that contains only general somatic sensory fibers (一般躯体感觉纤维). It carries impulses from the midface. The maxillary nerve emerges from the trigeminal ganglion, enters the lateral wall of the cavernous sinus and passes along its lower part. It then exits the maxillary division of the skull via the foramen rotundum and enters the upper part of the pterygopalatine fossa. The main branches are as follows: the infraorbital nerve, superior alveolar nerves, zygomatic nerve and pterygopalatine nerves. It supplies sensory innervation to the skin and mucosa of the lower eyelid, the nasal alar, the upper lip, the maxillary teeth, the gingiva and maxillary sinus mucosa, the palate, the nasal mucosa and the palatine tonsil. It is responsible for the conduction of sensation in these areas.

(3) **The mandibular nerve** (下颌神经) (CN V3). It is the last of the three trigeminal branches. As the largest component of CN V, it carries both general somatic sensory fibers (一般躯体感觉纤维) and special visceral motor fibers (特殊内脏运动纤维). The motor fibers inneroate to the muscles that originate from the first pharyngeal arch. The sensory fibers supply sensation to the lower third of the face, excluding the angle of the mandible (supplied by the second and the third cervical segments). As it descends from the foramen ovale, it is divided into auriculotemporal nerve (耳颞神经) that supplies sensation to the tragus and part of the adjoining auricle of the ear and the posterior part of the temple, buccal nerve (颊神经) that supplies sensation to the skin over the anterior part of the buccinator, as well as the corresponding buccal mucous membrane along the outside of the buccinator, lingual nerve (舌神经) that supplies sensory innervation to the mucosa of the floor of the mouth, and mucosa of the presulcal part of the tongue, as a conduit for the chorda tympani (a branch of CN VII), which carries taste, inferior alveolar nerve (下牙槽神经) that supplies the mandibular teeth and gums, skin and mucous membrane of the chin and lower lip, and nerve of muscles of mastication (咀嚼肌神经) that innervates the masticatory muscles.

The three branches of the trigeminal nerve exhibit distinct regional distribution patterns across the head and facial skin. These regions are demarcated by the ophthalmic fissure and oral fissure. The area above the ophthalmic fissure is the distribution area of the ophthalmic nerve, the region between the ophthalmic fissure and oral fissure is the distribution area of the maxillary nerve, and the area below the fissure is the distribution area of the mandibular nerve. In the event of injury to one side of the trigeminal nerve, sensory loss occurs in the ipsilateral head, the skin of face and eyes, oral and nasal mucosa. Additionally, general sensory loss, and the absence of corneal reflex are observed, The ipsilateral masticatory muscle was paralyzed, and the jaw was tilted to the affected side when the mouth was opened.

6. Abducent Nerve

The abducens nerve (展神经) is a motor cranial nerve composed of general somatic motor fibers (一般躯体运动纤维). It originates from the abducent nucleus located at the base of the fourth ventricle. The fibers exit the brain ventrally from the medial line of the pontomedullary sulcus, and then sharply curve over the upper border of the petrous part of the temporal bone to enter the cavernous sinus, where it lies lateral to the internal carotid artery. It then enters the orbit through the superior orbital fissure, within the common tendinous ring. It passes forward to enter the medial (ocular) surface of lateral rectus, typically in the posterior one-third of the muscle. Damage to the abducent nerve can cause paralysis of the external rectus muscle, leading to esotropia.

7. Facial Nerve (面神经)

The facial nerve is a mixed cranial nerve with four fibrous components.

Special visceral motor fibers (特殊内脏运动纤维) originate from the nucleus of facial nerve (面神经核)in the tegmentum ponticus, mainly innervate the muscles of facial expression.

General visceral motor fibres (一般内脏运动纤维) in the facial nerve arise from preganglionic parasympathetic neurons located in the superior salivatory nucleus (上泌涎核). These fibers travel through the chorda tympani to the submandibular ganglion, where postganglionic fibers are distributed to the submandibular glands and the sublingual glands. Alternatively, the fibers travel via the greater petrosal nerve to the pterygopalatine gangliong, and postgang-lionic fibers are distributed to the lacrimal glands and mucosal glands of nasal cavity and palate.

The special visceral sensory fibers (特殊内脏感觉纤维), also known as taste fibers, whose cellular bodies are located in the genicular ganglion (膝神经节) around the bend of the facial nerve canal in the petrous part of the temporal bone, and the peripheral process carry taste from the anterior two-thirds of the tongue, with the central process terminating in the upper part of the solitary nucleus (孤束核上部) in the brain stem.

General somatic sensory fibers (一般躯体感觉纤维), whose cellular bodies are located in the geniculate ganglion. These fibers carry cutaneous sensation from the ear and the proprioception of the muscles of facial expression to the sensory nucleus of the trigeminal nerve (三叉神经感觉核) in the brain stem.

The facial nerve consists of two roots: The larger motor root of the facial nerve located at the cerebellar triangle, exits from the lateral part of the bulbopontine sulcus; the smaller mixed roots, also called intermediate nerves(中间神经), exit the brain from the lateral of the motor roots. These two roots typically merge after entering the internal acoustic meatus, accompanied by the vestibulocochlear nerve. They pass through the fundus of the internal acoustic meatus into the facial nerve canal which is adjacent to the tympanum. The facial nerve exits the skull through the stylomastoid foramen and enters the infratemporal fossa, then passes forward through the superficial and deep parts of the parotid gland to the face, supplying the muscles with facial expression. At the bend of the facial nerve canal, there is an enlarged geniculate ganglion, where the cell body of sensory neurons are located.

The facial nerve gives off many branches, which are mainly located in the facial nerve canal and outside the facial nerve canal respectively, called the branches that arise within the facial canal and the extracranial branch.

(1) Extracranial branch

The facial nerve emerges from the base of the skull through the stylomastoid foramen and almost immediately gives off the nerves to supply the posterior belly of digastric, stylohyoid, the occipital belly of occipitofrontalis and some of the intrinsic auricular muscles. The nerve then enters the parotid gland where it forms a parotid plexus. Five main terminal branches arise from the plexus, diverge within the gland. These branches exit its anteromedial surface, medial to its anterior margin, to supply the muscles with facial expression. The branches are as follows (Fig.10-14).

1) Temporal branches (颞支) diverge within the parotid gland and exit through its upper margin, usually in two or three branches. They supply the frontal belly with occipitofrontalis and orbicularis oculi.

2) Zygomatic branches (颧支) are generally multiple, diverging within the parotid gland and exiting through its anteromedial margin. They supply orbicularis oculi and Zygomatic muscle.

3) Buccal branches (颊支) originate above or below the parotid duct in the anterior margin of the parotid gland, these branches typically consist of with three to four branches, supply the buccinator、orbicularis oris and other perioral muscles.

4) Marginal mandibular branches (下颌缘支) originate from the lower part of the anterior margin of the parotid gland and passes along the lower margin of the mandible, supply the muscles of the lower lip.

5) Cervical branches (颈支) emerge from the lower part of the parotid gland and run anteroinferiorly under platysma to the anterior neck. They supply platysma.

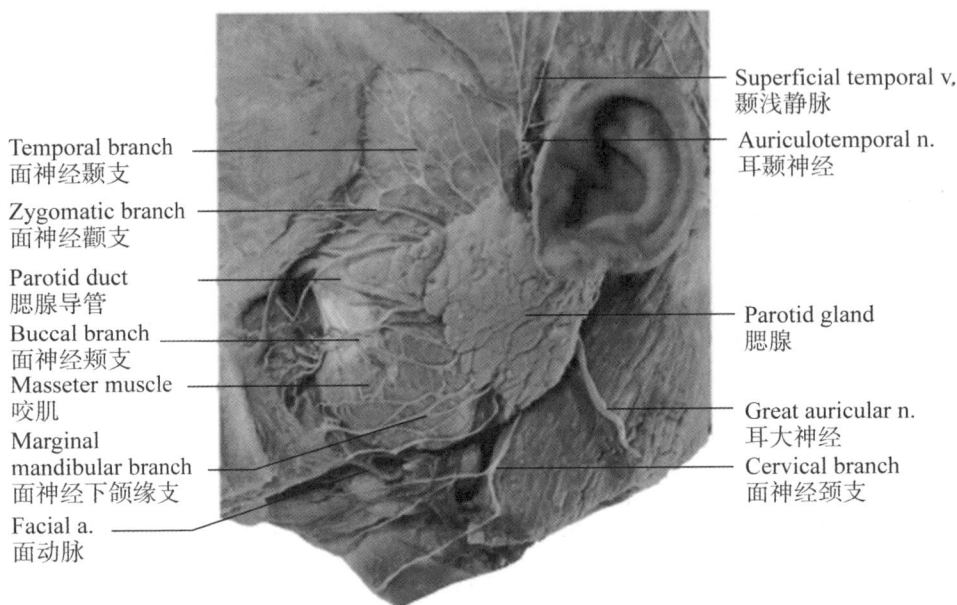

Superficial temporal v,
颞浅静脉

Auriculotemporal n.
耳颞神经

Temporal branch
面神经颞支

Zygomatic branch
面神经颧支

Parotid duct
腮腺导管

Buccal branch
面神经颊支

Masseter muscle
咬肌

Marginal
mandibular branch
面神经下颌缘支

Facial a.
面动脉

Parotid gland
腮腺

Great auricular n.
耳大神经

Cervical branch
面神经颈支

Fig.10-14   Superficial nerves of the face

(2) Within the facial canal branch

In the facial canal, the facial nerve initially runs anterolaterally. After making a sharp turn, it passes through the lateral wall of the tympanic cavity above the fenestra vestibuli and reaches the posterior wall of the tympanic cavity. The stapedial nerve arises from the upper segment of the vertical part, and the chorda tympani arises from the junction of the middle and lower segments of the vertical part, about 6 mm above the stylomastoid foramen.

1) Stapedial nerve (镫骨肌神经) supplies the stapedius in the tympanic cavity.

2) Greater petrosal nerve (岩大神经) is also known as the superficial petrosal nerve (岩浅神经). As the main branch from the geniculate ganglion, the greater petrosal verve contains the general visceral motor nerve, traverses a hiatus on the anterior surface of the petrous part of the temporal bone, and then exits the middle cranial fossa to the base of skull through the foramen lacerum, and continues forward through the pterygopalatine fossa. It then enters the pterygopalatine ganglion (翼腭神经节), where the postganglion fibers are distributed to the lacrimal glands, palatal and nasal mucosa glands, innervating their secretion.

3) Chorda tympani (鼓索) exits the facial nerve 6 mm above the stylomastoid foramen and enter the tympanic cavity via the posterior canaliculus. It travels along the inside of the tympanic membrane, and crosses medial to the upper part of the handle of the malleus to the anterior wall of the tympanic cavity. It exits the tympanic cavity and enters the infratemporal

fossa by passing through the petrotympanic fissure. Chorda tympani joins the posterior aspect of the lingual nerve, and distributes with the branches of lingual nerve. The chorda tympani contains two fiber components: Special visceral sensory fibers carry taste fibres from the anterior two-thirds of the tongue, conducting taste. General visceral motor fibers (parasympathetic fibers) enter the submandibular ganglion below the lingual nerve, and postganglionic fibers are distributed to the submandibular gland and the sublingual gland, regulating the secretion of the glands (Fig.10-15).

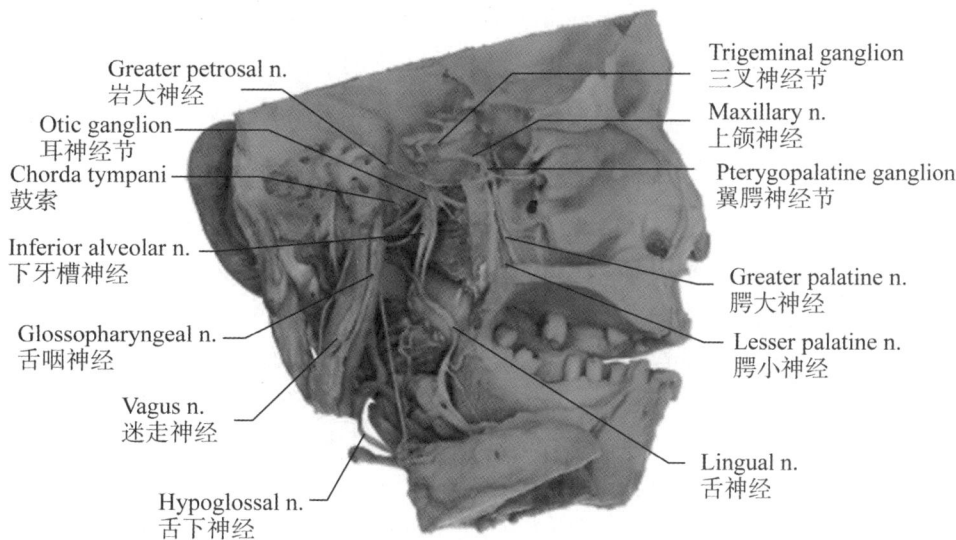

Fig.10-15   Chorda tympani, pterygopalatine ganglion and auricular ganglion

The pterygopalatine ganglion (翼腭神经节), also known as sphenopalatine ganglion (蝶腭神经节), is located in the upper of the pterygopalatine fossa. It is flattened and reddish-grey in colour and lies just below the maxillary nerve. It has three roots. First comes the parasympathetic root (副交感根). The parasympathetic fibers arise from the greater petrosal nerve, exchanging neurons within the pterygo-palatine ganglion. Second, the sympathetic root (交感根) arises from the deep petrosal nerve (岩深神经), which gives out the internal carotid plexus. Third, the sensory root (感觉根) arises from several short pterygopalatine nerves (翼腭神经) clescending from the maxillary nerve. Postganglionic fibres are distributed to the lacrimal gland, palatine, pharyngeal and nasal mucous glands, conducting mucosal general sensation and regulating glandular secretion.

The submandibular ganglion (下颌下神经节) is located superior to the deep part of the submandibular gland and inferior to the lingual nerve. It has three roots. First, the parasympathetic root (副交感根) conveys preganglionic fibres from the superior salivatory nucleus in the brainstem via the facial, chorda tympani (鼓索) and lingual nerves to the ganglion, where synapse occurs. Second, the sympathetic root (交感根) is derived from the plexus on the facial artery. Third comes the sensory root (感觉根). The Sensory fibres are derived from the lingual nerve, suppling sensory innervation to the submandibular gland and the sublingual gland, conducting general sensation and controlling glandular secretion.

As mentioned above, the parasympathetic preganglionic fibers in the facial nerve, arise from the superior salivertory nucleus, distribute to the glands in the head and face via the greater petrosal nerve and chorda tympani. These preganglion fibers synapse in the corresponding parasympathetic ganglion before reaching the innervated gland. The parasympathetic ganglia associated with the preganglionic fibers of the facial nerve are the pterygopalatine ganglion and the submandibular ganglion.

Facial nerve injury and clinical manifestations (面神经损伤及临床表现)

The clinical manifestations of facial nerve injury differ significantly depending on whether the injury occurs within the facial canal or in the extracranial branch due to the different fiber components involved. When the extracranial branch of the facial nerve is injured (面神经在面神经管外损伤时), only the facial muscle on the affected side is paralyzed. This includes an the inability to frown and close the eyes, the shallow nasolabial groove, the inability to drum the cheek, the angle of the mouth tending to the healthy side when laughing, the saliva flowing from the angle of the mouth when speaking, and difficulty in closing eyes. When the facial nerve was injured in the facial nerve canal (面神经在面神经管内损伤时), in addition to the above symptoms of paralysis of the facial muscle on the injured side, the taste of the anterior two-thirds of the affected tongue was impaired. The secretion of lacrimal glands and salivary glands on the injured side was impaired.

8. Vestibulocochlear Nerve (前庭蜗神经)

The vestibulocochlear nerve, also known as the auditory nerve (听神经), is a special somatic sensory cranial nerve. It consists of two components, the vestibular nerve (前庭神经), responsible for balance, the cochlear nerve, and hearing.

(1) Vestibular nerve

The somata of the bipolar neurons that form the vestibular nerve are the vestibular ganglion (前庭神经节), located in the end of the internal acoustic meatus, conducting the sense of balance. The peripheral processes of the vestibular ganglion cells pass through the end of the internal acoustic meatus and supply the macula of the saccule, the macula of the utricle, the hair cells in the ampullary crest. The central processes of the vestibular ganglion cells form the vestibular nerve, which passes through the internal acoustic meatus and the internal acoustic pore into the cranial cavity, enters the brainstem at the cerebellopontine angle and terminates in the vestibular nuclear complex and the flocculonodular lobe of the cerebellar.

(2) Cochlear nerve

The somata of the bipolar neurons forming the cochlear nerve (蜗神经) are the cochlear ganglion (蜗神经节), located in the modiolus of cochlea, conducting hearing. The peripheral processes of the cochlear ganglion cells supply the hair cells in the cochlear spiral canal. The central processes of the cochlear ganglion cells form the cochlear nerve which follows the vestibular nerve through the internal acoustic meatus and enters the cranial cavity. It enters the brainstem at the cerebellopontine angle through the lateral part of the bulbopontine sulcus, and ultimately terminates in the dorsal (posterior) and ventral (anterior) cochlear nuclei.

9. Glossopharyngeal Nerve

The glossopharyngeal nerve (舌咽神经) is a mixed cerebral nerve, which contains the most fiber among the 12 pairs of cerebral nerves, and 5 distinct fiber components. i) General visceral motor fibers (一般内脏运动纤维): The parasympathetic fibers, derived from the inferior salivatory nucleus (下泌涎核), exchange neurons in the otic ganglion (耳神经节), postganglionic to the parotid gland. ii) Special visceral motor fibers (特殊内脏运动纤维): The nucleus ambiguus (疑核) contributes special visceral efferent fibers to the stylopharyngeus. iii) General visceral sensory fibers (一般内脏感觉纤维): The somata of the neurons is located in the inferior ganglion of glossopharyngeal nerve (舌咽神经下神经节) at the jugular foramen. The peripheral processes are distributed to the tympanic cavity, pharyngotympanic tube, fauces, tonsils, naso-pharynx, uvula and posterior 1/3 of the tongue, carotid sinus, carotid glomus. The central process terminate in the lower part of the nucleus of the solitary tract (孤束核下部), conducting general visceral sensation. iv) Special visceral sensory fibers (特殊内脏感觉纤维). The somata of these neurons are located in the inferior ganglion of glossopharyngeal nerve (舌咽神经下神经节), and the peripheral processes are distributed to the taste buds of the posterior 1/3 of the tongue. The central process terminates in the upper part of nucleus of the solitary tract (孤束核上部). v) General somatic sensory fibers (一般躯体感觉纤维). The somata of these neurons are located in the superior ganglion of glossopharyngeal nerve (舌咽神经上神经节), and the peripheral process is distributed to the skin behind the ear. The central process terminates in the spinal nucleus of trigeminal nerve (三叉神经脊束核).

The roots of the glossopharyngeal nerve are attached to the upper part of the posterior lateral sulci of the medulla oblongata (retroolivary sulcus). The glosso-pharyngeal nerve exits the skull through the anteromedial part of the jugular foramen, anterior to the vagus and accessory nerves, and is enclosed in a separate dural sheath. The main branches are as follows: The lingual branch is distributed to the mucosa and taste buds of the posterior 1/3 of the tongue; the pharyngeal branch(咽支) conducts sensory of the pharyngeal mucosa and participating in the pharyngeal reflex activities; the tympanic nerve (鼓室神经) supplies the mucosa of the tympanic cavity, pharyngotympanic tube and mastoid air cells, conducting general visceral sensation; the lesser petrosal nerve (岩小神经) exits the middle cranial fossa via the foramen ovale to join the otic ganglion (耳神经节), and its postganglionic fibers innervate the parotid gland; the branch of the carotid sinus (颈动脉窦支)to the wall of the carotid sinus (颈动脉窦) and the carotid glomus (颈动脉小球). It carries the stimulation of changes in arterial pressure and carbon dioxide concentration in the blood into the center, reflexively regulating blood pressure and respiration; the tonsillaris plexus (扁桃体丛) is formed by the tonsillar branches (扁桃体支)and the stylopharyngeal branch (茎突咽肌支), which supplies the stylopharyngeus.

10. Vagus Nerve (迷走神经)

The vagus nerve is a large mixed nerve with a more extensive distribution than any other cranial nerves, running through the neck, the thorax and the abdomen. It contains five fiber components. i) General visceral motor fibers (一般内脏运动纤维). The parasympathetic fibers originate from the dorsal nucleus of the vagus nerve (迷走神经背核) in the medulla oblongata. They travel to the pulmonary, cardiac, oesophageal, gastric and intestinal branches, synapse in minute ganglia in the visceral walls. ii) Special visceral motor fibers (特殊内脏运动纤维) arise from the nucleus ambiguus in the medulla oblongata and are distributed to the muscles of the pharynx. iii) General visceral sense fibers (一般内脏感觉纤维) carry sensation from thoracic and abdominal viscera and end in the nucleus solitarius of the medulla. Their cell bodies are located in the inferior ganglion of vagus nerve (迷走神经下神经节) below the jugular foramen. iv)General somatic sense fibers (一般躯体感觉纤维). Their cell bodies are in the superior ganglion of the vagus nerve (迷走神经上神经节). The central process terminates in the spinal nucleus of the trigeminal nerve (三叉神经脊束核). The peripheral process is distributed to the dura, behind the auricle and the skin of the external acoustic meatus along with the branches of the vagus nerve, conducting general sensation.

The vagus nerve is attached to the middle of the retroolivary sulcus of the medulla oblongata and exits the skull through the jugular foramen located behind the glossopharyngeal nerve. The vagus descends vertically in the neck within the carotid sheath, situated between the internal jugular vein and the internal carotid artery or common carotid artery, reaching the root of the neck, and continuing into the thorax through the thoratic inlet. The course of the vagus nerve differs between the two sides in the thorax. The left vagus (左迷走神经) enters the thorax between the left common carotid and subclavian arteries. It crosses the left side of the aortic arch, and then passes posterior to the left lung hilum. It continues descending anteriorly on the oesophagus, gives off many branches which join with a ramus from the left pulmonary plexus (左肺丛) and the anterior oesophageal plexus (食管前丛). In the lower part of the esophagus, the anterior vagal trunk (迷走神经前

干), which contains nerve fibers from both vagus nerves, leaves the plexus and passes inferiorly on the posterior surface of the oesophagus. It enters the abdomen by passing through the oesophageal hiatus in the respiratory diaphragm, and is distributed in the anterior wall of the stomach, as well as liver and gallbladder. The right vagus nerve (右迷走神经) desends along the right side of the trachea through the right subclavian artery and the vein, and reaches behind the esophagus behind the right lung hilum. It gives off branches to form the right pulmonary plexus (右肺丛) and the posterior oesophageal plexus (食管后丛). In the lower part of the esophagus, the posterior vagal trunk (迷走神经后干), containing nerve fibres from both vagus nerves, passes inferiorly on the anterior surface of the oesophagus and enters the abdomen through the oesophageal hiatus, and distributes in the posterior wall of the stomach. The terminal branches of the vagus nerve are the celiac branches, together with the sympathetic nerve, forms the coeliac plexus (腹腔丛). These branches distribute in the abdominal organ. The vagus nerve gives off many branches along the way. The main branches are as follows:

(1) **Vagus nerve in the neck**

1) The superior laryngeal nerve (喉上神经) originates from the inferior vagal ganglion. The superior laryngeal nerve descends toward the internal carotid artery, and is divided into internal and external branches at the greater cornu of the hyoid. The small external branches are motor branches with special visceral motor fibers. It descends alongside the superior thyroid artery and innervates the cricothyroid. The internal branch, also known as the internal laryngeal nerve, is the sensory branch. It enters the larynx, and is distributed to the base of the tongue, the epiglottis, the pharynx and the laryngeal mucosa above the vocal folds, conducting general visceral sensation.

2) The cervical cardiac branches (颈心支) consists of the superior cervical cardiac branches (颈上心支) and the inferior cervical cardiac branches (颈下心支), which descend into the thorax on both sides of the larynx and trachea. They form the cardiac plexuses (心丛) in conjunction with the branches of the cervical sympathetic trunk toregulate cardiac activity. The superior cervical cardiac branches has a small branch called the aortic nerve (主动脉神经) or the aortic depressor nerve (减压神经), which is located in the wall of the aortic arch and senses changes in blood pressure and blood chemistry.

3) The auricular branch (耳支) (Arnold's nerve) arises from the superior vagal ganglion, contains general somatic sensory fibers. It is distributed to the skin of part of the ear and to the external acoustic meatus.

4) The pharyngeal branch (咽支) arises from the inferior vagal ganglion, contains general visceral sensory and special visceral motor fibers. Together with the phary-ngeal branch of glossopharyngeal nerve and the sympathetic trunk, it forms the pharyngeal

plexus, which supplies all the muscles of the soft palate and all the muscles and mucosa of the pharynx.

5) The meningeal branches (脑膜支) originate from the superior vagal ganglion and pass through the jugular foramen to be distributed to the dura mater in the posterior cranial fossa.

(2) Vagus nerve in the thorax

1) The recurrent laryngeal nerve (喉返神经). The nerve differs in origin and course on the two sides. The right recurrent laryngeal nerve (右喉返神经) almost always arises from the right vagus trunk in front of the right subclavian artery, and then loops down and backward around this artery to ascend and return to the neck. The left recurrent laryngeal nerve (左喉返神经) arises from the vagus on the left of the aortic arch, curves below the aortic arch and rises back to the neck. On both sides, the recurrent laryngeal nerve ascends along or near the tracheo-oesophageal groove, reaching the deep side of the lateral lobe of the thyroid gland and enters the throat behind the cricothyroid joint. The terminal branch is called the inferior laryngeal nerve (喉下神经), which carries special visceral motor fibers supply all the laryngeal muscles except cricothyroid. The generalvisceral sensory fibers are distributed in the laryngeal mucosa below the vocal folds. The recurrent laryngeal nerve also sends out the cardiac (心支), the tracheal branch (气管支) and the oesoph-ageal branch (食管支) during its course, which are involved in the formation of the cardiac, pulmonary and esophageal plexus respectively.

During thyroid surgery, the recurrent laryngeal nerve should be protected when the inferior thyroid artery is clamped or ligation. Damage to one side recurrent laryngeal nerve leads to hoarseness; Simultaneous damage to both recurrent laryngeal nerves causes loss of voice, an difficulty in breathing, and even asphyxia.

2) The tracheal branch and the oesophageal branch (支气管支和食管支) are small branches of both the left and the right vagus nerves in the thorax. Together with the branches of the sympathetic nerves, they form the pulmonary plexus (肺丛)and the esophageal plexus (食管丛). Thin branches given out from the plexuses are distributed in the trachea, the bronchus, the lungs, and the esophagus. These branches contain the general visceral sensory fibers and the general visceral motor fibers, conducts the corresponding organs and pleura sensation, controls smooth muscle activity and gland secretion.

(3) Vagus nerve in the abdomen

After entering the abdominal cavity, the vagus nerve contains only general visceral motor fibers (parasympathetic fibers) and general visceral sensory fibers. The left vagal trunk is divided into anterior gastric branches and hepatic branches near the front of the cardia. The right vagal trunk is divided into the posterior gastric branches and the celiac branches near the rear of the cardiac.

1) Anterior gastric branches (胃前支) arise from the anterior vagal trunk near the cardia and run to the right along the lesser curvature of the stomach. Along the way gives out the cardia branch, and anterior wall gastric branches are distributed to the anterior wall of the stomach. The terminal branch contributes to the anterior wall of the pyloric part with a "crow's foot" shape.

2) Hepatic branches (肝支). The anterior vagal trunk gives off a hepatic branch, which passes to the right between the two layers of the lesser omentum. It joins with the branch of the sympathetic nerve to form the heaptic plexus. The hepatic plexus gives out branch innervates the liver and the gallbladder along with the branches of the proper hepatic arteries.

3) Posterior gastric branches (胃后支) arise from the posterior vagal trunk near the cardia and run along the back of the lesser curvature of the stomach towards the pylorus. Along the way, the fundus of stomach branch is given off and posterior wall gastric branches are distributed to the posterior wall of the stomach. The terminal branch contributes to the anterior wall of the pyloric part with a "crow's foot" shape.

4) Celiac branches (腹腔支) are the terminal branch of the posterior vagal trunk. They run to the right near the celiac trunk and form the coeliac plexus (腹腔丛)together with the sympathetic nerve. The coeliac plexus gives off branches that are distributed to the liver, the gallbladder, the pancreas, the spleen, the kidney, and above the left curvature of the colon along with the branches of the celiac trunk, the superior mesenteric artery and the renal artery.

The vagus nerve is an important part of the parasympathetic nervous system with a more extensive course and distribution than any other cranial nerves. The damage to the vagus nerve trunk can disrupt visceral function, manifesting as pulse speed, palpitations, nausea, vomiting, deep and slow breathing, and even suffocation. Because one side of the palatine muscle is paralyzed, the uvula may be biased to the unaffected side.

11. Accessory Nerve (副神经)

The accessory nerve is a motor cranial nerve composed of special visceral motor fibers and consists of two parts: the cranial root (颅根) and the spinal root (脊髓根). The cranial root arises from the lower part of the nucleus ambiguous of the medulla oblongata. It exits the brain from the post-olivary groove below the vagus nerve roots, and then travels the skull through the jugular foramen together with the spinal root of the accessory nerves. The cranial roots then join the vagus nerve, its branches innervate the throat muscles. It is now believed that the nerve fibers that make up the extracranial segment of the accessory nerve mainly originate from the spinal roots. The spinal root arises from the accessory nucleus of the cervical segments of the spinal cord. It exits from the spinal cord between the anterior and posterior roots of the spinal nerve. The spinal root ascends within the vertebral canal and enters the skull via the foramen magnum. The cranial and spinal roots join, either before or within the jugular foramen, forming a bundle that divides into internal and external branches on leaving the jugular foramen. It runs posterolaterally and passes either medial or lateral to the internal jugular vein, reaches the upper part of sternocleido-mastoid and enters its deep surface. The final branch which passes above the posterior margin of the sternocleidomastoid, enters the deep surface of the trapezius at a point on the anterior border of trapezius above the clavicle, where it innervates the trapezius.

An injury to the spinal root of the accessory nerve results in paralysis of the sternocleidomastoid muscle, causing inability to bend the head ipsilateral to the affected side, and inability to turn the face contralateral. Additionally, due to the loss of the great suspensory muscle, trapezius, the scapula drops down and away from the spinal column.

Jugular foramen syndrome (颈静脉孔综合征): Because the glossopharyngeal, vagus and accessory nerve all exit the skull through the jugular foramen, the lesions at the jugular foramen often involve the above three pairs of cranial nerves, so that their function is impaired, resulting in the jugular foramen syndrome

Accessory nerve transplantation (副神经移植术): Due to the relatively constant position of the accessory nerve from the sternocleidomastoid posterior margin superior, the middle 1/3 junction to the junction of the middle and lower 1/3 of the trapezius anterior edge, and without muscle or important blood vessels on the surface, a part of the accessory nerve fiber bundle is often collected. This portion can be anastomosied with the facial nerve to treat facial nerve injury.

12. Hypoglosal Nerve (舌下神经)

The hypoglossal nerve is a motor cranial nerve composed of general somatic motor fibers. The hypoglossal nerve arises from the hypoglossal nucleus located in the medulla oblongata, and exits the brain from the anterolateral sulci of the medulla oblongata with a number of filaments. The nerve exits the skull laterally through the hypoglossal tube, then moves forward and down in the arch between the internal jugular vein and the internal carotid artery. It reaches the superficial surface of the hyoglossus across the internal and external carotid arteries. The hypoglossal nerve penetrates the genioglossus below the lingual nerve and the submandibular duct, and enters the tongue. The hypoglossal nerve is motor to all the muscles of the tongue except palatoglossus.

If one side of the hypoglossal nerve is completely damaged, it results in unilateral lingual paralysis, the protruded tongue to deviate towards the paralyzed side. If the lingual muscle is paralyzed for a long time, atrophy will eventual be caused.

Cerebral nerve components, including initial-terminatal nuclei, distribution, and post-injury symptoms are summarized in Table 10-2.

Table 10-2 Cerebral nerve components, initial-terminatal nuclei, distribution, and post-injury symptoms

Name	Composition	Initial nucleus	Terminating nucleus	Distribution	Post-injury symptom
I Olfactory nerve	Special visceral sensory fibers		Olfactory bulb	Olfactory mucosa of nasal cavity	Olfactory disturbance
II Optic nerve	Special somatic sensory fibers		Lateral geniculate body	Retina	Visual impairment
III Oculomotor nerve	General somatic motor fibers	Nucleus of oculomotor nerve		Superior, inferior and medial rectus and inferior oblique levator palpebrae superioris	Ptosis, pupil oblique outward and lower
	General visceral motor fibers (parasympathetic fibers)	Accessory oculomotor nucleus (E-W nucleus)		Aphincter pupillae, ciliary muscle	Pupil dilation, light reflection disappeared, Lens regulation disorders
IV Trochlear nerve	General somatic motor fibers	Nucleus of trochlear nerve		superior oblique	The eyes shouldn't strabismus outward or downward
V Trigeminal nerve	General somatic sensory fibers		Spinal nucleus of trigeminal nerve, mesencephalic nucleus oftrigeminal nerve, pontine nucleus oftrigeminal nerve	Cephalic and facial skin, oral and nasal mucosa, teeth and teeth Gingival, eyeball, dura mater	Cephalic and facial dysesthesia
	Special visceral motor fibers	Motor nucleus of trigeminal nerve		Masticatory muscles, tensor tympani, tensor veli palatini, mylohyoid and the anterior belly of digastric	Paralysis of the masticatory muscles

(To be continued)

333

Table 10-2

Name	Composition	Initial nucleus	Terminating nucleus	Distribution	Post-injury symptom
VI Abducens nerve	General somatic motor fibers	Nucleus of abducent nerve		External rectus muscle	Esotropia
	General somatic sensory fibers		Spinal nucleus of trigeminal nerve	Skin of the ear	Sensory disturbance
	Special visceral motor fibers	Nucleus of facial nerve		Posterior belly of digastric, stylohyoid, stapedius, facial muscles, platysma,	Absence of the frontal striae on the injured side, inability to close the eyes, the shallow nasolabial groove, the angle of the mouth tends to the unaffected side
VII Facial nerve	General visceral motor fibres	Superior salivatory nucleus		Mandibular gland, sublingual gland, lacrimal gland, palatine, pharyngeal and nasal mucous glands	Gland secretion disorders
	Special visceral sensory fibers		Upper part of the nucleus of the solitary tract	Taste buds from the anterior two-thirds of the tongue	Taste disorders from the anterior two-thirds of the tongue
VIII Vestibulocochlear nerve	Special somatic sensory fibers		Vestibular nuclei	Macular sacculi, macular utriculi, crista ampullaris	Vertigo, nystagmus
	Special somatic sensory fibers		Cochlear nuclei	The spiral organ	Hearing impairment

(To be continued)

Table 10-2

Name	Composition	Initial nucleus	Terminating nucleus	Distribution	Post-injury symptom
IX Glossopharyngeal nerve	Special visceral motor fibers	Nucleus ambiguus	Nucleus of solitary tract	Stylopharyngeus	Gland secretion disorders
	General visceral motor fibers (parasympathetic fibers)	Inferior salivertory nucleus		The parotid gland	
	General visceral sensory fibers			Tympanic cavity, pharyngotympanic tube, fauces and mucosa of the posterior (postsulcal) third of the tongue, carotid sinus, carotid glomus	Sensory disturbances in fauces and 1/3 of the posterior region of the tongue, Disappearance of pharyngeal reflex
	Special visceral sensory fibers		Upper part of nucleus of solitary tract	Taste buds of the posterior 1/3 of the tongue	Loss of taste in 1/3 of the posterior region of the tongue
	General somatic sensory fibers		Spinal nucleus of trigeminal nerve	Skin behind the ear	Sensory disturbances in the distribution area

(To be continued)

Table 10-2

Name	Composition	Initial nucleus	Terminating nucleus	Distribution	Post-injury symptom
X Vagus nerve	General visceral motor fibers (parasympathetic fibers)	Dorsal nucleus of vagus n.		Smooth muscle, myocardial and gland in the neck, thorax and abdomen.	Rapid heartbeat, dysfunction of internal organs
	Special visceral motor fibers	Nucleus ambiguus		Laryngeal muscle	Dysphonia, hoarseness, swallowing disorders
	General visceral sensory fibers		Nucleus of solitary tract	Organs in the neck, thorax and abdomen. throat mucosa	Sensory disturbances in the distribution area
	General somatic sensory fibers		spinal nucleus of trigeminal nerve	The dura, behind the auricle and the skin of the external acoustic meatus	Sensory disturbances in the distribution area
XI Accessory nerve	Special visceral motor fibers	Nucleus ambiguous (brain), accessory nucleus (Spinal cord)		Laryngeal muscle, Sternocleidomastoid, trapezius	Laryngeal muscle dysfunction, sternocleidomastoid paralysis, head weakness to turn to the contralateral; Trapezius paralysis, shoulder droop, shoulder lift weakness
XII Hypoglossal nerve	General somatic motor fibers	Nucleus of hypoglossal nerve		All the muscles of the tongue except palatoglossus	Tongue muscles paralysis and atrophy, the protruded tongue deviates to the paralysed side

（浙江中医药大学　付笑笑）

10.3 Visceral Nerve

The visceral nervous system (内脏神经系统) is a component of the peripheral nervous system (周围神经系统) that controls the glands, cardiac and smooth muscle of all the internal organs (viscera) unconsciously. For this reason, it is called the autonomic nervous system (自主神经系统) or the vegetative nervous system (植物神经系统) (Fig.10-15). It contains two components: the sensory nerve and the motor nerve. Visceral sensory nerves (内脏感觉神经) are distributed in visceral and cardiovascular visceral receptors, and the primary neurons are in the brain ganglia and spinal ganglia. These visceral receptors can receive various stimuli and transmit them to visceral sensory centers through visceral sensory nerves.

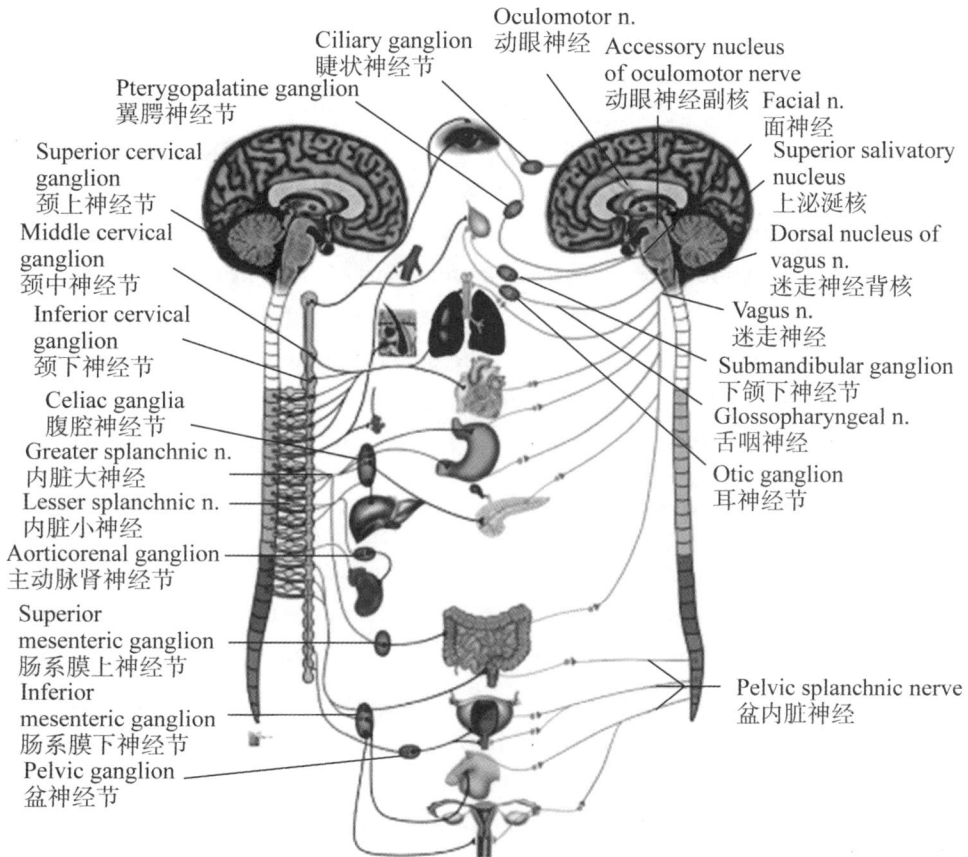

Fig.10-15 Autonomic nerve

There are many differences between the visceral motor nerve and the somatic motor nerve both in morphology and function. The differences in morphology and structure are mainly shown in the following aspects. i) The difference in the objects of innervation: The somatic motor nerve innervates the skeletal muscle, whereas the visceral motor nerve innervates the smooth muscle, myocardium and glands. ii) The difference in fiber components: The somatic motor nerve has only one fiber component, whereas the visceral motor nerve consist of two fiber components: sympathetic and parasympathetic. Most visceral organs are both receive sympathetic and parasympathetic innervation. iii) The difference in the number of neurons: The somatic motor nerve consists of only one neuron from the anterior horn of the spinal cord, while the visceral motor nerve involves two neurons from the lower center to the effector: The first neuron is located in the visceral efferent nuclei of the brainstem and in the lateral horn of the spinal cord which is called preganglionic neuron (节前神经元), their axons are called preganglionic fiber (节前纤维). The second neuron is located in the peripheral vegetative ganglion which is called the postganglionic neuron(节后神经元), their axons are called the postganglionic fiber (节后纤维). iv) The diffe-rence in distribution forms: The somatic motor nerve is distributed directly in the effector in the form of nerve trunk, whereas the postganglionic fibers of the visceral motor nerve are often attached to organs or blood vessels to form a nerve plexus, which then branches out to innervate in the smooth muscle, myocardium and glands. v) The differences in fiber types: The somatic motor nerves typically consist of thick myelinated fibers, while the visceral motor nerves comprise thin myelinated (preganglionic fibers) and unmyelinated (postganglionic fibers) fine fibers. vi) The different degrees of consciousness control: The somatic motor nerve often controls the effector under the control of human consciousness, whereas the visceral motor nerve is unconsciously.

Visceral Motor Nerves

Visceral motor nerves (内脏运动神经) are traditionally divided into the sympathetic nerve (交感神经) for the fight, and the parasympathetic nerve (副交感神经) for the rest (digest). There are some significant differences between the sympathetic and parasympathetic nerves in terms of their nerve origins, morphological structure, distribution area, and function. i) The differences of low centers: The low centers of sympathetic nerves are located in the lateral nuclei of T1—L3 spinal cord. In contrast, the lower centers of parasympa-thetic nerves are located in the general visceral motor nucleus of the brainstem and in the sacral parasympathetic nucleus of the S2—S4 spinal cord. ii) Differences in the locations of the peripheral ganglia: Sympathetic ganglia divides into paravertebral and prevertebral ganglia, which are located at the sides of the spine and anterior to the spine, respectively. Parasympathetic ganglia are divided into parasympathetic and intra-organ ganglia, which are located near the innervated organ or within the organ wall, respectively. Thus, the preganglionic fibers of the parasympathetic nerve are longer than those of the sympathetic nerve, while the postganglionic fibers of the parasympathetic nerve are shorter. iii) The difference in the ratios of preganglionic to postganglionic neurons: The axon of a sympathetic preganglionic neuron constitutes synapse with several postganglionic neurons, whereas the axon of a parasympathetic preganglionic neurons constitutes synapses with a fewer postganglionic neuron. Thus, sympathetic nerves have a broader range of innervation, whereas parasympathetic nerves have a limited range of innervation. iv) Differences in distribution: The distribution of the sympathetic nerveshave more extensive distribution, affecting the head, neck, the thoracic and abdominal organs, but also in the blood vessels, glands, and erector spinae of the body. The parasym-pathetic nerves, however, are less widespread, with most of the blood vessels, sweat glands, erector pili muscles and adrenal medulla lacking parasympathetic nerves fibers. v) Different effects on the same organ: The sympathetic and parasym-pathetic nerves have both antagonistic and unifying effects on the same organ. For example, during a in "fight or flight" response, the sympathetic nervous system is excited, while the parasympathetic nerve (rest and digest) is inhibited causing an increased heart rate, blood pressure, bronchial dilation, pupil dilation, while digestive activity is inhibited, indicating that the body's metabo-lism is increased and energy expenditure is accelerated to adapt to the drastic changes in the environment. Conversely, in a resting or sleeping state, the parasympathetic nerves are excited while the sympathetic nerves are inhibited, resulting in a slower heartbeat, lower blood pressure, bronchial constriction, narrowed pupils and enhanced digestive activity, which are conducive to physical recovery and energy storage.

1. Sympathetic Nerve

The lower center of the sympathetic nerve (交感神经) is located in the medial lateral nucleus of the gray matter lateral in (T1—L3) spinal cord segments, from which pregang-lionic fibers emanate. The peripheral part of the sympathetic nerve consists of the communicating branch, the sympathetic trunk, the sympathetic ganglion, the branches from the sympathetic ganglion and the sympathetic plexus.

According to the position of the sympathetic ganglia, it can be divided into the paravertebral ganglia (椎旁神经节) and the prevertebral ganglion (椎前神经节). There are 19 to 24 paravertebral ganglia which are connected by two sympathetic trunks (交感干), also called ganglion of the sympathetic trunk (交感干神经节). The left and right sympathetic trunks travel along both sides of the spine and merge in front of the coccyx. The sympathetic trunk can divides into the cervical, thoracic, lumbar, sacral, and caudal regions, containing a number of ganglia as follows: 3—4 ganglia in the cervical region, 10—12 ganglia in the thoracic region, 4 ganglia in the lumbar region, 2—3 ganglia in the sacral region, and 1 ganglion in the caudal region. The prevertebral ganglia mainly consists of the celiac ganglion (腹腔神经节), the superior mesenteric ganglion (肠系膜上神经节), the inferior mesenteric ganglion (肠系膜下神经节) and the aorticorenal ganglion (主动脉肾神经节). The preganglionic fibers emanate from the lower sympathetic center as splanchnic nerve, then cross the paravertebral ganglion to end in these prevertebral ganglia (Fig.10-16).

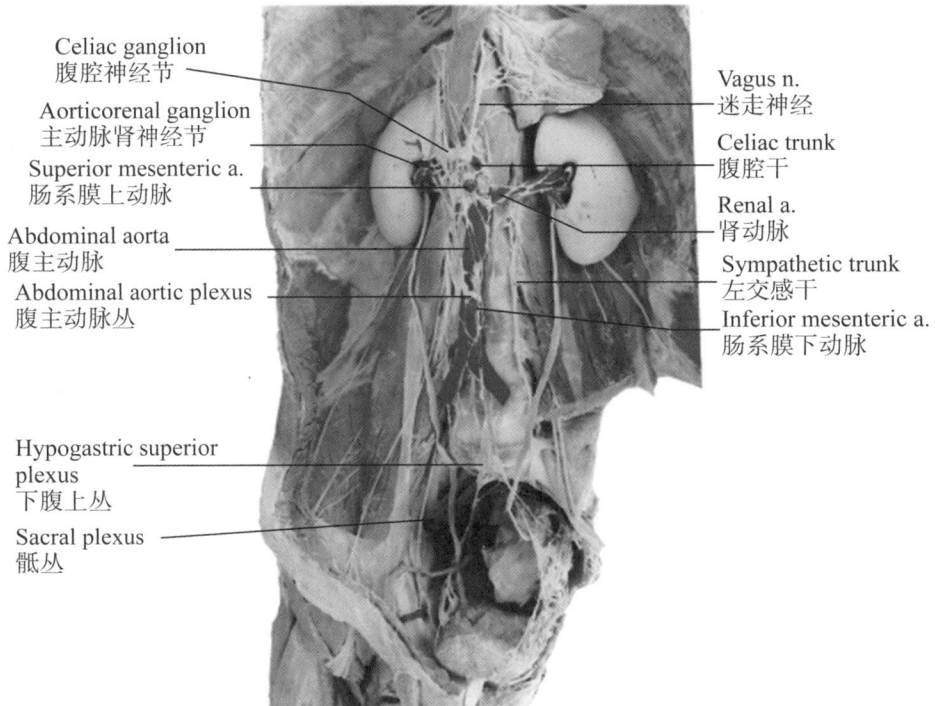

Celiac ganglion 腹腔神经节
Aorticorenal ganglion 主动脉肾神经节
Superior mesenteric a. 肠系膜上动脉
Abdominal aorta 腹主动脉
Abdominal aortic plexus 腹主动脉丛
Hypogastric superior plexus 下腹上丛
Sacral plexus 骶丛
Vagus n. 迷走神经
Celiac trunk 腹腔干
Renal a. 肾动脉
Sympathetic trunk 左交感干
Inferior mesenteric a. 肠系膜下动脉

Fig.10-16　The ganglion of the abdominal cavity

The communicating branches connect between the ganglia with the correspon-ding spinal nerve. They are classfied into white communicating branches (白交通支)and grey communicating branches (灰交通支). The white communicating branches consist of preganglionic fibers, which mainly composed of myelinated fibers (pregang-lionic fibers). These branches exist between the anterior branch of the T1－L3 spinal nerve and the corresponding sympathetic ganglion. The gray communicating branch is the postganglionic fibers, which composed by unmyelinated fibers. These branches connect the sympathetic trunk and 31 pairs of anterior branches of spinal nerves.

(1) Destination of preganglionic nerve fibers and postganglionic nerve fibers

The white communicating branches (preganglionic nerve fibers) originate from the lateral horn of the spinal cord. These fibers enter the sympathetic trunk through the anterior root of the spinal nerve, the spinal nerve trunk and the communicating branch. After entering the sympathetic trunk, they have three different destinations: terminating at the corresponding ganglion of the sympathetic trunk, ascending or descending in the sympathetic trunk, and then terminating at the upper or the lower paravertebral ganglion of the sympathetic trunk. It is generally believed that pregang-lionic fibers from the middle lateral nucleus of the upper thoracic segment of the spinal cord (T1—T5) ascend within the sympathetic trunk to the cervical region and preganglionic fibers from the lower thoracic and lumbar segments (T11—L3) descend within the sympathetic trunk to exchange neurons within sympathetic ganglia in the lumbosacral region. These fibers pass through the paravertebral ganglia to constitute greater splanchnic nerve (T5—T9 thoracic sympathetic ganglia which terminates at the celiac ganglia and the lesser splanchnic nerve (T10—T11 thoracic sympathetic ganglia) terminating in the aorticorenal or superior mesenteric ganglia. The least splanchnic nerves (T11—T12 thoracic sympathetic ganglia) join the renal ganglia, contributing to the sympathetic innervation for the renal plexus.

The grey communicating branches (postganglionic nerve fibers) from the sympa-thetic ganglion also have various destinations. These fibers return to the spinal nerve through the gray communication branches, and are distributed to the blood vessels, sweat glands and arrector pili muscles of the trunk and limbs along with the spinal nerve. Additionally, the nerve plexus is composed of the winding arteries, which distribute to the innervated organs along with the artery branches and the sympa-thetic ganglia branch is given out to distribute directly to the organs they innervate.

The distribution of preganglionic and postganglionic nerve fibers of the sympathetic nerve has a certain pattern, which can be summarized as follows: Preganglionic fibers originate from the lateral horn of the T1—T5 segment of the spinal cord, and their postganglionic fibers are distributed in the head, cervical, thoracic organs and upper limbs; preganglionic fibers originate from the lateral horn of the T5—T12 segment of the spinal cord, their postganglionic fibers are distributed in the liver,the pancrea, the kidney, the spleen and the digestive tract above the left curvature of the colon and thoracoabdominal wall; preganglionic fibers originate from the lateral horn of L1—L3 segment of the spinal cord, their postganglionic fibers are distributed in the digestive tract below the left curvature of the colon, the pelvic viscera and the lower extremities.

(2) Parasympathetic nerve

The lower centers of the parasympathetic nerve are located in the parasym-pathetic nucleus in the brainstem and the gray matter of S2—S4 of the sacral parasympathetic nucleus in the spinal cord, and their postganglionic fibers reach the innervated organ.

Parasympathetic ganglia are mostly located near or within the walls of the organs which are called parasympathetic ganglia (器官旁节) and intra-organ ganglia(器官内节), respectively. The parasympathetic ganglia located in the cranial region is larger, such as the ciliary ganglia, the submandibular ganglia, the pterygopalatine ganglia and the otic ganglia. In contrast, the parasympathetic ganglia in other parts of the body are smaller and difficult to distinguish with the naked eye and can only be seen under a microscope, which include the parasympathetic ganglia located in the cardiac plexus, pulmonary plexus, bladder plexus, utero-vaginal plexus, and the intra-organ ganglia located in the walls of the bronchi and digestive tubes.

1)Cranial parasympathetic nerve. The preganglionic fibers of cranial parasympathetic nerves originate from the parasympathetic nucleus of the brainstem and participate in the composition of CN - Ⅲ , Ⅶ , Ⅸ and Ⅹ pairs of cerebral nerves. Edinger-Westphal nucleus (accessory oculomotor nucleus) sends preganglionic fibers into oculomotor nerve, arrives in the ciliary ganglion in the orbit where they synapse. The postganglionic fibers enter the eyes, innervating pupillary sphincter that constricts the pupil and ciliary muscle that controls the shape of the lens in the eye. Stimulation of these muscles causes, the lens "balls up", bending light to focus on close objects. This process is called accommodation. The superior salivary nucleus sends preganglionic fibers into facial nerve, then travels through the greater petrosal nerve to the pterygopalatine ganglion where they synapse. The postganglionic fibers then innervate in the lacrimal gland and the glands of the nasal, oral and palatal mucosa. Some preganglionic fibers join the lingual nerve to the submandibular ganglion, and their postganglionic fibers are distributed in the submandibular and sublingual glands. The inferior salivary nucleus sends preganglionic fibers into glossopharyngeal nerve, which projects to the otic ganglion. Then, the postganglionic fibers of this ganglion project to the salivary parotid gland on which they have a secretory effect. The dorsal nucleus of the vagus nerve sends preganglionic fibers into the vagus nerve and follows its branches to reach numerous parasympathetic ganglia around and within the organs of the thorax and abdomen. The postganglionic fibers are distributed in the thoracic and abdominal organs (the lungs, the heart, the liver, the spleen, the pancreas, and the gastrointestinal tract up to the splenic flexure of the large intestine).

2) Sacral parasympathetic nerves originate from the sacral parasympathetic nucleus in S1 — S4 segments of the spinal cord, and they exit the presacral foramen with the sacral nerve. After leaving the sacral nerve, they form the pelvic visceral nerve, which is added to the pelvic plexus and distributed with the pelvic plexus in the pelvic organs. These fibers synapse in the parasympathetic ganglia near or in the organ wall, and its postganglionic fibers innervate the digestive tract below the left curvature of the colon and pelvic organs.

(3) Visceral sensory nerves

1) Distribution of visceral sensory nerves (内脏感觉神经). General visceral afferent (GVA) which transmit sensory information from the viscera to the central nervous system

(CNS) goes together with the visceral efferent (sympathetic and parasympathetic) fibers. They are primarily pseudounipolar neurons. The cell bodies of GVA fibers are typically located in the dorsal root of the spinal cord or within the cranial nerves. These GVA cell bodies are, for the most part, extracranial, except for the GVA fibers of the trigeminal nerve, whose nucleus lies with in the brainstem. The cell body controls all neuronal functions and allows information to pass between the receptive distal part and the centrally projecting part. The peripheral processes of GVA fibers are myelinated or unmyelinated fibers and varyin thickness. The vast majority of the visceral afferent fibers are thin Aδ and C fibers. In general, fibers conducting signals from visceral nociceptors follow the sympathetic nerves, whereas the parasympathetic nerves contain fibers conducting from other kinds of receptors. The center can regulate the activity of the visceral organs directly through the visceral motor nerves or indirectly through the humoral regulation. These afferent fibers connect directly or via intermediate neurons with visceral motor neurons, completing visceral-visceral reflexes. They can also synapse with somatic motor neurons, forming visceral-somatic reflexes.

2) Characteristics of visceral nociception. High pain threshold: The number of visceral sensory fibers is small and most of them are fine fibers, therefore, the pain threshold is high and it is difficult to produce subjective sensation for stimuli of general intensity. Visceral nerves are not sensitive to cutting or burning stimuli. However, visceral sensation can be produced when the organ undergoes more intense activity. Conscious sensations arising from the viscera, in addition to pain, include organ filling, bloating and distension, dyspnea, and nausea, whereas somatic afferent activity gives rise to sensations such as touch, pinch, heat, cutting, crush, and vibration. Both sensory systems can detect chemical stimuli.

Inaccurate localization: The afferent pathway of visceral sensation is relatively decentralized, meaning that sensory fibers from one organ enter the center through multiple segments of spinal nerves. Moreover, a single spinal nerve contains sensory fibers from several organs. As a result, visceral pain is often diffuse and inaccurate. For example, nociceptive fibers from the heart enter the spinal cord along with sympathetic nerves (mainly the central and subcardiac nerves) via the first to the fifth thoracic nerves, while nociceptive fibers from the kidney, ureter and some pelvic organs enter the spinal cord along with sympathetic nerves via the T11－L2 spinal nerves.

Finally, visceral pain is commonly accompanied by greater emotional valence and exaggerated autonomic reflexes. The emotional response is a central pheno-menon and should not be confused with nociception.

3) Referred pain (牵涉性痛). Referred pain is a sensation of hypersensitivity or pain in a specific area of the body's surface when certain internal organs are diseased. Spinal

neurons that receive visceral input also receive convergent input from skin or deeper structures (including other viscera), producing referred pain. For example, cardiac pain (angina) is typically referred to the left arm and shoulder (but skin, joint, or muscle pain is not referred from shoulder to heart). Referred pain can occur in the area of the skin adjacent to the diseased organ, or in the area of the skin far from the diseased organ. For example, in angina pectoris, pain is often felt in the anterior thoracic region and the skin of the left medial arm, and in hepatobiliary disease, pain is often felt in the right shoulder.

Current knowledge indicates that referred pain occurs because multiple primary sensory neurons converge on a single ascending tract in the spinal cord. When painful stimuli activate visceral receptors, the brain is unable to distinguish between the visceral signals and somatic signals; the brain interprets that the pain is coming from somatic regions (e. g., skin, skeletal musculature, and bones) of the body rather than the visceral regions (i.e., spleen, kidney, and heart). For example, patients with angina pectoris, a type of cardiac pain, experience referred pain in the chest and the upper left arm.

(杭州市第一人民医院　徐麟皓)

Exercise

1. A 6-year-old girl was diagnosed with pneumonia. Penicillin sodium was injected in the upper outer quadrant of the buttock. Which of the following nerves should be avoided injuring?

(A) The femoral nerve.

(B) The lateral femoral cutaneous nerve.

(C) The obturator nerve.

(D) The sciatic nerve.

(E) The superior gluteal nerve.

2. A 47-year-old man complains that his scrotum was unconscious. Which of the following nerves was most likely affected?

(A) The genitofemoral nerve.

(B) The iliohypogastric nerve.

(C) The ilioinguinal nerve.

(D) The lateral cutaneous nerve.

(E) The pudendal nerve.

Answer

1. The correct answer is D.

The sciatic nerve (Choice D) is the longest and largest branch of the sacral plexus. It exists the pelves through the infrapiriform foramen, and travels beneath the middle point of the line between the ischial tuberosity and the greater trochanter of femur down to the posterior thigh. In order to prevent damage to the sciatic nerve, intragluteal injection is given in the upper, outer quadrant of the buttocks. The other nerves, including the femoral nerve (Choice A), the lateral femoral cutaneous nerve (Choice B), the obturator nerve (Choice C) and the superior gluteal nerve (Choice E), are not vulnerable to be injured during intragluteal injection.

2. The correct answer is C.

The ilioinguinal nerve (Choice C) distributes sensory filaments to the skin of the scrotum and the medial thigh.

The genitofemoral nerve (Choice A) consists of the first and the second lumbar nerve roots which distribute motor fibers to the cremaster muscle and a small area of skin on thigh.

The cutaneous branches of the iliohypogastric nerve (Choice B) distributes to the skin of the anterior lower abdominal wall. The muscular branches of the iliohypo-gastric nerve innervate the abdominal muscles.

The lateral cutaneous nerve (Choice D) of the thigh distributes to the skin over the lateral surface of the thigh. The pudendal nerve (Choice E) gives off branches that distribute to the external anal the sphincter.

Chapter 11 Neural Pathways of Nervous System

CNS communicates with body structures via pathways. Neural pathways that connect the spinal cord and the brain are called the ascending which carry sensory information from the peripheral to the brain and descending tracts which transmit motor information from the brain or brainstem to the spinal cord. For example, how sensation from your fingertips reaches your brain and how conscious and reflexive actions return to your fingers.

11.1 General Introduction

The general senses include touch (ranging from light to discriminative), pressure, vibration, pain, thermal sensation and proprioception (perception of posture and movement). Stimuli from the external and internal environments activate a diverse range of receptors in the skin, fascia, viscera, muscles, bones, tendons and joints. Afferent impulses from the trunk and limbs are conveyed to the spinal cord in spinal nerves, while those from the head are carried to the brain in cranial nerves.

Ascending (somatosensory) pathway carry impulses from pain, thermal, tactile, muscle and joint receptors to the brain. Some of this information finally reaches a conscious level (the cerebral cortex) while some is destined for subconscious centres (e.g. the cerebellum). The somatosensory system includes multiple types of sensation from the body — light touch, pain, pressure, temperature, fine touch and joint and muscle position sense (also called proprioception).

Generally, there are three types of sensation. The first sensation is called discriminative touch (fine touch), which includes touch, pressure, and vibration perception, and enables us to "read" raised letters with our fingertips, or describe the shape and texture of an object without seeing it. The second sensation is pain and temperature, which is just what it sounds like, and also includes the sensations of itch and tickle. The third sensation is called proprioception, which includes receptors for what happens below the body's surface: muscle stretch, joint position, tendon tension, and so on.

Ascending pathway that carries information to a conscious level shares certain common characteristics.

1) There is a sequence of three neurons between the peripheral receptor and the cerebral cortex.

2) The first neurons' cell body lies in the dorsal root ganglion.

3) The second-order neurons' cell body lies in the spinal cord or medulla ob-longata. Its axon crosses over (decussates) to the opposite side of the CNS and ascends to the thalamus, where it terminates upon the third neuron.

4) The third-order neurons' cell body lies in the thalamus. Its axon passes to the somatosensory cortex of the parietal lobe of the cerebral hemisphere.

11.2   Ascending Pathway

1. Proprioceptive and Fine Touch (Deep Sensation, 深感觉) Pathways of Trunk and Limbs (Fig. 11-1)

Sensory Pathways of trunk and limbs can be seen in Fig.11-1.

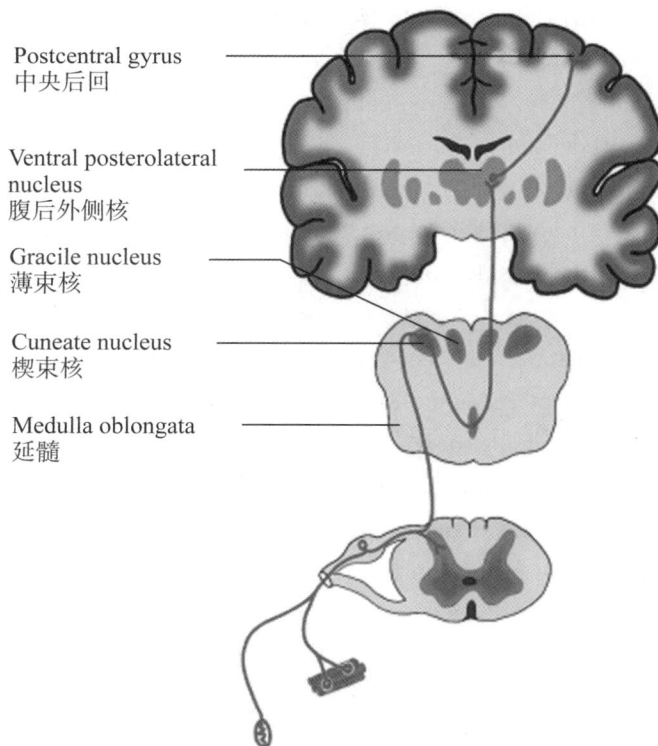

Postcentral gyrus
中央后回

Ventral posterolateral nucleus
腹后外侧核

Gracile nucleus
薄束核

Cuneate nucleus
楔束核

Medulla oblongata
延髓

Fig.11-1   Sensory pathways of trunk and limbs

The action potential [proprioceptive information and fine (discriminative) touch] from the trunk and limbs is generated by a mechanoreceptor in the tissue, the impulse travels along the peripheral axons of the first-order neuron in the dorsal root ganglion. The input will travel along its axon, through the dorsal root and into the posterior horn, then ascending in the dorsal columns (fasciculus gracilis and fasciculus cuneatus on the same side). The gracilis fasciculus carries tactile and proprioceptive information from the lower half of the body (T7 to the first coccygeal nerve), while the fasciculus cuneatus carries input from C1 and T6 spinal cord levels. They end by synapsing on second-order neurons in the medulla oblongata nuclei (nucleus gracilis and nucleus cuneatus respectively) . Axons of second-order neurons cross over to the other side of the medulla and are named internal arcuate fibers. This crossing is known as medial lemniscus decussation, eventually form the medial lemniscus to the third - order neurons of the ventral posterolateral nucleus in the contralateral thalamus. Axons of third-order neurons pass through the posterior limb of internal capsule as central thalamic radiation and terminate in the upper part of primary somatosensory cortex.

Lesions of the medial lemniscus results in loss of two points discrimination, vibration and conscious proprioception from the contralateral side of the body.

2. Pain, Temperature and Simple Touch (Superficial Sensation) Pathways of Trunk and Limbs

Primary afferent fibers carrying pain, temperature and light touch/ pressure information from the trunk and limbs travel along the peripheral axons of the first-order neuron in the dorsal root ganglion. The input will travel along its axon, through the dorsal root and into the posterior horn, then terminate in second-order neurons (nucleus propria) and are located in either the dorsal horn. Their axons decussate and ascend as contralateral spino - thalamic tract, that synapse on the cell bodies of third-order neurons (the ventral posterolateral nucleus) in the thalamus. Axons of third - order neurons pass through the posterior limb of the internal capsule as central thalamic radiation to reach the cerebral cortex, terminating in the the upper part of the primary somatosensory cortex.

Lesions of the spino-thalamic lemniscus results in loss of pain, temperature and simple touch from the contralateral side of the body.

3. Sensory Pathways of Head and Face

The principal regulator of the sensory modalities of head and face is the trigeminal nerve (Fig.11-2). This is the fifth of twelve pairs of cranial nerves that are responsible for transmitting numerous motor, sensory, and autonomous stimuli to structures of the head and neck. The first-order neurons are located in the trigeminal ganglion, whose peripheral processes join the sensory branches of the trigeminal nerve and terminate in the superficial receptors in the skin and mucosa of the head and face. The central process enters the pons to terminate in the second-order neurons. They are spinal nucleus of trigeminal nerve with pain and thermal sensations, the pontine nucleus of trigeminal nerve with tactile and pressure sensation and mesencephalic nucleus of the trigeminal nerve with proprioceptive impulses. Their axons then decussate at multiple levels. They coalesce to form the ventral trigeminothalamic tract, which moves cranially, adjacent to the medial lemniscus pathway as the trigeminal lemniscus tract. The fibers access the third order neurons (ventral posteromedial nucleus) of the thalamus. Axons of third-order neurons pass through the internal capsule to reach the cerebral cortex, terminating in the the inferior part of the primary somatosensory cortex.

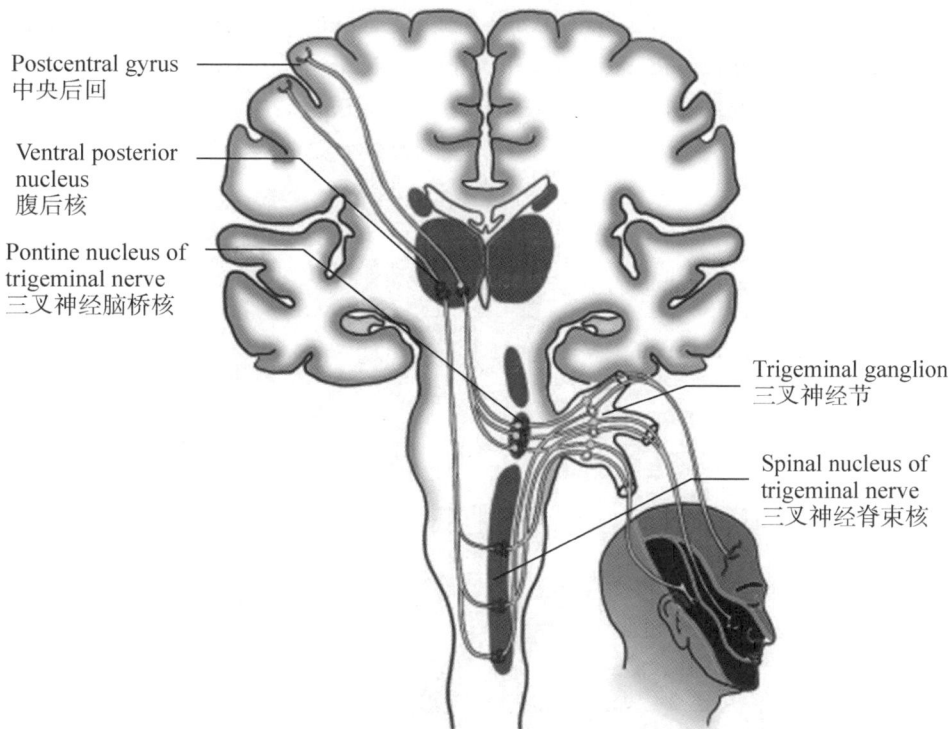

Postcentral gyrus
中央后回

Ventral posterior
nucleus
腹后核

Pontine nucleus of
trigeminal nerve
三叉神经脑桥核

Trigeminal ganglion
三叉神经节

Spinal nucleus of
trigeminal nerve
三叉神经脊束核

Fig.11-2　The sensory pathway of head and face

Lesions of the trigeminothalamic lemniscus results in loss of all sensory from the contralateral side of the head and face.

4. Acoustic (Auditory) Pathways

Hearing is an essential process that enables us to communicate with each other. It is composed of a number of nuclei and is dependent on a range of functional areas. The first-order neurons are bipolar cells in the cochlear. Their peripheral processes run to the spiral organ (of Corti) in the internal ear, whose central processes join the cochlear nerve and pass through the internal acoustic meatus to the cochlear nuclei, which are the second-order neurons. Some axons of the second-order neurons course medially along the ventral border of the pontine tegmentumt form the trapezoid body, which passes through or ventrally to the medial leminiscus. They next cross the midline to the opposite to form a longitudinal ascending bundle known as the lateral lemniscus. Most of the lemniscal fibers are crossed fibers that ascend from the contralateral auditory apparatus to synapse in the inferior colliculus: they include fibers relayed from the superior olivary nucleus and trapezoid body. Some lateral lemniscal fibers carry information from the ipsilateral cochlea that has passed through the ipsilateral superior olivary nucleus. The fibers of the lateral lemniscus terminate directly or indirectly in the medial geniculate body, whose cells are the third-order neurons. The axons join the acoustic radiation. The fibers of the acoustic radiation course via the posterior limb of the internal capsule (the inferior thalamic radiation) to the auditory area (transverse temporal gyri)(Fig.11-3).

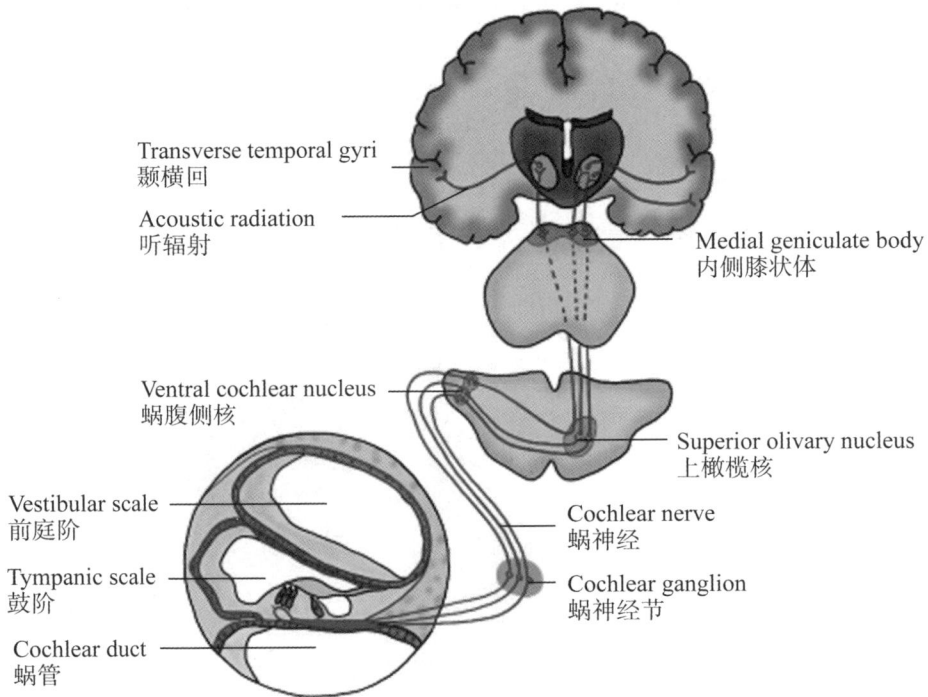

Fig.11-3　Acoustic(auditory) pathways

Because the acoustic center on one side receives fibers from the bilateral cochlear nuclei, damage to ipsilateral paths does not cause a hearing defect.

5. Visual Pathways and Pupillary Reflex

Vision is generated by photoreceptors in the retina, a layer of cells at the back of the eye. The first-order neurons are bipolar cells in retina. The ganglionic cells in the innermost layer of the retina are the second-order neurons. Their axons leave the eye by way of the optic nerve, and there is a partial crossing of axons at the optic chiasm that temporal fibers arising from the retina do not decussate, as well as nasal fibers originating from the retina decussate to the contralateral side. After the chiasm, the axons are called the optic tract. The optic tract is paired. Each is made up from the majority of these fibers to the lateral geniculate body of the thalamus, where they synapse on the dorsal lateral geniculate nucleus. However, a minority of these fibers will bypass the lateral geniculate body to terminate in the pretectal nucleus (to participate in the pupillary light reflex) and the superior colliculus (regulation of saccadic eye movements). However, there are fibers that leave the lateral geniculate body to form the optic radiation (geniculocalcarine tract) and ultimately travel to primary visual cortex in calcarine sulcus.

Light shining on the retina of one eye causes both pupils to constrict normally. The response in the eye stimulated is called the direct pupillary light reflex, while that in the opposite eye is known as the indirect pupillary light reflex. Pathways involved in the pupillary light reflex are not entirely known, but the follows are invloved: i) axons of retinal ganglion cells which pass via the optic nerve, optic tract and branchium of superior colliculus to the pretectal area, ii) axons of pretectal neurons which partially cross in the posterior commissure and presumably terminate bilaterally in Edinger-Westphal neuclus, iii) preganglionic fibers from the E-W neuclus course with fibers of the oculomotor nerve and synapse in the ciliary ganglion, and iv) postganlionic fibers from the ciliary ganglion innervate to the sphincter of the iris to regulate the contraction of the pupil (Fig.11-4).

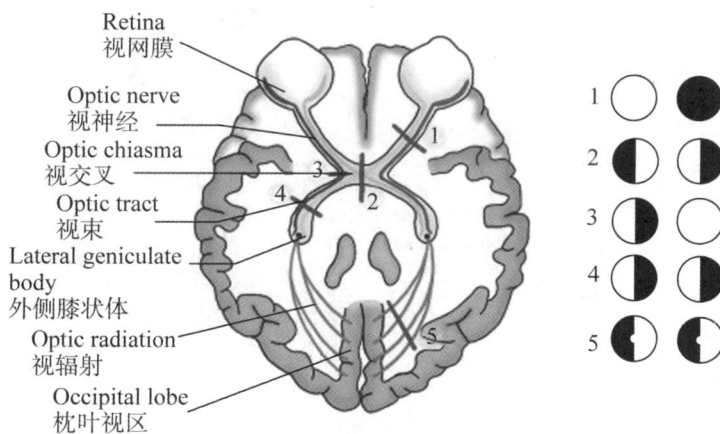

Fig.11-4   The visual pathways and pupillary reflex

Light shining on the retina of one eye whose optic nerve is injured could not cause both pupils to constrict, but light shone on the healthy one cause both pupils to constrict. The pupil on the side of which the oculomotor nerve is damaged, does not constrict when light shines on either pupil.

11.3 Descending Pathway

Unlike the sensory pathways, the descending motor tracts have the upper motor neurons (UMN) in the brain and the lower motor neurons (LMN) in the spinal cord or brain stem.

Muscular contraction are dependent on action potentials generated by the spinal motor neurons of the anterior horn in order to produce a movement. Both conscious and unconscious regulation of these lower motor neurons of the anterior grey horn is achieved by numerous upper motor neurons in cerebral cortex, cerebellum, etc. The motor pathways include pyramidal and extrapyramidal systems.

1. The Pyramidal Tract

This tract is a descending white matter tract of the central nervous system that provides voluntary control of striated muscle movement. It is composed of two distinct tracts:

The corticospinal tract, which mainly arises from upper motor neurons of the primary motor cortex in the brain, then to the lower motor neurons of the spinal cord, which further relay them to the muscles of the trunk and limbs; the corticonuclear tract, which also arises from upper motor neurons in the primary motor cortex in the brain, then to the lower motor neurons in the motor cranial nerve nuclei of the brainstem, which innervate the muscles of the head, the face and the neck (Fig.11-5).

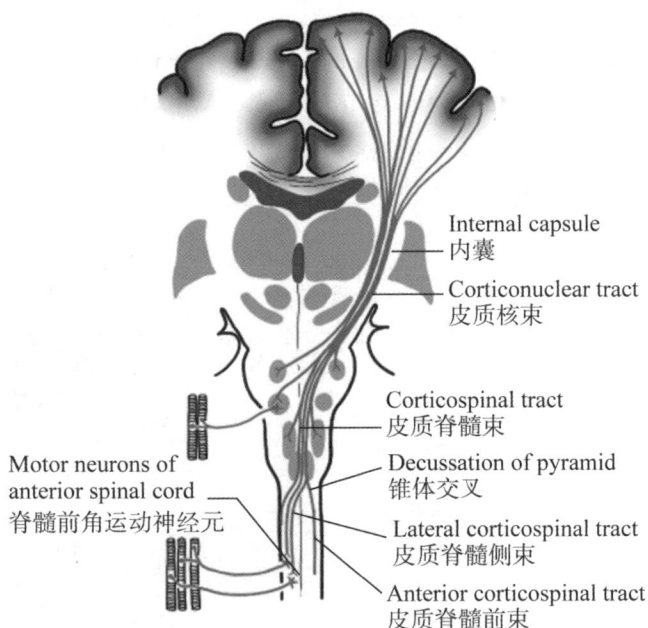

Fig.11-5　The pyramidal tract

(1) **The corticcospinal tract**

The tract is a motor pathway that carries efferent information from the cerebral cortex to the spinal cord for the voluntary movements of the limbs and trunk.

The upper motor neurons are called the pyramidal cells of Betz. Axons of Betz cells descend and pass inferiorly through the anterior two-thirds of the posterior limb of the internal capsule, through the cerebral peduncles of the midbrain, the pons into the medulla. The majority (70% — 90%) of corticospinal fibers decussate (pyramidal decussation) in the medulla. The crossed fibers form the lateral corticospinal tract (providing voluntary motor information to the muscles of the limbs) while the uncrossed fibers enter the anterior corticospinal tract (supplies the axial muscles of the trunk). Both tracts run along the spinal cord, synapsing with lower motor neurons in the anterior gray horn on the same side. The lower motor neurons leave the spinal cord through the ventral root and form spinal nerves which innervate the musculature of the body.

(2) **The corticonuclear tract**

This tract originates from upper motor neurons located in the inferior part of the primary motor cortex. The arising fibers converge to pass within the knee "genu" of the internal capsule, and then continue inferiorly through the cerebral peduncle of the midbrain, to reach the brainstem and terminate on the lower motor neurons (LMNs) in the nuclei of certain cranial nerves within the midbrain, pons and medulla. After relay, they carry efferent fibers directly to the muscles of the face, head and neck. In the midbrain, LMNs are the nuclei of oculomotor and trochlear nerves. In the pons, LMNs are the facial nuclei, the motor nuclei of the trigeminal and abducens nerves. In the medulla oblongata, LMNs are the nucleus ambiguus, accessory nerves motor nuclei and hypoglossal nucleus. However, the corticonuclear tract gives rise to the bilateral oculomotor, trochlear, trigeminal motor, ambiguus, accessory nuclei, the superior part of the facial nucleus, and to the contralateral hypoglossal nucleus and the inferior part of the facial nucleus.

1) Lesion of corticospinal tracts (upper motor neurones, hard paralysis). Lesion above the decussation of the pyramid results in impairment of contralateral muscles of the upper and low limbs, below the decussation of the pyramid results in impair-ment of ipsilateral hard paralysis of muscles of the upper and low limbs.

2) If damage happens to the right internal capsule, then results in serious neurologic deficits will be resulted in.

Corticospinal tract injury: left lesion of voluntary motor paralysis (upper and lower limbs)

Corticobulbar tract injury: left lesion of voluntary motor paralysis including facial expression and tongue muscles. The rest motor nuclei function in brainstem are not lost for the bilateral innervation.

Supranuclear paralysis (*spastic / hard paralysis*): damage of upper motor neurones.

Infrannuclear paralysis (*flaccid / soft paralysis*): damage of lower motor neurones.

2. Extrapyramidal System

The extrapyramidal system (Fig. 11-6) is actively involved in the initiation and selective activation of voluntary movements, along with their coordination, whose fibers pass through the tegmentum rather than the medullary pyramid, therefore distinguished from the pyramidal motor system.

The main components of the extrapyramidal motor system are the nuclei of the basal ganglia. Other structures involved include the nuclei of the cerebellum and brainstem, as well as the mesencephalic reticular formation. All these structures share intricate connections that modulate the motor activity of the body, which is why the extrapyramidal system is also often described as the motor-modulation system. The four main pathways are the reticulospinal, vestibulospinal, rubrospinal and tecto-spinal tracts. Main functions of the extrapyramidal system are as follows: regulating the tonicity of the muscles, coordination of the muscular activities and maintaining the normal body posture and producing habitual and rhythmic movements.

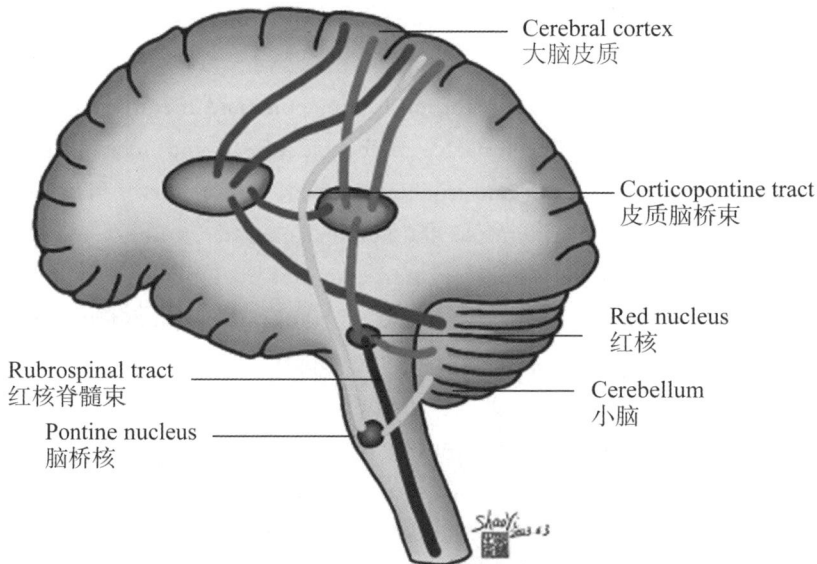

Fig.11-6   The extrapyramidal system

1) The reticulospinal tract is one of the pathways of the corticoreticulospinal system. This system gathers all the pathways that receive the impulses from the cerebral cortex, starts within the reticular formation of the brainstem and terminates within the spinal cord. It influences their reflexes and muscle tone.

2) The vestibulospinal tract also originates from the medulla and pons. Depending on its nucleus of origin, it is divided into medial and lateral vestibulo-spinal tracts. They control the extensor musculature and enable the erect body posture.

3) The rubrospinal tract originates from neurons of the caudal part of the red nucleus, located centrally in the midbrain tegmentum. This tract mainly transmits signals that arrive in the red nucleus from the motor centers in the cortex and cerebellum. The main

function is to maintain the muscle tone of these muscles and to modulate their movements that are directed by the pyramidal system.

4) The tectospinal tract (colliculospinal tract) originates from the superior colliculus located in the dorsal midbrain. It projects inferiorly to the cervical and upper thoracic portions of the spinal cord. The tectospinal tract represents the crucial link between the visual and auditory stimuli and the muscle movements.

（浙江大学医学院　韩曙）

Chapter 12 Meninges and Blood Vessels of Central Nervous System, and Cerebrospinal Fluid

12.1 Meninges of Central Nervous System

The meninges are the three connective tissue membranes that envelop the brain and the spinal cord, and separate them from walls of the skull and the vertebral column to support and protect the delicate tissues. Based on their location, meninges are referred to as the cranial meninges which envelop the brain, and spinal meninges which envelop the spinal cord. There are three meningeal layers. From superficial to deep are the dura mater (硬膜, outer layer), the arachnoid mater (蛛网膜, middle layer), and the pia mater (软膜, inner layer).

12.1.1 Spinal Meninges

1. The Spinal Dura Mater

The spinal dura mater (硬脊膜)(Fig. 12-1) is a thick, tough, fibrous membrane that encloses the spinal cord in a sac. It receives blood and nerve supply from the meningeal arteries, veins and nerves. The upper end is firmly attached to the margin of the foramen magnum and other intracranial foramen, and the lower end becomes thinner at the level of the second sacral vertebra, encloses the filum terminalis, and attaches to the coccyx. In the spinal cord, only one layer of dura mater is found. Unlike in the cranium, the dura is not closely integrated with the overlying bones. Instead, a space exists between the dura and periosteum in the vertebral canal known as the epidural space, which contains loose conjunctival tissue, fat, lymphatic vessels, spinal venous plexus and spinal nerve roots. There is slight negative pressure in the cavity, and epidural anesthesia is often performed here clinically.

2. The Spinal Arachnoid Mater

The spinal arachnoid matter (脊髓蛛网膜) is located between the dura mater and the pia mater and directly continues with the cerebral arachnoid. The potential space between the arachnoid and the dura is called the subdural space. The space between the arachnoid and the pia is called the subarachnoid space that communicates with the subarachnoid space of the brain. It is filled with the cerebrospinal fluid (CSF). The lower part of this space extends from the lower end of the spinal cord to the level of the second sacral vertebra into the terminal cistern, which contains the cauda equina. Therefore, puncture (lumbar puncture) is usually performed between the L3—L4 or L4—L5 vertebrae in clinical practice to extract cerebrospinal fluid or inject drugs without endangering the spinal cord.

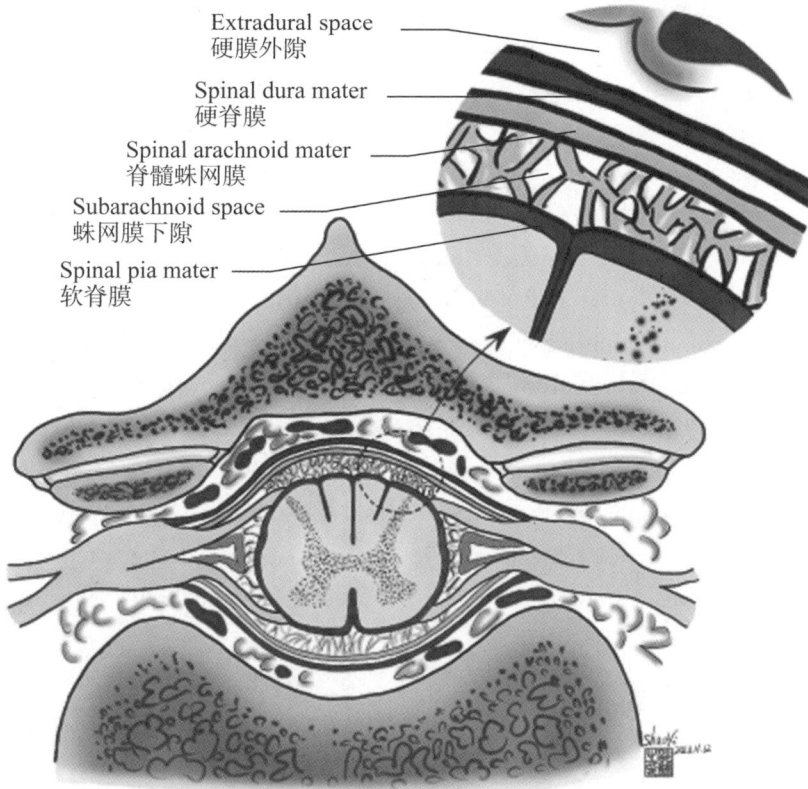

Fig.12-1   The capsule of the spinal cord

3. The Spinal Pia Mater

The pia mater (spinal pia mater)(软脊膜) is a thin, delicate membrane with abundant blood vessels that tightly envelop the surface and enter the grooves and fissures of the spinal cord, forming terminal filaments at the lower end of the spinal cord. Between the anterior and posterior roots of the spinal nerves on both sides, the pia mater forms a denticulate ligament. The shape and position of the denticulate ligaments change during the spinal movement to maintain the relative stability of the spinal cord.

12.1.2　Brain Meninges

1. The Cerebral Dura Mater

The cerebral dura mater (硬脑膜, Figs.12-2 & 12-3) is a thick, tough outermost meningeal layer of the brain with dense irregular connective tissue. It is composed of two layers: The superficial layer is the periosteal cranial dura that overlies the inner table of the cranial vault bones, acting like the periosteal layer of the cranium, and the meningeal cranial dura, which lies superficial to the arachnoid mater. In some parts, the two layers of the dura mater are separated from each other, and the dural sinuses are lined with endothelial cells, which contain venous blood, lack valves and their walls are devoid of muscular tissue. It is difficult to stop bleeding when it is injured, and easy to cause intracranial hematoma. The fibrous septa of the dura mater that partially separates the cranial cavity within the cranium are as follows. i) Falx cerebri, which extends across the midline on the inner surface of the calvaria, from crista galli to the internal occipital protuberance. It separates the left and right cerebral hemispheres and houses the superior sagittal and inferior sagittal sinuses. Posteriorly, the falx blends with tentorium cerebelli. ii) Tentorium cerebelli, which separates the cerebrum from the cerebellum, spans in a transverse plane from the inner surface of the occipital bone. It contains the transverse, straight and superior petrosal sinuses. iii) Falx cerebelli, which projects from the midline of the occipital bone. It separates the hemispheres of the cerebellum and houses the occipital sinus. iv) Diaphragma sellae, which is a flat membrane that surrounds the pituitary stalk, contains the anterior and posterior intercavernous sinuses. The meningeal dura mater overlies the trigeminal ganglion, enclosing it in a compartment known as the trigeminal cave.

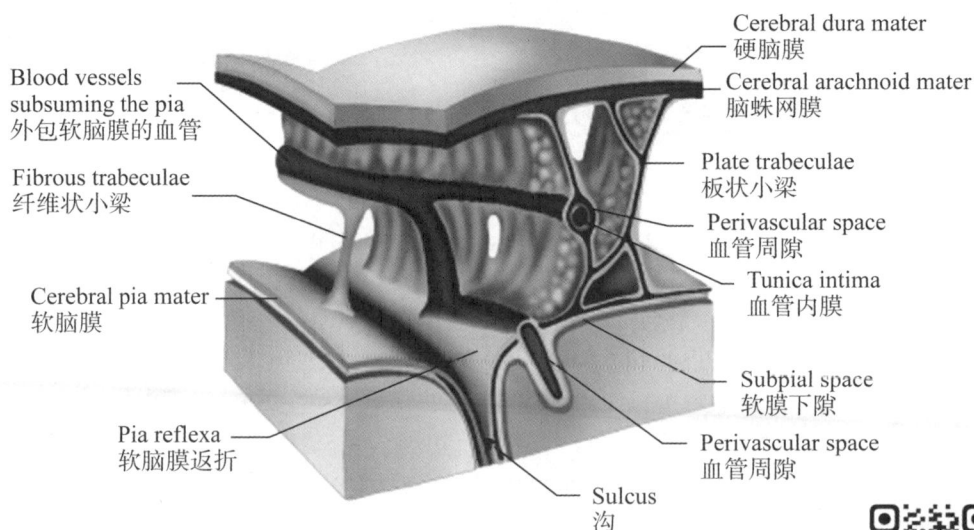

Blood vessels subsuming the pia
外包软脑膜的血管

Fibrous trabeculae
纤维状小梁

Cerebral pia mater
软脑膜

Pia reflexa
软脑膜返折

Cerebral dura mater
硬脑膜

Cerebral arachnoid mater
脑蛛网膜

Plate trabeculae
板状小梁

Perivascular space
血管周隙

Tunica intima
血管内膜

Subpial space
软膜下隙

Perivascular space
血管周隙

Sulcus
沟

Fig.12-2　The capsule of the brain

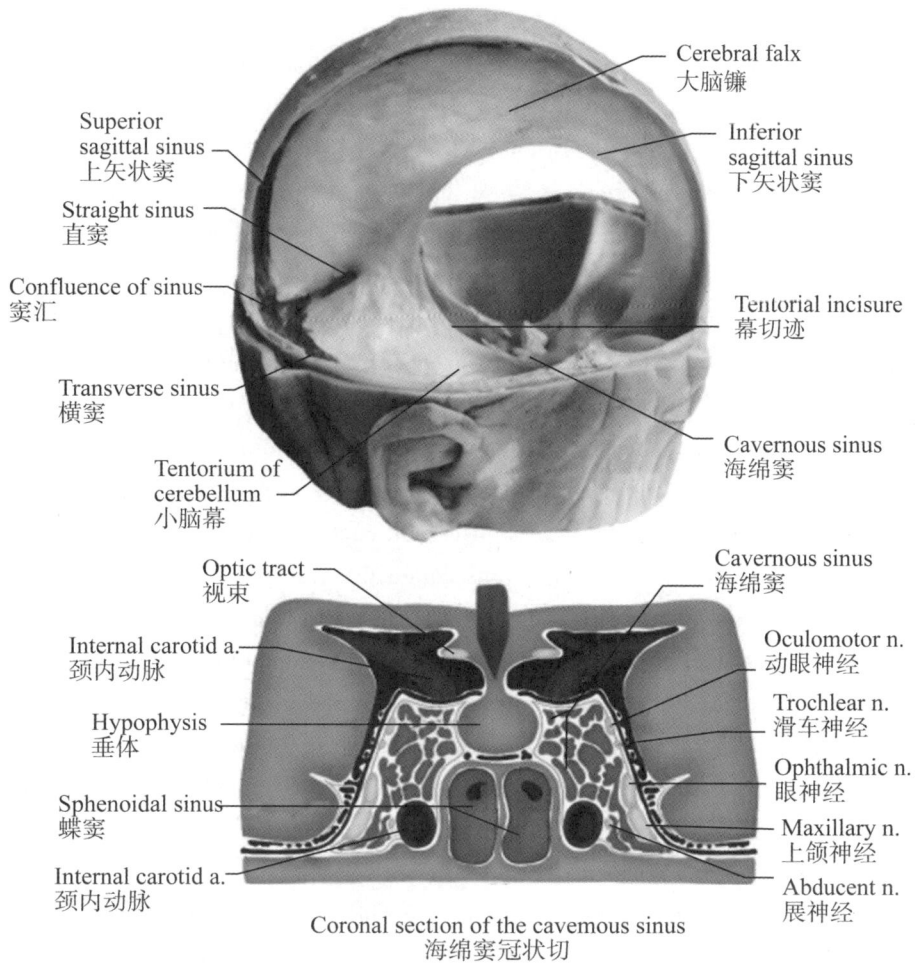

Coronal section of the cavemous sinus
海绵窦冠状切

Fig.12-3 The cerebral dura mater

The superior sagittal sinus is contained in the superior margin of the Falx cerebri, the inferior sagittal sinus is contained in the lower margin, and the straight sinus is connected with the tentorial cerebellum. The confluence sinus formed by the confluence of the superior sagittal sinus and the straight sinus at the occipital carina. It passes laterally into the transverse sinus. At the medial surface of the occipital, the transverse sinus is located at the transverse sinus groove; the sigmoid sinus is located at the sigmoid sinus groove, and the cavernous sinus is located on both sides of the sella turcica. Several cranial nerves run forward through the cavernous sinus to enter the orbit via the superior orbital fissure. The internal carotid artery and abducens nerve pass through the cavernous sinus, and the oculomotor nerve, trochlear nerve, ophthalmic nerve, and maxillary nerve pass through its lateral wall from top to bottom. The front of the cavernous sinus communicates with the facial vein through the ophthalmic vein, connects to the apterygial plexus through the foramen ovals. The superior and inferior petrological sinuses are located at the upper and lower margins of the petrous part of the temporal bone, pass backward to the transverse sinus ,sigmoid sinus and inject into the jugular vein at the jugular foramina.

2. The Cerebral Arachnoid Mater

The cerebral arachnoid mater (脑蛛网膜) is a spiderweb-like meningeal layer between the dura and the pia, and directly continues with the spinal cord arachnoid mater. The potential space between the arachnoid and the dura is called the subdural space. The space between the arachnoid and pia is called the subarachnoid space and it is filled with the cerebrospinal fluid (CSF). The outer surface of the arachnoid attaches to the dura mater forming a barrier that prevents the leakage of CSF into the subdural space. At the sites where dura forms the venous sinuses, the arachnoid shows mushroom-like protrusions called the arachnoid granulations that mostly near the superior sagittal sinus. CSF can seep through it into the dural sinuses and back into the veins. The inner surface of arachnoid shows thin fibrous projections called the arachnoid trabeculae that traverse the subarachnoid space and attach to the outer surface of the pia mater. Some parts of the subarachnoid space are enlarged and called the subarachnoid cistern, including the Cisterna magna (cerebellomedullary cistern), the pontine cistern, the chiasmatic cistern, the quadrigeminal cistern, the interpeduncular cistern, the ambient cistern, the crural and carotid cisterns, the cistern of lateral cerebral fossa (the sylvian cistern), the cerebellopontine cistern and the cistern of lamina terminalis.

3. The Cerebral Pia Mater

The cerebral pia mater (软脑膜) is thin and highly vascular membrane, close to the surface of the brain, and extends into the fissure of the brain. In a certain part of the ventricle, the pia mater and its blood vessels are in contact with the ependymal epithelium. Together they form the choroid plexus which produces cerebrospinal fluid. The function of the pia mater is to physically separate the neural tissue from the blood vessels in the subarachnoid space, adding to the efficacy of the blood-brain barrier. Furthermore, it contributes to the degradation of the neurotransmitters, preventing their prolonged action on the nervous tissue.

12.2　Blood Vessels of Central Nervous System

12.2.1　Blood Vessels of the Spinal Cord

1. Arteries of the Spinal Cord (脊髓的动脉)

The vertebral arteries are the main source of blood to the spinal cord. The anterior and two posterior spinal arteries are direct branches of the two vertebral arteries.

Similarly, the radicular arteries have their origin from spinal branches of the vertebral arteries and spinal branches of ascending cervical arteries, deep cervical arteries, intercostal arteries, lumbar arteries and sacral arteries. The arteries of the spinal cord from longitudinal and transverse arteries anastomose with each other.

2. Longitudinal Arteries

One anterior spinal artery (脊髓前动脉) and two posterior spinal arteries (脊髓后动脉) from the vertebral artery run longitudinally on both sides of the anterior median fissure of the spinal cord and the back of the spinal cord respectively. The posterior spinal arteries supply the posterior 1/3 of the spinal cord (posterior cord and posterior horn) and the dorsal part of the medulla bulbar. Transverse arteries are from some segmental arteries, such as posterior intercostal arteries, lumbar arteries, and spinal branches of lateral sacral arteries. These vessels pass directly to the longitudinal arteries, reinforcing them.

3. Veins of the Spinal Cord (脊髓的静脉)

The veins of the spinal cord are more numerous and thicker than the arteries. The small veins in the spinal cord are collected and finally synthesized into the anterior and posterior spinal cord veins, which are injected into the intravertebral venous plexus of the epidural space through the anterior and posterior root veins. It communicates with the medulla oblongata vein in the upward direction, with the thoracic azygos vein and the superior vena cava in the thoracic segment, and with the inferior vena cava, portal vein and pelvic vein in the abdomen. There is no venous valve in the vertebral venous plexus, and the internal pressure is very low. The direction of blood flow often changes with the changes of chest and abdominal pressure (such as weight lifting, cough, defecation, etc.), which is a possible route of infection and malignant tumor metastasis into the skull.

12.2.2 Blood Vessels of the Brain

1. Arteries of Brain

The brain has a high metabolic rate that reflects the energy requirements of constant neural activity. It is only 2% body weight ratio which receives about 15% of the cardiac output and utilizes 25% of the total oxygen consumption of the body. Owing to the high oxygen and nutrient demand of the organ, it is supplied by two arterial systems: the internal carotid artery (anterior circuit) and the vertebrobasilar artery system(posterior circuit). The supply areas of the two are roughly bounded by the parieto-occipital groove, which are called the internal carotid artery system and the vertebral-basilar artery system. The internal carotid artery mainly supplies the anterior 2/3 of the cerebral hemisphere and the anterior part of the diencephalon. The two vertebral arteries merge into one basilar artery, which mainly supplies the posterior 1/3 of the brain (occipital lobe, lower temporal lobe, and medial surface), diencephalon, brainstem, cerebellum, and the spinal cord (Fig.12-4).

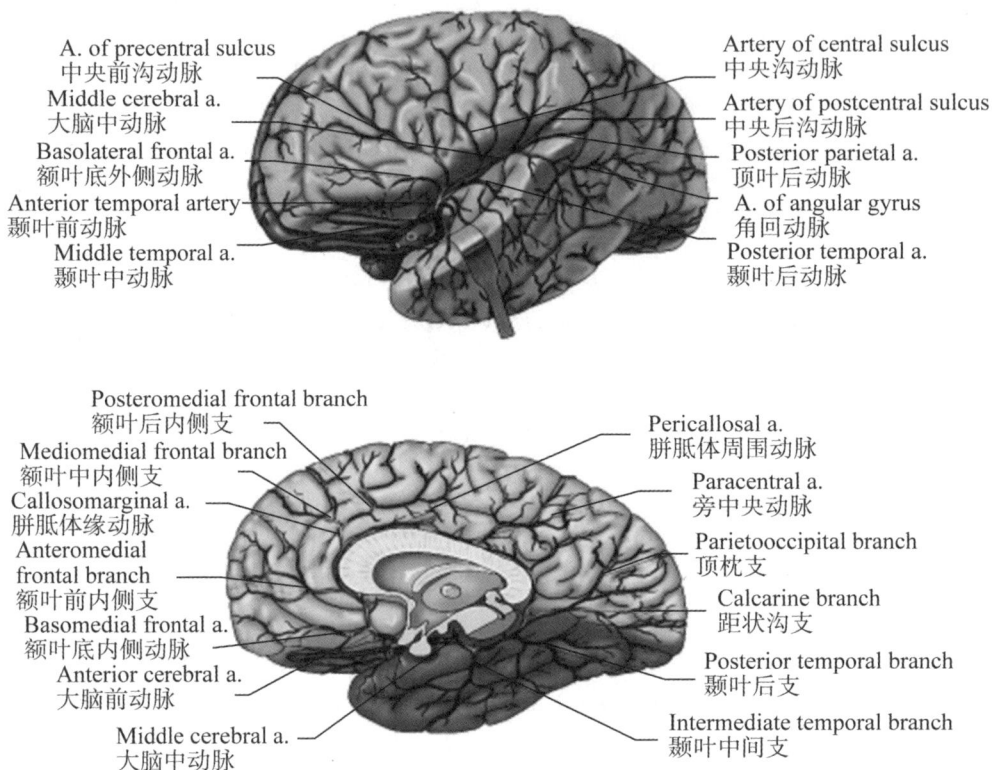

A. of precentral sulcus 中央前沟动脉
Middle cerebral a. 大脑中动脉
Basolateral frontal a. 额叶底外侧动脉
Anterior temporal artery 颞叶前动脉
Middle temporal a. 颞叶中动脉

Artery of central sulcus 中央沟动脉
Artery of postcentral sulcus 中央后沟动脉
Posterior parietal a. 顶叶后动脉
A. of angular gyrus 角回动脉
Posterior temporal a. 颞叶后动脉

Posteromedial frontal branch 额叶后内侧支
Mediomedial frontal branch 额叶中内侧支
Callosomarginal a. 胼胝体缘动脉
Anteromedial frontal branch 额叶前内侧支
Basomedial frontal a. 额叶底内侧动脉
Anterior cerebral a. 大脑前动脉
Middle cerebral a. 大脑中动脉

Pericallosal a. 胼胝体周围动脉
Paracentral a. 旁中央动脉
Parietooccipital branch 顶枕支
Calcarine branch 距状沟支
Posterior temporal branch 颞叶后支
Intermediate temporal branch 颞叶中间支

Fig.12-4   The arteries of the brain

Internal carotid artery (颈内动脉)

The internal carotid artery is separated from the common carotid artery at the plane of the upper edge of the thyroid cartilage, ascends in the neck and enters the skull cavity through the carotid canal, then passes through the cavernous sinus along the carotid groove on the lateral side of the Sella turcica. After reaching the lower part of the anterior clinoid process, it bends upward and enters the subarachnoid space, thus forming a forward convex curve. After reaching the upper part of the posterior clinoid process, it turns to the upper lateral side and reaches the bottom of the brain. Therefore, the course of the internal carotid artery is divided into four segments: cervical segment, petrous segment, cavernous segment, and anterior clinoid segment. The branches of the internal carotid artery are as follows.

1) Ophthalmic artery (眼动脉). Given off immediately after the internal carotid artery, the ophthalmic artery leaves the cavernous sinus, supplies blood to the eyes, eye muscles, and other structures in or near the bony area around each eye. During

an ophthalmic artery occlusion, the artery becomes partially or completely blocked. This is a medical emergency and can lead to permanent vision loss if it isn't treated right away.

2) Anterior cerebral artery (大脑前动脉). Above the optic nerve, the anterior cerebral artery enters the interhemispheric fissure, connects with the contralateral artery of the same name via the anterior communicating artery, and then runs upward and posteriorly along the sulcus of the corpus callosum. The cortical branches are distributed on the anteromedial surface of the parieto-occipital groove and the upper and outer edges of the two frontal and parietal lobes; the central branch penetrates the precibarium (the anterior perforated substance) and enters the brain parenchyma, supplying the caudate nucleus, the anterior part of the lenticular nucleus, and the forelimb of the internal capsule.

3) Middle cerebral artery (大脑中动脉). The middle cerebral artery is a larger terminal branch of the internal carotid artery, which runs outward and backward along the lateral sulcus of the brain, and is divided into several cortical branches and a central branch. The cortical branch supplies most of the dorsolateral surface of the cerebral hemisphere and Insula (before parieto-occipital groove). The middle cerebral artery gives off a thin central branch that penetrates vertically into the brain parenchyma and supplies the caudate nucleus, putamen, genu and hind limbs of the internal capsule. Among them, the lenticulostriate artery ascending from the outside of the lenticular nucleus to the internal capsule is relatively curved, which is prone to rupture in the case of arteriosclerosis and hypertension (hence also called hemo-rrhagic artery), leading to cerebral hemorrhage (stroke).

4) Posterior communicating artery (后交通动脉). The posterior communicating artery anastomoses with the posterior cerebral artery and is the anastomotic branch of the internal carotid artery system and the vertebral-basilar artery system.

5) Anterior choroidal artery (脉络丛前动脉). The anterior choroid plexus artery generally originates from the terminal end of the internal carotid artery and runs behind the optic tract, between the cerebral peduncle and the sulci, and enters the lower part of the choroid fissure backward, finally entering the choroid plexus of the lateral ventricle and anastomosing with the posterior choroid plexus artery. The cortical branch mainly supplies the choroid plexus of the lateral ventricle, the lateral geniculate body, the hippocampus and the uncus, and the central branch feeds the lower hind limbs of the inner capsule and the globus pallidus. This artery is small and long, which is easy to embolize and cause the lesions of globus pallidus and hippocampus.

2. Vertebral Artery

The paired vertebral artery (椎动脉) originates from the first part of each subclavian artery, passes through the transverse foramen of the up six cervical vertebrae, and enters the cranial cavity through the foramen magnum (Fig.12-5). At the junction of the pons and the medulla oblongata, the left and right vertebral arteries synthesize a basilar artery, which ascends along the basilar sulcus on the ventral surface of the pons, and is divided into two terminal branches at the upper border of the pons: the left and right posterior cerebral arteries which the cerebral artery circle. The vertebral-basilar artery gives rise to three additional branches before joining with its companion vessel to form the basilar artery (基底动脉).

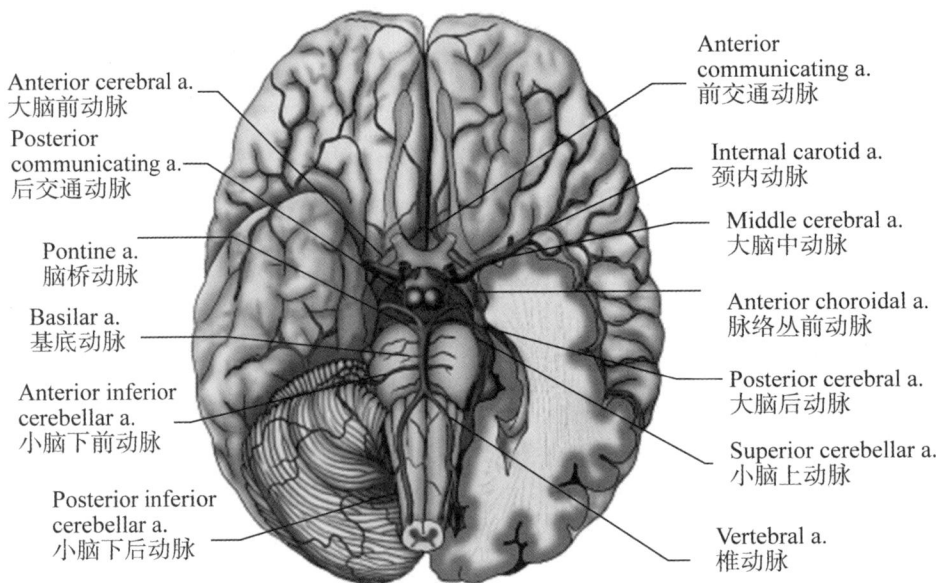

Fig.12-5　Arteries at the bottom of the brain

(1) **Anterior and posterior spinal arteries**

The anterior and posterior spinal arteries (脊髓前、后动脉) originate from the vertebral artery (see Section 12.2.1)

(2) **Posterior inferior cerebellar artery**

The posterior inferior cerebellar artery (小脑下后动脉) is the largest branch of the intracranial segment of the vertebral artery, originating before the basilar artery from the two vertebral arteries; it supplies the lower posterior part of the cerebellum and the posterolateral part of the medulla.

The basilar artery travels in a rostral direction along the anterior aspect of the pons, the branches includes:

(3) **Anterior inferior cerebellar artery**

The anterior inferior cerebellar artery (小脑下前动脉) arises from the basilar artery and supplies the lower front of the cerebellum.

(4) **Labyrinthine artery**

Also known as the internal auditory artery, the labyrinthine artery (迷路动脉)

originates from the basilar artery and is very thin, supplying the labyrinth of the inner ear.

(5) Pontine arteries

The pontine arteries (脑桥动脉) are small branches that supply the pons.

(6) Superior cerebellar artery

The superior cerebellar artery (小脑上动脉) originates near the end of the basilar artery, goes around the cerebral peduncle, and supplies the upper part of the cerebellum.

(7) Posterior cerebral artery

The posterior cerebral artery (大脑后动脉) originates near the superior border of the pons, goes back around the peduncles, and turns along the parapocampus gyrus to the medial surface of the temporal and occipital lobes. The cortical branch is distributed on the medial and bottom surfaces of the temporal lobe and the occipital lobe; the central branch originates from the root, enters the brain parenchyma through the posterior perforation, and supplies the dorsal thalamus, posterior thalamus, hypothalamus, and subthalamus. The posterior cerebral artery communi-cates with the internal carotid artery through the posterior communicating artery. There is an oculomotor nerve between the posterior cerebral artery and the superior cerebellar artery. Any cause of arterial displacement, compression and traction of the oculomotor nerve result in eye movement paralysis.

(8) Cerebral arterial circle

The cerebral artery circle (大脑动脉环), also known as Willis circle, is located above the sella and surrounds the optic chiasm, cinder tubercle and mammillary body. It is jointly formed by the anterior communicating artery (前交通动脉), the initial segment of the bilateral anterior cerebral artery (大脑前动脉), the terminal end of the bilateral internal carotid artery (颈内动脉), the bilateral posterior communi-cating artery (后交通动脉), and the initial segment of the bilateral posterior cerebral artery (大脑后动脉). Under normal circumstances, the blood on both sides of the arterial circle is not mixed. When a certain feeding artery is stenotic or occluded, the blood can be redistributed and compensated through the cerebral arterial circle to a certain extent to maintain the blood supply to the brain. The junction between the posterior communicating artery and the internal carotid artery, and the junction between the anterior communicating artery and the anterior cerebral artery, are the common sites of aneurysms.

Cerebral veins (Fig. 12-6) are not accompanied by arteries and can be divided into superficial and deep groups, both of which are widely connected in the brain and outside the brain. The superficial veins are divided into superior cerebral vein, middle cerebral vein and inferior cerebral vein, and there are abundant anastomoses between them, which collect venous blood from the cortex and the subcortical medulla, and are directly injected into the dural venous sinus; the deep veins collect venous blood from the medulla, the basal ganglia, the diencephalon and the ventricular choroid plexus in the deep part of the brain, finally merge into the great cerebral vein, which pours into the straight sinus posteriorly and inferiorly to the splenium of the corpus callosum, and eventually leads to the internal jugular veins.

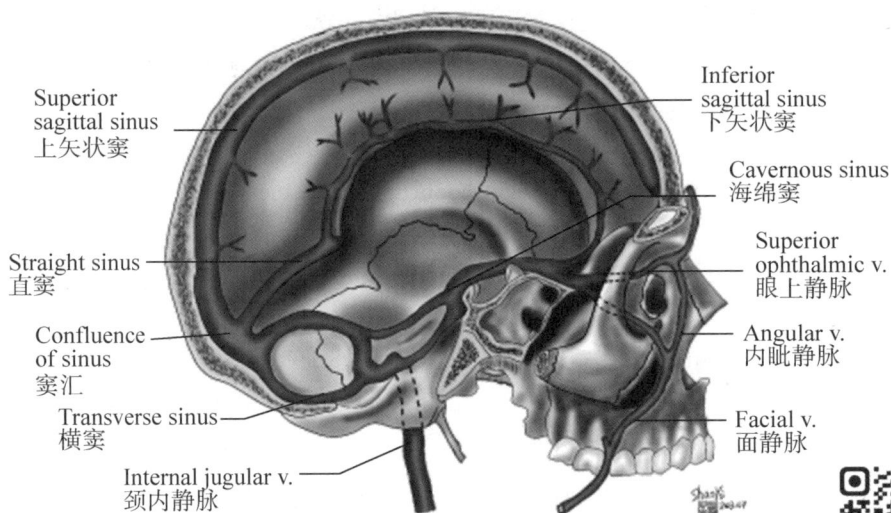

Fig.12-6 Superficial veins of the brain

12.3 Ventricular System, Cerebrospinal Fluid and Its Circulation

The ventricular system consists of a series of interconnected spaces and channels within the brain derived from the central lumen of the embryonic neural tube and the brain vesicles it generates. Each cerebral hemisphere has a large lateral ventricle that is connected to the third ventricle near its rostral end through the interventricular foramina (foramen of Monro). The third ventricle is a midline suture space between the left and right thalamus and the hypothalamus. Communicating with the fourth ventricle through the cerebral aqueduct, there is a wide cavity between the brain stem and the cerebellum, which enters the subarachnoid space of the cisterna magna through the foramen median (Magendie's foramen) and the foramen lateral on both sides (Luscgha's foramen). The caudal side is attached to the degenerated central canal of the spinal cord (Fig.12-7).

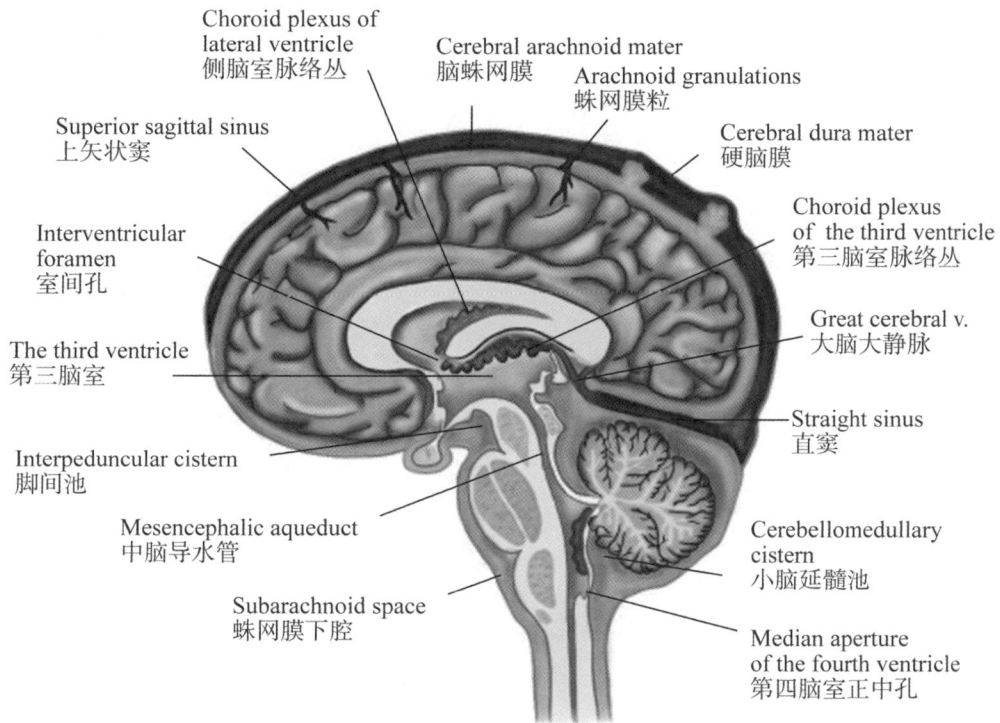

Fig.12-7   Cerebrospinal fluid and its circulation

The ventricle contains the choroid plexus, which produces cerebrospinal fluid that fills the ventricle and infuses the subarachnoid space to nourish the nerve tissue, acting as a buffer medium to protect the brain tissue from shock. Cerebrospinal fluid is a colorless, transparent liquid that fills the ventricular system, central canal of the spinal cord, and subarachnoid space. In the central nervous system, cerebrospinal fluid plays a role in buffering, protecting, nourishing, transporting metabolites, and maintaining intracranial pressure. Cerebrospinal fluid is continuously produced by the choroid plexus of the ventricular system, circulates through the ventricular system and the subarachnoid space, and finally flows back into the dural venous sinus through the arachnoid granules to maintain the dynamic balance of cerebrospinal fluid. If a part of the ventricular system is obstructed, obstructive hydrocephalus occurs. The circulation of cerebrospinal fluid is as follows:

Left and right ventricle (generated by choroid plexus) → interventricular foramen → third ventricle (generated by choroid plexus) → midbrain aqueduct → fourth ventricle (generated by choroid plexus) → median foramen, two lateral foramen → subarachnoid space → spider web Membrane → superior sagittal sinus → sinus confluence → sigmoid sinus → internal jugular vein.

（浙江大学医学院　韩曙）

367